United Health Foundation

United Health Foundation
P.O. Box 1459, Minneapolis, MN 55440-1459

July, 2003

Dear Colleague,

We at United Health Foundation are pleased once again to provide you with a complimentary copy of the BMJ's increasingly relevant publication, *Clinical Evidence*. This ninth edition continues to demonstrate that *Clinical Evidence* is the international resource of the best available evidence for effective health care. We are proud that *Clinical Evidence* benefits from considerable input by leading clinical experts from the United States.

Issue 9 continues the publication of *Clinical Evidence* in a concise format that is supplemented by an enclosed CD-ROM containing the full text. The BMJ Publishing Group's experience with this new format, and feedback to United Health Foundation from numerous American clinicians, indicates that this is a convenient format for providing timely access to information that is essential to medical decision making. As medicine benefits from an ever increasing amount of new clinically relevant scientific knowledge, we think that the concise version will become even more practical in the future and will facilitate the translation of evidence based information at the point of care delivery. In addition, we continue to be encouraged by the growing number of physicians and health professionals who are accessing Clinical Evidence through the Internet. Please note that as a recipient of the United Health Foundation distribution you have free access to the online version of *Clinical Evidence*. To make use of this feature go to www.clinicalevidence.com. Once there, register as a recipient of the UHF distribution program.

Our goal at United Health Foundation is to support you in making the best possible medical decisions with and for your patients. We are convinced that we can achieve our shared goals by using the best evidence based literature in formats that can be conveniently accessed at anytime, and in particular when you are making your clinical decisions. We look forward to working with you, and the BMJ Publishing Group, in the future.

Sincerely,

Bill McGuire

William W. McGuire, M.D.
Chairman
United Health Foundation

9 ISSUE
JUNE 2003

clinical evidence concise

The international source of the best available evidence for effective health care

BMJ Publishing Group

Editorial Office
BMJ Publishing Group, BMA House, Tavistock Square, London, WC1H 9JR, United Kingdom.
Tel: +44 (0)20 7387 4499 • Fax: +44 (0)20 7383 6242 • CEfeedback@bmjgroup.com •
www.bmjpg.com

Subscription prices for *Clinical Evidence*
Clinical Evidence and *Clinical Evidence Concise* (with companion CD-ROM) are both published six monthly (June/December) by the BMJ Publishing Group.The annual subscription rates for both publications (June, Issue 9 and December, Issue 10) are:

Personal: £85 • €135 • US$135 • Can$200
Institutional: £175 • €280 • US$280 • Can$420
Student/nurse: £40 • €65 • US$65 • Can$95

The above rates are for either the full print or the concise formats. The combined rates, for both formats, are:

Personal: £120 • €190 • US$190 • Can$285
Institutional: £235 • €375 • US$375 • Can$560
Student/nurse: £65 • €105 • US$105 • Can$155

All individual subscriptions (personal, student, nurse) include online access at no additional cost. Institutional subscriptions are for full print/concise version only. Institutions may purchase online site licences separately. For further subscription information please visit the subscription pages of our website www.clinicalevidence.com or email us at CEsubscriptions@bmjgroup.com (UK and ROW) or clinevid@pmds.com (Americas). You may also telephone us or fax us on the following numbers:

UK and ROW Tel: +44 (0)20 7383 6270 • Fax: +44 (0)20 7383 6402
Americas Tel: +1 800 373 2897/240 646 7000 • Fax: +1 240 646 7005

Bulk subscriptions for societies and organisations
The Publishers offer discounts for any society or organisation buying bulk quantities for their members/specific groups. Please contact Miranda Lonsdale, Sales Manager (UK) at mlonsdale@bmjgroup.com or Maureen Rooney, Sales Manager (USA) at mrooney@bmjgroup.com.

Contributors
If you are interested in becoming a contributor to *Clinical Evidence,* please contact us at clinicalevidence@bmjgroup.com.

Rights
For information on translation rights, please contact Daniel Raymond-Barker at draymond-barker@bmjgroup.com.

British Library Cataloguing in Publication Data. A catalogue record for this book is available from the British Library. ISSN 1462-3846 ISBN 0-7279-18044

Permission to reproduce
Please contact Josephine Woodcock at jwoodcock@bmjgroup.com when requesting permission to reprint all or part of any contribution in *Clinical Evidence*.

Printed by Quebecor World, Kingsport, USA
Designed by Pete Wilder, The Designers Collective Limited, London UK

Team

Executive Editor Fiona Godlee **Acting Editors** Anna Donald, Vivek Muthu **Clinical Editors** Mike Bedford, Luis Gabriel Cuervo Amore, Anjana Patel **Quality Assurance Editor** James Woodcock **Content Editor** Karen Pettersen **Assistant Content Editor** Polly Brown **North American Editor** David Goldmann **Managing Editor** Josephine Woodcock **Production Editors** Samantha Bedser, Alan Thomas **Editorial/Production Assistants** Claire Folkes, Rachael Kriefman **Freelance Editors** Bazian Ltd **Technical Editors** Andy Baker, Anne Lawson, Pamela Morley, Andrea Porter, Jane Tozer **Indexer** Angela Cottingham **Digital Production** Cassara Burgess, Karen Caillé, Kourosh Mojar, BMJ Electronic Production **Print Production** Charlotte Pestridge **Information Specialist Manager** Sam Vincent **Information Specialists** Mick Arber, Olwen Beaven, Sarah Greenley, Jane McHugh **Information Specialist Administrator** Varsha Mistry **Business Manager** Paula McQuillan **Technical Manager** Peter Hearn **Department Administrator** Hannah Lawrence **Marketing and Sales** Jaspal Chaggar, Diane Harris, Miranda Lonsdale, Daniel Raymond-Barker

Section Advisors

Cardiovascular disorders Nick Hicks, UK **Child health** Mary Rudolf, UK and Virginia Moyer, Professor, USA **Digestive system disorders** David Cave, Professor of Medicine, USA, John McDonald, Canada and David Metz, Associate Professor, USA **Ear, nose, and throat disorders** George Browning, Professor, UK **Endocrine disorders** Shereen Ezzat, Professor of Medicine, Canada and Victor Montori, Assistant Professor, Canada **Eye disorders** Andrew Dick, Professor and Liam Smeeth, General Practitioner, UK **Infectious diseases** Paul Garner, Professor, UK **Kidney disorders** Fred Coe, Professor of Medicine and Physiology and Michael Conlin, Associate Professor, USA **Men's health** Peter Schlegal, Chairman of Department of Urology, USA and Robyn Webber, Consultant Urological Surgeon, UK **Mental health** John Geddes, Professor of Epidemiological Psychiatry, UK **Musculoskeletal disorders** Troels Mork Hansen, Chief Consultant, Denmark and John Stothard, UK **Neurological disorders** Tony Marson, Lecturer in Neurology, UK **Oral health** Aubrey Sheiham, Professor, UK **Perioperative care** Andrew Smith, Consultant Anaesthetist, UK and Valerie Palda, Assistant Professor of Medicine, USA **Poisoning** Robin Ferner, Consultant Physician and Allister Vale, Director of National Posions Information Service (Birmingham Centre), UK **Pregnancy and childbirth** Metin Gulmezoglu, Scientist, WHO, Switzerland **Respiratory disorders** John Cunnington, Associate Professor of Medicine, Canada **Sexual health** George Schmid, Epidemiologist, USA **Skin disorders** Hywel Williams, Professor or Dermato-Epidemiology and Jane McGregor, Senior Lecturer and Consultant in Dermatology, UK **Sleep disorders** Michael Hensley, Professor of Medicine, Australia **Women's health** Mike Dixon, Senior Lecturer in Surgery, UK **Wounds** Nicky Cullum, Director of Centre for Evidence-Based Nursing, UK

Editorial Board

Acknowledgements

The BMJ Publishing Group thanks the following people and organisations for their advice and support: The Cochrane Collaboration, and especially Iain Chalmers, Mike Clarke, Phil Alderson, Peter Langhorne, and Carol Lefebvre; the National Health Service (NHS) Centre for Reviews and Dissemination, and especially Jos Kleijnen and Julie Glanville; the NHS, and especially Tom Mann, Sir John Patteson, Ron Stamp, Veronica Fraser, Muir Gray, Nick Rosen, and Ben Toth; the British National Formulary, and especially Dinesh Mehta, Eric Connor, and John Martin; Martindale: The Complete Drug Reference, and especially Sean Sweetman; the Health Information Research Unit at McMaster University, and especially Brian Haynes and Ann McKibbon; the United Health Foundation (UHF), and especially Dr Reed Tuckson and Yvette Krantz; Bazian Ltd, and especially Anna Donald and Vivek Muthu for their content delivery and management responsibilities; Dr Paul Dieppe, Dr Tonya Fancher, and Professor Richard Kravitz who are working closely with *Clinical Evidence* to explore ways of presenting evidence on the usefulness of diagnostic tests; the clinicians, epidemiologists, and members of patient support groups who have acted as peer reviewers.

The BMJ Publishing Group values the ongoing support it has received from the global medical community for *Clinical Evidence*. In addition to others, we wish to acknowledge the efforts of the UHF and the NHS who have provided educational funding to support the wide dissemination of this valuable resource to many physicians and health professionals in the USA (UHF) and UK (NHS). We are grateful to the clinicians and patients who spare time to take part in focus groups, which are crucial to the development of *Clinical Evidence*. Finally, we would like to acknowledge the readers who have taken the time to send us their comments and suggestions.

Contents

Welcome to Issue 9

Welcome to Issue 9 of *Clinical Evidence*, the international source of the best available evidence on the effects of common clinical interventions. *Clinical Evidence* summarises the current state of knowledge and uncertainty about the prevention and treatment of clinical conditions, based on thorough searches and appraisal of the literature. It is neither a textbook of medicine nor a set of guidelines. It describes the best available evidence, and if there is no good evidence it says so.

Clinical Evidence undergoes a continual process of updating, expansion, and improvement, to include new evidence, cover new questions, and respond to user feedback. New and updated topics are posted on the website as soon as they are ready for publication. We encourage readers to access the site regularly (www.clinicalevidence.com) to see what is new and to view the "web extra" tables and figures. Old paper or CD-ROM issues of *Clinical Evidence* should be discarded or treated as a historical curiosity.

The content published in *Clinical Evidence* Issue 9 is a snapshot of all content that was ready for publication in February 2003. Seven new topics have been added since Issue 8: varicose veins, pancreatic cancer, seasonal allergic rhinitis, bronchiectasis, insomnia, raynauds phenomenon (primary), and non-Hodgkin's lymphoma. In addition, 80 topics have been updated and a further 10 updates will be posted on the website by the time the paper issue is in circulation.

The aim of the updating process is to minimise the interval between literature search date and publication. The most recent search date for topics included in this issue is December 2002. Figure 1 shows a distribution of the search dates for each topic.

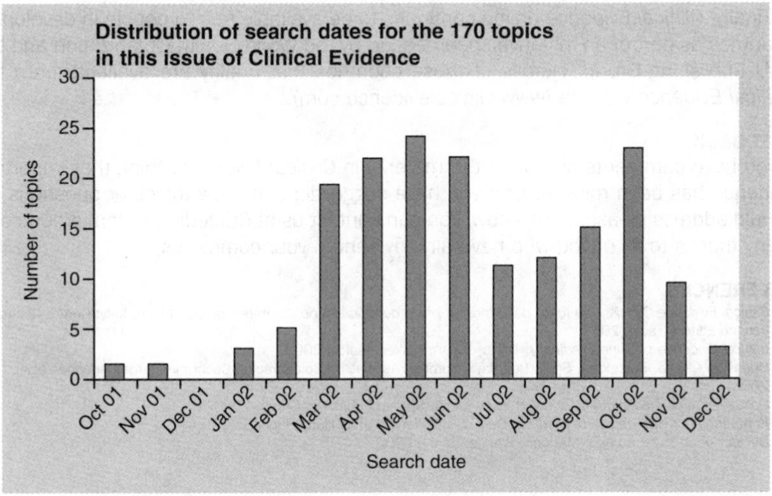

Contributors and editors incorporate the results of a rigorous update search every 8 months, as well as taking on feedback from users. This process sometimes involves substantial revisions. Stress incontinence and croup have been temporarily withdrawn while we restructure the content around revised questions; they will be posted on the website as soon as possible.

CONTRIBUTORS AND ADVISORS

We are extremely grateful to our contributors, peer reviewers, and editorial advisors. As expected in an ongoing project such as this, some contributors have stepped down and new ones have signed up. Former contributors are acknowledged in chronological order at the end of each topic. We also now list the titles and affiliations of our section advisors and editorial board members on the team page.

INTERNATIONAL REACH

Clinical Evidence has an international circulation. Thanks to the United Health Foundation in America, over 500,000 doctors and healthcare professionals in the United States receive *Clinical Evidence Concise* every six months and free access to the website. Thanks to the UK National Health Service, *Clinical Evidence* is available free to everyone in England via the National Electronic Library for Health (www.nelh.nhs.uk), and *Clinical Evidence Concise* is sent to 50,000 doctors and healthcare professionals every six months. In addition, 14,000 student members of the BMA now receive a copy of the full edition.

In May 2003, 300,000 Italian doctors received a copy of *Clinical Evidence Conciso*[1] and CD-ROM, both translated into Italian. This second Italian edition is based on Issue 7 of the English version and has been funded by the Italian Ministry of Health in the framework of their programme for independent health information. The scientific responsibility for the translation and adaptation to the Italian context has been assumed by the Italian Cochrane Centre, assisted by Editore Zadig.

Clinical Evidence is also available in other non-English language editions. The full text is available in Japanese (second edition), Spanish, and Russian (seven broad speciality editions). The *Concise* edition is available in German (with CD-ROM in English), Spanish, and French (second edition, with CD-ROM in English). We are pleased to be working closely with the Cochrane Centres in Italy and Spain, which have taken responsibility for these translations

Finally, *Clinical Evidence* online continues to be available free to people in developing countries as part of an initiative spearheaded by the World Health Organization and the BMJ Publishing Group. Details of those countries that qualify are available from the *Clinical Evidence* website (www.clinicalevidence.com).

FEEDBACK

If you have comments on any of the material in *Clinical Evidence*, think that important evidence has been missed, or if you have suggestions for new topics or questions we should address please let us know. You can contact us at CEfeedback@bmjgroup.com. Many thanks to all of you who have already sent in your comments

REFERENCES

1. *Clinical Evidence Conciso: La fonte delle migliori prove de efficacia per la pratica clinica.* Milan, Italy: Centro Cochrane Italiano/Editore Zadig, 2003.
2. *Clinical Evidence (Japanese edition).* Tokyo, Japan: Nikkei Medical 2002.
3. *Evidencia Clinica.* Barcelona, Spain/Bogotá, Colombia: Asociación Colaboración Cochrane Iberoamericana/Legis, 2003.
4. *Dokazatel'naya meditsina.* Moscow, Russia: Media Sphera Publishing Group, 2003.
5. *Kompendium evidenzbasierte Medizin.* Bern, Switzerland: Verlag Hans Huber, 2003.
6. *Décider pour traiter abrégé.* Meudon, France: RanD, 2002.

A Guide to Clinical Evidence Concise

Clinical Evidence Concise is an index of the summary information from each chapter in *Clinical Evidence* Issue 9.

Clinical Evidence Concise contains evidence relating to hundreds of therapeutic or preventative interventions, derived from thousands of original studies, and presents it in under 500 pages. For each condition, interventions are categorised according to whether they have been found to be effective or not. The full evidence detail behind these summaries, including clinical questions, figures, tables, and appendices, are featured on the accompanying CD-ROM, along with quantified, referenced, and up to date information about each condition.

Making summaries involves discarding detail, and users of *Clinical Evidence Concise* need to be aware of the limitations of the evidence that is presented. It is not possible to make global statements that are both useful and apply to every patient or clinical context that occur in practice. For example, when stating that we found evidence that a drug is beneficial, we mean that there is evidence that the drug has been shown to deliver more benefits than harms, when assessed in at least one subgroup of people, using at least one outcome at a particular point in time. It does not mean that the drug will be effective in all people given that treatment or that other outcomes will be improved, or even that the same outcome will be improved at a different time after the treatment.

MEASURE OF TREATMENT EFFECTS

The dilemma is how to present summaries that are useful but not misleading. We have experimented with providing statements with no numerical information at all, with NNTs only, with a batch of absolute and relative risks, or with just the odds ratio. Each measure has its advantages and disadvantages, and not all are available from the included studies. Quantitative results may be misleading in the absence of discussion of their precision, reliability, and applicability. In *Clinical Evidence Concise*, we present non-numerical information only. Detailed quantitative results are presented on the CD-ROM, where we are able to discuss their interpretation in more detail. Your suggestions on improvements are welcome and will be read with interest.

USING CLINICAL EVIDENCE CONCISE AND COMPANION CD-ROM

Clinical Evidence Concise is intended to be used as a first point of call when trying to decide what the options for treatment might be. A detailed exploration of the evidence will require looking up the detail on the CD-ROM, the full print version, or *Clinical Evidence* online. The electronic versions link, whenever possible, to abstracts of the original research in PubMed or published online versions. In this way, *Clinical Evidence* is also designed to act as a pointer, connecting the clinician rapidly to the relevant original evidence.

INDEX PAGE

Each topic on the CD-ROM contains an index page listing interventions within their assigned categories of whether they have been found to be effective or not. Key messages summarising the evidence for each intervention are listed below the categorisation table. The full evidence detail supporting the categorisation, consisting of the question, a summary statement, benefits, harms, and a comment can be accessed by a hyperlink from the categorisation table. We would value your feedback on the presentation of interventions in future issues.

CATEGORISATION

We have developed these categories of effectiveness from one of the Cochrane Collaboration's first and most popular products, *A guide to effective care in pregnancy and childbirth*.[1] The categories we now use are explained in the table below.

TABLE	Categorisation of treatment effects in *Clinical Evidence*
Beneficial	Interventions for which effectiveness has been demonstrated by clear evidence from RCTs, and for which expectation of harms is small compared with the benefits.
Likely to be beneficial	Interventions for which effectiveness is less well established than for those listed under "beneficial".
Trade off between benefits and harms	Interventions for which clinicians and patients should weigh up the beneficial and harmful effects according to individual circumstances and priorities.
Unknown effectiveness	Interventions for which there are currently insufficient data or data of inadequate quality.
Unlikely to be beneficial	Interventions for which lack of effectiveness is less well established than for those listed under "likely to be ineffective or harmful".
Likely to be ineffective or harmful	Interventions for which ineffectiveness or harmfulness has been demonstrated by clear evidence.

Fitting interventions into these categories is not always straightforward. For one thing, the categories represent a mix of several hierarchies: the level of benefit (or harm), the level of evidence (RCT or observational data), and the level of certainty around the finding (represented by the confidence interval). Another problem is that much of the evidence that is most relevant to clinical decisions relates to comparisons between different interventions rather than to comparison with placebo or no intervention. Where necessary, we have indicated the comparisons. A third problem is that interventions may have been tested, or found to be effective, in only one group of people, such as those at high risk of an outcome. Again, we have indicated this where possible. But perhaps most difficult of all has been trying to maintain consistency across different topics. We are working on refining the criteria for putting interventions under each category.

REFERENCES

Full references to the individual studies cited in *Clinical Evidence Concise* are available on the accompanying CD-ROM.

References cited in the definition, incidence/prevalence, aetiology/risk factors, and prognosis sections are listed in the text but are available as hyperlinks from the equivalent section on the CD-ROM.

TOPIC GLOSSARY

Topics may contain glossary listings; these are available in full on the CD-ROM and can be accessed from the index page of each topic or as hyperlinks from the equivalent section on the CD-ROM. Terms with corresponding CD-ROM definitions will be flagged up with a symbol Ⓖ.

MAIN GLOSSARY

Words and terms that are used throughout *Clinical Evidence* are listed in the main glossary on the companion CD-ROM. One example is the use of the word "significant", which, when used without qualification, is being used in the statistical sense; however, the term "clinically significant" indicates a finding that is clinically important.

TABLES AND FIGURES

The presence of figures and tables on the CD-ROM are flagged up in a similar way to the glossary with the use of Ⓕ for figures and Ⓣ for tables.

FEEDBACK

We would like feedback from CD-ROM users, in order to improve future releases. Simply follow the guidance on the CD-ROM welcome page. This process should take up just 10 minutes of your time.

The design of *Clinical Evidence Concise* will change progressively over the next few years. We will perform evaluation studies ourselves to measure the relevance of the material to the questions that are being asked in practice, the ease of use, and to check that the message extracted from the summary corresponds closely with that intended. If you have any comments, suggestions, or detect any errors, please let us know at CEfeedback@bmjgroup.com.

For more information on any of our methods or processes, please visit our website at www.clinicalevidence.com.

Please refer to the CD-ROM for more information about *Clinical Evidence*.

REFERENCES

1. Enkin M, Keirse M, Renfrew M, et al. *A guide to effective care in pregnancy and childbirth*. Oxford: Oxford University Press, 1998.

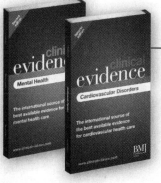

Non-Hodgkin's lymphoma

Search date October 2002

Graham Mead, James Woodcock, and Charles Young

Effects of treatments for early stage aggressive non-Hodgkin's lymphoma (NHL) in younger adults New

LIKELY TO BE BENEFICIAL

Short schedule CHOP plus radiotherapy versus longer schedule CHOP alone

One RCT found that short schedule CHOPⒼ plus radiotherapy significantly improved 5 year survival with the addition of radiotherapy compared with longer schedule CHOP alone. It included many older people. Longer schedule CHOP increased the risk of congestive heart failure and possibly the risk of myelosuppression.

UNKNOWN EFFECTIVENESS

ACVBP versus m-BACOD

One RCT, mostly in people with early stageⒼ disease, found no significant difference in 5 year survival between ACVBPⒼ and m-BACODⒼ.

Chemotherapy versus radiotherapy

We found no systematic review or RCTs of chemotherapy compared with radiotherapy.

CVP versus BACOP

Subgroup analysis in one RCT found no significant difference in complete remission between CVPⒼ and BACOPⒼ.

Effects of treatments for advanced stage aggressive NHL in younger adults New

LIKELY TO BE BENEFICIAL

CHOP versus BCOP

One RCT compared CHOP with BCOPⒼ. Subgroup analysis of people with advanced stageⒼ disease found significantly higher complete response with CHOP. Subgroup analysis in people younger than 60 years found similar results but the difference was not significant. However, 20% of people were excluded for poorly defined reasons.

CHOP versus HOP

One poorly reported RCT, including people with all grades of NHL, found significantly higher complete response with CHOP with HOPⒼ. However, 20% of people were excluded for a variety of reasons.

CHOP versus MEV

One RCT, including some older people and people who relapsed after treatment for early stage disease, found weak evidence of a survival benefit with CHOP compared with MEVⒼ. Subgroup analysis in people with advanced disease found that more people achieved complete response with CHOP. ▶

Non-Hodgkin's lymphoma

TRADE OFF BETWEEN BENEFITS AND HARMS

CHOP versus MACOP-B

One RCT, including some people aged over 65 years, found no significant difference in 3 year survival between four chemotherapy regimens: CHOP, MACOP-B**G**, m-BACOD**G**, and ProMACE-CytaBOM**G**. It found limited evidence of greater toxicity with MACOP-B and m-BACOD compared with CHOP and ProMACE-CytaBOM. A second RCT, including some people with early disease and some older people, found no significant difference in complete response. Subgroup analysis in younger people found significantly improved 5 year survival with MACOP-B. A third RCT, including people with stage II disease, found no significant difference in complete response. Subgroup analysis from one centre found better quality of life and physical function with MACOP-B compared with CHOP. These two RCTs found a different range of adverse events with CHOP compared with MACOP-B.

UNKNOWN EFFECTIVENESS

CHOP versus CHOP-B

One RCT in a population of mixed ages found no significant difference in 5 year mortality between CHOP and CHOP-B**G**.

CHOP versus CHOP-M

One poorly reported RCT in a population of mixed ages and disease stages found similar mortality at 36 months with CHOP and CHOP-M**G**.

CHOP versus CHOP plus interferon

We found no systematic review or RCTs of CHOP versus CHOP plus interferon.

CHOP versus CHOP plus monoclonal antibodies

We found one systematic review, which found no RCTs of CHOP versus CHOP plus monoclonal antibodies.

CHOP versus CHOP/VIA

One RCT, including people with stage II disease, found no significant difference in 3 year survival between CHOP and CHOP/VIA**G**.

CHOP versus CIOP

One RCT of people with Kiel classification intermediate grade lymphoma, including some people with stage II disease and some people over 65 years of age, found similar overall survival at 42 months with CHOP and CIOP**G**.

CHOP versus m-BACOD

We found one RCT comparing four different chemotherapy regimens (see CHOP versus MACOP-B above). A second RCT comparing CHOP with m-BACOD, including older adults and with a high withdrawal rate, found no significant difference in mortality at 4 or 5.3 years.

CHOP versus PACEBOM

One RCT of people with intermediate grade lymphoma, including some people with stage II disease, found no difference in 5 or 8 year mortality in the total population. Subgroup analysis found mortality was lower with PACEBOM**G** than CHOP in people with stage IV disease at 8 years' follow up, but the difference was not significant.

CHOP versus ProMACE-CytaBOM

We found one RCT comparing four different chemotherapy regimens (see CHOP *v* MACOP-B above). A second RCT, including some people with stage II disease and some people over 65 years of age, found longer median survival with CHOP compared with ProMACE-CytaBOM, but significance was not assessed.

Non-Hodgkin's lymphoma

DEFINITION NHL consists of a complex group of cancers arising mainly from B lymphocytes and occasionally from T lymphocytes (15% of cases). NHL usually develops in lymph nodes but can arise in other tissues almost anywhere in the body. NHL is divided according to histology and stage (spread). **Histology:** Historically histology was divided into aggressive and low grade disease. This chapter focuses on the most common aggressive lymphoma — diffuse large B cell lymphoma in the WHOⓉ,[1] and REAL classification systemsⒼ. Interpretation of older studies is complicated by changes in classification systems and diagnostic techniques. We have included studies using older systems if they are primarily in people with the following types of aggressive lymphoma: Working Formulation classification — primarily intermediate grades (grades E–HⓉ);[2] Kiel classification — centroblastic, immunoblastic, and anaplasticⓉ;[3] Rappaport classification — diffuse histiocytic, diffuse lymphocytic poorly differentiated, and diffuse mixed (lymphocytic and histiocyticⓉ).[4] There is no direct correspondence between the terms used in the different classification systems and attempts to generalise results must be treated with caution.[1–4] **Stage:** Historically, NHL has been staged according to disease spread using the Ann ArborⒼ systemⓉ.[5] Ann Arbor stages I and II correspond to early disease, whereas stages III and IV are advanced disease. However, people with bulky disease will usually be treated as having advanced disease even if the stage is only I or II. There is also substantial variation in prognosis within each stage. More recent studies assess stage using a prognostic indicator. We excluded RCTs that were primarily in children (< 16 years old), older people (> 65 years old), people with HIV infection, and people who had received prior treatment except local radiotherapy. We also excluded RCTs of maintenance treatment and RCTs with fewer than 50 people in each arm. In RCTs of mixed populations we have reported subgroup analysis in the population of interest, if available.

INCIDENCE/ PREVALENCE NHL occurs more commonly in males than females, and is increasing in incidence in the Western world at about 4% a year. It is the seventh most common cancer in the UK consisting of 8680 new cases in 1998 (3% of cancers) and causing 4500 deaths in 2000.[6]

AETIOLOGY/ RISK FACTORS Unknown for most people. Surveys have implicated pesticides and hair dyes. Incidence is higher in people who are immunosuppressed.

PROGNOSIS Relates to histological type, stage, age, performance status, and lactate dehydrogenase levels. High grade lymphomas, particularly diffuse large B cell lymphoma and Burkitt's lymphoma, have a high cure rate, with both initial and salvage (high dose) chemotherapy.[7] CHOP is the standard treatment for aggressiveⒼ NHL and placebo controlled trials would be considered unethical.

Please refer to CD-ROM for full text and references.

Acute myocardial infarction

Search date June 2002

Nicolas Danchin, Edoardo De Benedetti, and Philip Urban

What treatments improve outcomes in acute myocardial infarction?

BENEFICIAL

Angiotensin converting enzyme inhibitors

One overview and one systematic review in people (treated within 36 h to 14 days of acute myocardial infarction) have found that angiotensin converting enzyme inhibitors versus placebo significantly reduce mortality after 30 days. However, the overview also found that angiotensin converting enzyme inhibitors versus placebo significantly increase persistent hypotension and renal dysfunction. Whether angiotensin converting enzyme inhibitors should be offered to everyone presenting with acute myocardial infarction or only to people with signs of heart failure remains unresolved.

Aspirin

One systematic review in people with acute myocardial infarction has found that aspirin versus placebo significantly reduces mortality, non-fatal reinfarction, and non-fatal stroke at 1 month.

β Blockers

Two systematic reviews and one subsequent RCT have found that β blockers versus control given within hours of acute myocardial infarction significantly reduce both mortality and reinfarction. One RCT in people receiving thrombolytic treatment found that immediate versus delayed treatment with metoprolol significantly reduced rates of reinfarction and recurrent chest pain at 6 days, but had no significant effect on mortality at 6 days or at 1 year. One RCT comparing carvedilol versus placebo in people with recent myocardial infarction and left ejection fraction of 40% or less receiving thrombolytic treatment found no significant difference in the combined endpoint of all cause mortality and hospital admission for any cardiovascular event after a median of 1.3 years, although mortality alone and recurrent non-fatal myocardial infarction were significantly lower with carvedilol.

Primary percutaneous transluminal coronary angioplasty versus thrombolysis (performed in specialist centres)

Two systematic reviews have found that primary percutaneous transluminal coronary angioplasty versus primary thrombolysis significantly reduces mortality and reinfarction at 30 days in people with acute myocardial infarction. However, the trials were conducted mainly in specialist centres. The effectiveness of percutaneous transluminal coronary angioplasty versus thrombolysis in less specialist centres remains uncertain.

Thrombolysis

One overview of RCTs in people with acute myocardial infarction and ST elevation or bundle branch block on their initial electrocardiogram has found that prompt thrombolytic treatment (within 6 h and perhaps up to 12 h and longer after the onset of symptoms) versus placebo significantly reduces short term mortality. The overview found that thrombolytic treatment versus control significantly increased the risk of stroke or major bleeding. Meta-analysis of RCTs comparing different types of thrombolytic agents versus each other have found no significant difference in mortality.

▶

Clin Evid Concise 2003;9:4–7.

LIKELY TO BE BENEFICIAL

Nitrates in the absence of thrombolysis

One systematic review of the trials conducted in the prethrombolytic era found that nitrates versus placebo significantly reduce the risk of mortality in people with acute myocardial infarction.

UNLIKELY TO BE BENEFICIAL

Nitrates in addition to thrombolysis

Two RCTs from the thrombolytic era comparing nitrates versus placebo in people with acute myocardial infarction found no significant difference in mortality.

TRADE OFF BETWEEN BENEFITS AND HARMS

Glycoprotein IIb/IIIa inhibitors *New*

Two large RCTs have found that combined treatment with half dose thrombolysis plus abciximab does not reduce mortality at 1 month compared with full dose thrombolysis in people with acute myocardial infarction, but may prevent non-fatal cardiovascular events. However, the RCTs found that combined treatment with abciximab increased bleeding complications, particularly extracranial haemorrhage. Three RCTs found conflicting evidence about the benefits of adding abciximab to primary coronary angioplasty or stenting in people with acute myocardial infarction, although all found that adding abciximab increased bleeding risk.

LIKELY TO BE INEFFECTIVE OR HARMFUL

Calcium channel blockers

Nine RCTs in people within the first few days of an acute myocardial infarction have found that neither dihydropiridines nor verapamil reduce mortality compared with placebo. In people with left ventricular dysfunction one RCT found limited evidence that nifedipine given in the first few days after myocardial infarction may increase mortality compared with placebo.

Which treatments improve outcomes for cardiogenic shock after acute myocardial infarction?

BENEFICIAL

Early invasive cardiac revascularisation

One large RCT in people with cardiogenic shock within 48 hours of acute myocardial infarction has found that early invasive cardiac revascularisation**G** versus initial medical treatment alone significantly reduces mortality after 6 months and 12 months. A second smaller RCT found similar results, although the difference was not significant.

UNKNOWN EFFECTIVENESS

Intra-aortic balloon counterpulsation

One abstract of an RCT comparing intra-aortic balloon counterpulsation**G** plus thrombolysis versus thrombolysis alone in people with cardiogenic shock following acute myocardial infarction found no significant difference in mortality after 6 months.

Cardiac transplantation; early cardiac surgery; positive inotropes and vasodilators; pulmonary artery catheterisation; ventricular assistance devices

We found no evidence from RCTs about the effects of these interventions.

UNLIKELY TO BE BENEFICIAL

Thrombolysis

Subgroup analysis of people with cardiogenic shock after acute myocardial infarction from one RCT comparing thrombolysis versus no thrombolysis found no significant difference in mortality after 21 days.

DEFINITION **Acute myocardial infarction:** The sudden occlusion of a coronary artery leading to myocardial cell death. **Cardiogenic shock:** Defined clinically as a poor cardiac output plus evidence of tissue hypoxia that is not improved by correcting reduced intravascular volume.[1] When a pulmonary artery catheter is used, cardiogenic shock may be defined as a cardiac index below 2.2 litres/minute/m^2 despite an elevated pulmonary capillary wedge pressure (≥ 15 mm Hg).[1–3]

INCIDENCE/ PREVALENCE **Acute myocardial infarction:** One of the most common causes of mortality worldwide. In 1990, ischaemic heart disease was the world's leading cause of death, accounting for about 6.3 million deaths. The age standardised incidence varies among and within countries.[4] Each year, about 900 000 people in the USA experience acute myocardial infarction of whom about 225 000 die. About half of these people die within 1 hour of symptoms and before reaching a hospital emergency room.[5] Event rates increase with age for both sexes and are higher in men than in women and in poorer than richer people at all ages. The incidence of death from acute myocardial infarction has fallen in many Western countries over the past 20 years. **Cardiogenic shock:** Cardiogenic shock occurs in about 7% of people admitted to hospital with acute myocardial infarction.[6] Of these, about half have established cardiogenic shock at the time of admission to hospital, and most of the others develop it during the first 24–48 hours of their admission.[7]

AETIOLOGY/ RISK FACTORS **Acute myocardial infarction:** See aetiology/risk factors under primary prevention, p 000. The immediate mechanism of acute myocardial infarction is rupture of an atheromatous plaque causing thrombosis and occlusion of coronary arteries and myocardial cell death. Factors that may convert a stable plaque into an unstable plaque (the "active plaque") have yet to be fully elucidated. Shear stresses, inflammation, and autoimmunity have been proposed. The changing rates of coronary heart disease in different populations are only partly explained by changes in the standard risk factors for ischaemic heart disease (particularly fall in blood pressure and smoking). **Cardiogenic shock:** Cardiogenic shock after AMI usually follows a reduction in functional ventricular myocardium, and is caused by left ventricular infarction (79% of people with cardiogenic shock), more often than by right ventricular infarction (3% of people with cardiogenic shock).[8] Cardiogenic shock after acute myocardial infarction may also be caused by cardiac structural defects, such as mitral valve regurgitation due to papillary muscle dysfunction (7% of people with cardiogenic shock), ventricular septal rupture (4% of people with cardiogenic shock), or cardiac tamponade following free cardiac wall rupture (1% of people with cardiogenic shock). Major risk factors for cardiogenic shock after AMI are previous myocardial infarction, diabetes mellitus, advanced age, hypotension, tachycardia or bradycardia, congestive heart failure with Killip class II–III, and low left ventricular ejection fraction (ejection fraction < 35%).[7,8]

Acute myocardial infarction

◀ **PROGNOSIS** **Acute myocardial infarction:** Acute myocardial infarction may lead to a host of mechanical and cardiac electrical complications, including death, ventricular dysfunction, congestive heart failure, fatal and non-fatal arrhythmias, valvular dysfunction, myocardial rupture, and cardiogenic shock. **Cardiogenic shock:** Mortality rates for people in hospital with cardiogenic shock after AMI vary between 50–80%.[2,3,6,7] Most deaths occur within 48 hours of the onset of shock Ⓕ.[9] People surviving until discharge from hospital have a reasonable long term prognosis (88% survival at 1 year).[10]

Please refer to CD-ROM for full text and references.

Angina (unstable)

Search date April 2002

Madhu Natarajan

What are the effects of treatments?

BENEFICIAL

Aspirin

One systematic review has found that aspirin versus placebo significantly reduces the risk of death, myocardial infarction, and stroke at 6 months.

LIKELY TO BE BENEFICIAL

Adenosine diphosphate inhibitors

One RCT found that clopidogrel versus placebo reduced death, myocardial infarction, and stroke after 9 months. Clopidogrel increased the risk of major bleeding, but not haemorrhagic stokes. Another RCT found that ticlopidine versus conventional treatment reduced vascular deaths and non-fatal myocardial infarction after 6 months, but was associated with neutropenia.

Direct thrombin inhibitors

One systematic review has found that direct thrombin inhibitors versus heparin reduces death and myocardial infarction after 30 days.

Intravenous glycoprotein IIb/IIIa inhibitors

One systematic review has found that intravenous glycoprotein IIb/IIIa inhibitors reduce death or myocardial infarction compared with placebo, but increase the risk of major bleeding complications.

Low molecular weight heparins

One systematic review has found that low molecular weight heparin versus placebo or no treatment reduced death or myocardial infarction and did not increase bleeding complications in the first 7 days after onset of symptoms. It also found that longer term treatment with low molecular weight heparin versus placebo did not reduce death or myocardial infarction, and increased major bleeding. One systematic review found that low molecular weight heparin versus unfractionated heparin did not reduce death or myocardial infarction.

Unfractionated heparin added to aspirin

Two systematic reviews have found that adding unfractionated heparin to aspirin in people with unstable angina reduces death or myocardial infarction with no significant increase in major bleeding after 1 week of treatment. One systematic review found that adding unfractionated heparin to aspirin did not reduce death or myocardial infarction after 12 weeks.

UNKNOWN EFFECTIVENESS

Routine early invasive treatment

Four RCTs found conflicting evidence on the effects of early invative treatment versus conservative treatment.

β Blockers; nitrates

We found insufficient evidence of the effects of these interventions.

UNLIKELY TO BE BENEFICIAL

Calcium channel blockers

One systematic review found that calcium channel blockers versus placebo or versus standard treatment did not reduce death or myocardial infarction.

◀ **Warfarin**

Five RCTs found no significant difference in myocardial infarction or death with the addition of warfarin to standard treatment. One RCT found that warfarin was associated with an increase in major bleeding.

LIKELY TO BE INEFFECTIVE OR HARMFUL

Oral glycoprotein IIb/IIIa inhibitors

One systematic review found that oral glycoprotein IIb/IIIa inhibitors did not reduce mortality, myocardial infarction, or recurrent ischaemia but increased bleeding events.

DEFINITION Unstable angina is distinguished from stable angina, acute myocardial infarction, and non-cardiac pain by the pattern of symptoms (characteristic pain present at rest or on lower levels of activity), the severity of symptoms (recently increasing intensity, frequency, or duration), and the absence of persistent ST elevation on a resting electrocardiogram. Unstable angina includes a variety of different clinical patterns: angina at rest of up to 1 week's duration; angina increasing in severity to moderate or severe pain; non-Q wave myocardial infarction; and post-myocardial infarction angina continuing for longer than 24 hours.

INCIDENCE/PREVALENCE In industrialised countries the annual incidence of unstable angina is about 6/10 000 people in the general population.

AETIOLOGY/RISK FACTORS Risk factors are the same as for other manifestations of ischaemic heart disease: older age, previous atheromatous cardiovascular disease, diabetes mellitus, smoking cigarettes, hypertension, hypercholesterolaemia, male sex, and a family history of ischaemic heart disease. Unstable angina can also occur in association with other disorders of the circulation, including heart valve disease, arrhythmia, and cardiomyopathy.

PROGNOSIS In people taking aspirin, the incidence of serious adverse outcomes (such as death, acute myocardial infarction, or refractory angina requiring emergency revascularisation) is 5–10% within the first 7 days and about 15% at 30 days. Between 5% and 14% of people with unstable angina die in the year after diagnosis, with about half of these deaths occurring within 4 weeks of diagnosis. No single factor identifies people at higher risk of an adverse event. Risk factors include severity of presentation (e.g. duration of pain, rapidity of progression, evidence of heart failure), medical history (e.g. previous unstable angina, acute myocardial infarction, left ventricular dysfunction), other clinical parameters (e.g. age, diabetes), electrocardiogram changes (e.g. severity of ST segment depression, deep T wave inversion, transient ST elevation), biochemical parameters (e.g. troponin concentration), and change in clinical status (e.g. recurrent chest pain, silent ischaemia, haemodynamic instability).

Please refer to CD-ROM for full text and references.

Atrial fibrillation (acute)

Search date June 2002

Gregory Y H Lip, Sridhar Kamath, and Bethan Freestone

What are the effects of interventions to control heart rate?

LIKELY TO BE BENEFICIAL

Digoxin

We found no RCTs only in people with acute atrial fibrillation. Two RCTs found that digoxin versus placebo significantly reduced ventricular rate within 2 hours in people with atrial fibrillation of up to 7 days' duration.

Diltiazem

One RCT in people with atrial fibrillation or atrial flutter**G** found that intravenous diltiazem (a calcium channel blocker) versus placebo significantly reduced heart rate over 15 minutes. Another RCT in people with acute atrial fibrillation or atrial flutter found that intravenous diltiazem versus intravenous digoxin significantly reduced heart rate within 5 minutes.

Timolol

One small RCT in people with atrial fibrillation of unspecified duration found that intravenous timolol (a β blocker) versus placebo significantly reduced ventricular rate within 20 minutes.

Verapamil

Two RCTs found that intravenous verapamil (a calcium channel blocker) versus placebo significantly reduced heart rate at 10 or 30 minutes in people with atrial fibrillation or atrial flutter. One RCT found no significant difference in rate control or measures of systolic function with intravenous verapamil versus intravenous diltiazem in people with atrial fibrillation or atrial flutter, but verapamil caused hypotension in some people.

UNKNOWN EFFECTIVENESS

Amiodarone *New*

We found no RCTs examining effects of amiodarone alone on heart rate in people with acute atrial fibrillation.

What are the effects of interventions for conversion to sinus rhythm?

UNKNOWN EFFECTIVENESS

Amiodarone *New*

We found insufficient evidence from three RCTs about the effects of amiodarone as a single agent compared with placebo for conversion to sinus rhythm in people with acute atrial fibrillation. Four small RCTs have found no significant difference between amiodarone versus digoxin in rate of conversion to sinus rhythm at 24–48 hours, although the studies may have lacked power to exclude clinically important differences. We found insufficient evidence from one small RCT to compare amiodarone versus verapamil. We found no RCTs comparing amiodarone with either DC cardioversion or diltiazem.

DC cardioversion

We found no RCTs of DC cardioversion in acute atrial fibrillation. It may be unethical to conduct RCTs.

◀ **Digoxin**

Three RCTs found no significant difference in conversion to sinus rhythm with digoxin versus placebo in people with atrial fibrillation of up to 7 days' duration. Four small RCTs found no significant difference between amiodarone versus digoxin for conversion to sinus rhythm in people with acute atrial fibrillation, although the trials might have lacked power to exclude clincially important differences.

Timolol

One small RCT found no significant difference between intravenous timolol (a β blocker) versus placebo for conversion to sinus rhythm in people with atrial fibrillation of unspecified duration, but the study may have lacked power to detect a clinically important effect.

What are the effects of interventions to prevent embolism?

UNKNOWN EFFECTIVENESS

Antithrombotic treatment prior to cardioversion

We found no RCTs of aspirin, heparin, or warfarin as thromboprophylaxis prior to cardioversion in acute atrial fibrillation.

DEFINITION Acute atrial fibrillation is rapid, irregular, and chaotic atrial activity of less that 48 hours' duration. It includes both the first symptomatic onset of persistent atrial fibrillationⒼ and episodes of paroxysmal atrial fibrillationⒼ. It is sometimes difficult to distinguish episodes of new onset atrial fibrillation from long standing atrial fibrillation that was previously undiagnosed. Atrial fibrillation within 72 hours of onset is sometimes called recent onset atrial fibrillation. By contrast, chronic atrial fibrillationⒼ is a more sustained form of atrial fibrillation, which in turn can be described as paroxysmal, persistent, or permanent atrial fibrillationⒼ. Intermittent atrial fibrillation, with spontaneous recurrences/termination and with sinus rhythm between recurrences is known as paroxysmal atrial fibrillation. More sustained atrial fibrillation, which is considered amenable to cardioversion, is called persistent atrial fibrillation. If cardioversion is considered inappropriate, then the atrial fibrillation is known as "permanent". In this review we have excluded episodes of atrial fibrillation that arise during or soon after cardiac surgery, and we have excluded management of chronic atrial fibrillation.

INCIDENCE/ PREVALENCE We found limited evidence of the incidence or prevalence of acute atrial fibrillation. Extrapolation from the Framingham study[1] suggests an incidence in men of 3/1000 person years at age 55 years, rising to 38/1000 person years at 94 years. In women, the incidence was 2/1000 person years at age 55 years and 32.5/1000 person years at 94 years. The prevalence of atrial fibrillation ranged from 0.5% for people aged 50–59 years to 9% in people aged 80–89 years. Among acute emergency medical admissions in the UK, 3–6% have atrial fibrillation and about 40% were newly diagnosed.[2,3] Among acute hospital admissions in New Zealand, 10% (95% CI 9% to 12%) had documented atrial fibrillation.[4]

AETIOLOGY/ RISK FACTORS Paroxysms of atrial fibrillation are more common in athletes.[5] Age increases the risk of developing acute atrial fibrillation. Men are more likely to develop atrial fibrillation than women (38 years' follow up from the Framingham Study, RR after adjustment for age and known predisposing conditions 1.5).[6] Atrial fibrillation can occur in association with underlying disease (both cardiac and non-cardiac) or can arise in the absence of any other condition. Epidemiological surveys have found that risk factors for the development of acute atrial fibrillation include ischaemic heart disease, hypertension, heart failure, valve disease, diabetes, alcohol abuse, thyroid disorders, and disorders of the lung ▶

and pleura.[1] In a UK survey of acute hospital admissions with atrial fibrillation, a history of ischaemic heart disease was present in 33%, heart failure in 24%, hypertension in 26%, and rheumatic heart disease in 7%.[3] In some populations, the acute effects of alcohol explain a large proportion of the incidence of acute atrial fibrillation.

PROGNOSIS We found no evidence about the proportion of people with acute atrial fibrillation who develop more chronic forms of atrial fibrillation (e.g. paroxysmal, persistent, or permanent atrial fibrillation). Observational studies and placebo arms of RCTs have found that more than 50% of people with acute atrial fibrillation revert spontaneously within 24–48 hours, especially if atrial fibrillation is associated with an identifiable precipitant such as alcohol or myocardial infarction. We found little evidence about the effects on mortality and morbidity of acute atrial fibrillation where no underlying cause is found. Acute atrial fibrillation during myocardial infarction is an independent predictor of both short term and long term mortality.[7] Onset of atrial fibrillation reduces cardiac output by 10–20% irrespective of the underlying ventricular rate[8,9] and can contribute to heart failure. People with acute atrial fibrillation who present with heart failure have worse prognosis. Acute atrial fibrillation is associated with a risk of imminent stroke.[10–13] One case series used transoesophageal echocardiography in people who had developed acute atrial fibrillation within the preceding 48 hours; it found that 15% had atrial thrombi.[14] An ischaemic stroke associated with atrial fibrillation is more likely to be fatal, have a recurrence, and leave a serious functional deficit among survivors, than a stroke not associated with atrial fibrillation.[15]

Please refer to CD-ROM for full text and references.

Changing behaviour

Search date May 2002

Margaret Thorogood, Melvyn Hillsdon, and Carolyn Summerbell

What are the effects of interventions?

BENEFICIAL

Advice on cholesterol lowering diet

Systematic reviews have found that advice on cholesterol lowering diet (i.e. advice to lower total fat intake or increase the ratio of polyunsaturated to saturated fatty acid) leads to a small reduction in blood cholesterol concentrations in the long term (≥ 6 months).

Advice on diet and exercise supported by behavioural therapy for the encouragement of weight loss

Systematic reviews and subsequent RCTs have found that a combination of advice on diet and exercise supported by behavioural therapy is probably more effective than either diet or exercise advice alone in the treatment of obesity, and might lead to sustained weight loss.

Advice from physicians and trained counsellors to quit smoking

Systematic reviews have found that simple, one off advice from a physician during a routine consultation is associated with 2% of smokers quitting smoking and not relapsing for 1 year. Advice from trained counsellors (who are neither doctors nor nurses) increases quit rates compared with minimal intervention.

Advice on reducing sodium intake to reduce blood pressure

Systematic reviews have found that salt restriction significantly reduces blood pressure in people with hypertension, and have found limited evidence that salt restriction is effective in preventing hypertension. One RCT found limited evidence that advice on restricting salt intake was less effective than advice on weight reduction in preventing hypertension.

Bupropion as part of a smoking cessation programme

One systematic review of antidepressants used as part of a smoking cessation programme has found that bupropion increases quit rates at 1 year.

Counselling people at high risk of disease to quit smoking

Systematic reviews and subsequent RCTs have found that antismoking advice improves smoking cessation in people at higher risk of smoking related disease.

Counselling pregnant women to quit smoking

Two systematic reviews have found that antismoking interventions in pregnant women increase abstinence rates during pregnancy and reduce the risk of low birthweight babies. Interventions without nicotine replacement were as effective as nicotine replacement in healthy non-pregnant women.

Exercise advice to women over 80 years of age

One RCT found that exercise advice delivered in the home by physiotherapists increased physical activity and reduced the risk of falling in women over 80 years.

Nicotine replacement in smokers who smoke at least 10 cigarettes daily

One systematic review and one subsequent RCT have found that nicotine replacement is an effective additional component of cessation strategies in smokers who smoke at least 10 cigarettes daily. We found no clear evidence that any method of delivery of nicotine is more effective than others. We found limited evidence from three RCTs with follow up of 2–6 years that the additional benefit of nicotine replacement treatment on quit rates reduced with time.

Changing behaviour

LIKELY TO BE BENEFICIAL

Advice from nurses to quit smoking

One systematic review has found that advice to quit smoking versus no advice significantly increased the rate of quitting at 1 year.

Counselling sedentary people to increase physical activity

We found weak evidence from systematic reviews and subsequent RCTs that counselling sedentary people increases physical activity compared with no intervention. Limited evidence from RCTs suggests that consultation with an exercise specialist rather than a physician may increase physical activity at 1 year.

Self help materials for people who want to stop smoking

One systematic review found that self help materials slightly improve smoking cessation compared with no intervention. It found that individually tailored materials were more effective than standard or stage based materials and that telephone counselling increased the effectiveness of postal self help materials.

UNKNOWN EFFECTIVENESS

Physical exercise to aid smoking cessation

One systematic review found very limited evidence that exercise might increase smoking cessation.

Training health professionals to give advice on smoking cessation (increases frequency of antismoking interventions, but may not improve effectiveness)

One systematic review has found that training professionals increases the frequency of antismoking interventions being offered, but found no good evidence that antismoking interventions are more effective if the health professionals delivering the interventions received training. One RCT found that a structured intervention delivered by trained community pharmacists increased smoking cessation rates compared to usual care delivered by untrained community pharmacists.

LIKELY TO BE INEFFECTIVE OR HARMFUL

Acupuncture for smoking cessation

One systematic review has found no significant difference in rates of smoking cessation at 1 year with acupuncture versus control.

Anxiolytics for smoking cessation

One systematic review found no significant difference in quit rates with anxiolytics versus control.

*In terms of producing the intended behavioural change

DEFINITION Cigarette smoking, diet, and level of physical activity are important in the aetiology of many chronic diseases. Individual change in behaviour has the potential to decrease the burden of chronic disease, particularly cardiovascular disease. This topic focuses on the evidence that specific interventions lead to changed behaviour.

INCIDENCE/ PREVALENCE In the developed world, the decline in smoking has slowed and the prevalence of regular smoking is increasing in young people. A sedentary lifestyle is becoming increasingly common and the prevalence of obesity is increasing rapidly.

Please refer to CD-ROM for full text and references.

Heart failure

Search date October 2002

Robert McKelvie

What are the effects of treatments?

BENEFICIAL

Angiotensin converting enzyme inhibitors

Systematic reviews and RCTs have found that angiotensin converting enzyme inhibitors versus placebo significantly reduce ischaemic events, mortality and hospital admission for heart failure. Relative benefits are similar in different groups of people, but absolute benefits are greater in people with severe heart failure. RCTs in people with asymptomatic left ventricular systolic dysfunction have found that angiotensin converting enzyme inhibitors versus placebo significantly delay the onset of symptomatic heart failure and reduce cardiovascular events over 40 months.

β Blockers

Systematic reviews have found strong evidence that adding a β blocker to an angiotensin converting enzyme inhibitor significantly decreases mortality and hospital admission. Limited evidence from a subgroup analysis of one RCT found no significant effect on mortality in black people.

Digoxin (improves morbidity in people already receiving diuretics and angiotensin converting enzyme inhibitors)

One large RCT in people already receiving diuretics and angiotensin converting enzyme inhibitors found that digoxin versus placebo significantly reduced the number of people admitted to hospital for worsening heart failure at 37 months, but did not significantly reduce mortality.

LIKELY TO BE BENEFICIAL

Angiotensin II receptor blockers

One systematic review has found that angiotensin receptor blockers versus placebo reduced all cause mortality and hospital admission in people with New York Heart Association**G** class II–IV heart failure, although the difference was not significant. It found no significant difference in all cause mortality or hospital admission with angiotensin receptor blockers versus angiotensin converting enzyme inhibitors. It found that angiotensin receptor blockers plus angiotensin converting enzyme inhibitors versus angiotensin converting enzyme inhibitors alone reduced admission for heart failure but did not significantly reduce all cause mortality.

Exercise

One systematic review has found that exercise training improved physiological measures compared with control. One included RCT assessed clinical outcomes and found that exercise versus control improved quality of life and reduced cardiac events, mortality, and hospital readmission for heart failure at 12 months. One subsequent RCT found no significant difference for 3 months of supervised aerobic and resistance training followed by 9 months of home based training versus usual care in 6 minute walk distance or quality of life at 12 months.

▶

Implantable cardiac defibrillators (in people with heart failure and near fatal arrhythmia)

One RCT has found good evidence that an implantable cardiac defibrillator reduces mortality in people with heart failure who have experienced a near fatal ventricular arrhythmia.

Multidisciplinary interventions

One systematic review has found that multidisciplinary programmes significantly reduce admissions to hospital but did not significantly reduce mortality. The review found that telephone contact plus improved coordination of primary care had no significant effect on admission rate. Two included RCTs found that that home-based support versus usual care significantly reduced cardiovascular events at 3–6 years. Subsequent RCTs found that education and nurse led support reduced death and hospital readmission and improved quality of life at 12 weeks to 1 year.

Prophylactic use of implantable cardiac defibrillators in people at risk of arryhthmia

Two RCTs have found that implantable cardiac defibrillators versus medical treatment reduce mortality in people with heart failure and at high risk of arrhythmia, whereas one RCT found no significant difference in mortality.

Spironolactone in severe heart failure

One RCT in people with severe heart failure taking diuretics, angiotensin converting enzyme inhibitors, and digoxin has found that adding spironolactone versus placebo significantly reduces mortality after 2 years.

UNKNOWN EFFECTIVENESS

Amiodarone

Systematic reviews have found weak evidence suggesting that amiodarone versus placebo may reduce mortality. However, we were not able to draw firm conclusions about effects of amiodarone in people with heart failure.

Anticoagulation

A preliminary report from one RCT found no significant difference for warfarin versus no antithrombotic treatment or for warfarin versus aspirin for the combined outcome of death, myocardial infarction and stroke after 27 months. However, the study may have lacked power to detect a clinically important difference.

Antiplatelet agents

A preliminary report from one RCT found no significant difference for aspirin versus no antithrombotic treatment or for aspirin versus warfarin for the combined outcome of death, myocardial infarction and stroke after 27 months. However, the study may have lacked power to detect a clinically important difference.

Calcium channel blockers

One systematic review has found no significant difference in mortality with second generation dihydropyridine calcium channel blockers versus placebo. RCTs comparing other calcium channel blockers versus placebo found no evidence of benefit.

Treatments for diastolic heart failure

We found no RCTs in people with diastolic heart failure.

LIKELY TO BE INEFFECTIVE OR HARMFUL

Non-amiodarone antiarrhythmic drugs

Evidence extrapolated from one systematic review in people treated after a myocardial infarction suggests that other antiarrhythmic drugs (apart from β blockers) may increase mortality.

Positive inotropes (ibopamine, milrinone, vesnarinone)

RCTs found that positive inotropic drugs (other than digoxin) versus placebo significantly increased mortality over 6–11 months.

DEFINITION Heart failure occurs when abnormality of cardiac function causes failure of the heart to pump blood at a rate sufficient for metabolic requirements under normal filling pressure. It is characterised clinically by breathlessness, effort intolerance, fluid retention, and poor survival. It can be caused by systolic or diastolic dysfunction and is associated with neurohormonal changes.[1] Left ventricular systolic dysfunction (LVSD) is defined as a left ventricular ejection fraction below 0.40. It may be symptomatic or asymptomatic. Defining and diagnosing diastolic heart failure can be difficult. Recently proposed criteria include: (1) clinical evidence of heart failure; (2) normal or mildly abnormal left ventricular systolic function; and (3) evidence of abnormal left ventricular relaxation, filling, diastolic distensibility, or diastolic stiffness.[2] However, assessment of some of these criteria is not standardised.

INCIDENCE/ PREVALENCE Both the incidence and prevalence of heart failure increase with age. Studies of heart failure in the USA and Europe found that under 65 years of age the incidence is 1/1000 men a year and 0.4/1000 women a year. Over 65 years, incidence is 11/1000 men a year and 5/1000 women a year. Under 65 years the prevalence of heart failure is 1/1000 men and 1/1000 women; over 65 years the prevalence is 40/1000 men and 30/1000 women.[3] The prevalence of asymptomatic LVSD is 3% in the general population.[4–6] The mean age of people with asymptomatic LVSD is lower than that for symptomatic individuals. Both heart failure and asymptomatic LVSD are more common in men.[4–6] The prevalence of diastolic heart failure in the community is unknown. The prevalence of heart failure with preserved systolic function in people in hospital with clinical heart failure varies from 13–74%.[7,8] Less than 15% of people with heart failure under 65 years have normal systolic function, whereas the prevalence is about 40% in people over 65 years.[7]

AETIOLOGY/ RISK FACTORS Coronary artery disease is the most common cause of heart failure.[3] Other common causes include hypertension and idiopathic dilated congestive cardiomyopathy. After adjustment for hypertension, the presence of left ventricular hypertrophy remains a risk factor for the development of heart failure. Other risk factors include cigarette smoking, hyperlipidaemia, and diabetes mellitus.[4] The common causes of left ventricular diastolic dysfunction are coronary artery disease and systemic hypertension. Other causes are hypertrophic cardiomyopathy, restrictive or infiltrative cardiomyopathies, and valvular heart disease.[8]

PROGNOSIS The prognosis of heart failure is poor, with 5 year mortality ranging from 26–75%.[3] Up to 16% of people are readmitted with heart failure within 6 months of first admission. In the USA, heart failure it is the leading cause of hospital admission among people over 65 years of age.[3] In people with heart failure, a new myocardial infarction increases the risk of death (RR 7.8, 95% CI 6.9 to 8.8). About a third of all deaths in people with heart failure are preceded by a major ischaemic event.[9] Sudden death, mainly caused by ventricular arrhythmias, is responsible for 25–50% of all deaths, and is the most common cause of death in people with heart failure.[10] The presence of asymptomatic LVSD increases an individual's risk of having a cardiovascular event. One large prevention trial found that for a 5% reduction in ejection fraction, the risk ratio for mortality was 1.20 (95% CI 1.13 to 1.29). For hospital admission for heart

Heart failure

failure, the risk ratio was 1.28 (95% CI 1.18 to 1.38) and the risk ratio of heart failure was 1.20 (95% CI 1.13 to 1.26).[4] The annual mortality of patients with diastolic heart failure varies in observational studies (1.3–17.5%).[7] Reasons for this variation include age, the presence of coronary artery disease, and variation in the partition value used to define abnormal ventricular systolic function. The annual mortality for left ventricular diastolic dysfunction is lower than that found in patients with systolic dysfunction.[11]

Please refer to CD-ROM for full text and references.

Peripheral arterial disease

Search date August 2002

Clinical Evidence freelance writers

What are the effects of treatments for chronic peripheral arterial disease?

BENEFICIAL

Antiplatelet treatment

Systematic reviews found that antiplatelet agents versus control treatments significantly reduce the rate of major cardiovascular events over about 2 years. Systematic reviews have found that antiplatelet agents versus placebo or no treatment significantly reduce the risk of arterial occlusion and reduce the risk of revascularisation procedures. The balance of benefits and harms is in favour of treatment for most people with symptomatic peripheral arterial disease, because as a group they are at much greater risk of cardiovascular events.

Exercise

Systematic reviews and one subsequent RCT in people with chronic stable claudication have found that regular exercise at least three times weekly versus no exercise significantly improves total walking distance and maximal exercise time after 3–12 months.

LIKELY TO BE BENEFICIAL

Bypass surgery (*v* thrombolysis in people with acute limb ischaemia)

One systematic review found that surgery versus thrombolysis significantly reduced the number of amputations and the number of people reporting ongoing ischaemic pain, but found no significant difference in mortality after 1 year.

Percutaneous transluminal angioplasty (transient benefit only)

Two small RCTs in people with mild to moderate intermittent claudication**Ⓖ** found limited evidence that angioplasty versus no angioplasty significantly improved walking distance after 6 months but found no significant difference after 2 or 6 years. Four RCTs in people with femoral to popliteal artery stenoses have found no significant difference with angioplasty alone versus angioplasty plus stent placement in patency rates, occlusion rates, or clinical improvement.

Smoking cessation (based on consensus of opinion)

We found no RCTs of smoking cessation in people with peripheral vascular disease. The consensus view is that smoking cessation improves symptoms in people with intermittent claudication. One systematic review has found observational evidence that continued cigarette smoking by people with intermittent claudication is associated with progression of symptoms, poor prognosis after bypass surgery, amputation, and need for reconstructive surgery.

TRADE OFF BETWEEN BENEFITS AND HARMS

Cilostazol

RCTs in people with intermittent claudication have found that cilostazol versus placebo significantly improves initial claudication distance**Ⓖ** and absolute claudication distance**Ⓖ** measured on a treadmill and significantly reduces the proportion of people with symptoms that do not improve. One RCT with a high withdrawal rate found that pentoxifylline versus cilostazol reduced initial and absolute claudication distance. Adverse effects are common and include headache, diarrhoea and palpitations.

Peripheral arterial disease

UNKNOWN EFFECTIVENESS

Bypass surgery (v percutaneous transluminal angioplasty)

One systematic review found that surgery versus percutaneous transluminal angioplasty significantly improved primary blood vessel patency after 12–24 months, but found no significant difference after 4 years. The review found no significant difference in mortality after 12–24 months. Although the consensus view is that bypass surgery is the most effective treatment for people with debilitating symptomatic peripheral arterial disease, we found inadequate evidence from RCTs reporting long term clinical outcomes to confirm this view.

Pentoxifylline

One systematic review and one subsequent RCT have found insufficient evidence to compare pentoxifylline versus placebo. One RCT found that pentoxifylline reduced absolute claudication distance compared with cilostazol.

DEFINITION Peripheral arterial disease arises when there is significant narrowing of arteries distal to the arch of the aorta. Narrowing can arise from atheroma, arteritis, local thrombus formation, or embolisation from the heart or more central arteries. This topic includes treatment options for people with symptoms of reduced blood flow to the leg that are likely to arise from atheroma. These symptoms range from calf pain on exercise (intermittent claudication), to rest pain, skin ulceration, or ischaemic necrosis (gangrene) in people with critical ischaemia.

INCIDENCE/ PREVALENCE Peripheral arterial disease is more common in people aged over 50 years than in younger people, and is more common in men than women. The prevalence of peripheral arterial disease of the legs (assessed by non-invasive tests) is about 3% in people under the age of 60 years, but rises to over 20% in people over 75 years.[1] The overall annual incidence of intermittent claudication is 1.5–2.6/1000 men a year and 1.2–3.6/1000 women a year.[2]

AETIOLOGY/ RISK FACTORS Factors associated with the development of peripheral arterial disease include age, gender, cigarette smoking, diabetes mellitus, hypertension, hyperlipidaemia, obesity, and physical inactivity. The strongest association is with smoking (RR 2.0–4.0) and diabetes (RR 2.0–3.0).[3] Acute limb ischaemia Ⓖ may result from thrombosis arising within a peripheral artery or embolic occlusion.

PROGNOSIS The symptom of intermittent claudication can resolve spontaneously, remain stable over many years, or progress rapidly to critical limb ischaemia Ⓖ. About 15% of people with intermittent claudication eventually develop critical leg ischaemia, which endangers the viability of the limb. The incidence of critical limb ischaemia in Denmark and Italy in 1990 was 0.25–0.45/1000 people a year.[4,5] Coronary heart disease is the major cause of death in people with peripheral arterial disease of the legs. Over 5 years, about 20% of people with intermittent claudication have a non-fatal cardiovascular event (myocardial infarction or stroke).[6] The mortality rate of people with peripheral arterial disease is two to three times higher than that of age and sex matched controls. Overall mortality after the diagnosis of peripheral arterial disease is about 30% after 5 years and 70% after 15 years.[6]

Please refer to CD-ROM for full text and references.

Primary prevention

Search date March 2002

Charles Foster, Cindy Mulrow, Michael Murphy, Andy Ness, Julian Nicholas, Michael Pignone, and Cathie Sudlow

What are the effects of interventions in asymptomatic people?

LIKELY TO BE BENEFICIAL

Eating more fruit and vegetables

Observational studies have found that consumption of fruit and vegetables reduces ischaemic heart disease and stroke. The size and nature of any real effect is uncertain.

Physical activity

Observational studies have found that moderate to high physical activity significantly reduces coronary heart disease and stroke. They also found that sudden death soon after strenuous exercise was rare, more common in sedentary people, and did not outweigh the benefits.

Smoking cessation

Observational studies have found a strong association between smoking and overall mortality and ischaemic vascular disease. Several large cohort studies have found that the increased risk associated with smoking falls after stopping smoking. The risk can take many years to approach that of non-smokers, particularly in those with a history of heavy smoking.

TRADE OFF BETWEEN BENEFITS AND HARMS

Anticoagulant treatment (warfarin)

One RCT found that the benefits and harms of oral anticoagulation among individuals without symptoms of cardiovascular disease were finely balanced, and that net effects were uncertain.

Aspirin in low risk people

We found insufficient evidence to identify which asymptomatic individuals would benefit overall and which would be harmed by regular treatment with aspirin. Benefits are likely to outweigh risks in people at higher risk.

UNKNOWN EFFECTIVENESS

Antioxidants (other than betacarotene)

Observational studies found insufficient evidence on the effects of vitamin C, vitamin E, copper, zinc, manganese, or flavonoids. Two RCTs found no significant difference in mortality after about 6 years with vitamin E supplements versus placebo.

LIKELY TO BE INEFFECTIVE OR HARMFUL

Betacarotene

RCTs found no evidence that betacarotene supplements are effective, and have found that they may be harmful.

What are the effects of interventions aimed at lowering blood pressure?

BENEFICIAL

Antihypertensive drug treatments in people with hypertension

Systematic reviews have found that initial treatment with diuretics, angiotensin converting enzyme inhibitors, or β blockers reduce morbidity and mortality, with minimal adverse effects. The biggest benefit was seen in those with the highest baseline risk. We found limited evidence from two systematic reviews that diuretics, β blockers, and angiotensin converting enzyme inhibitors reduced coronary heart disease and heart failure more than calcium channel antagonists. However, calcium channel antagonists reduced risk of stroke more than the other agents. One RCT found no significant difference in coronary heart disease outcomes with α blockers versus diuretics, but found that α blockers significantly increased cardiovascular events, particularly congestive cardiac failure at 4 years.

Diuretics in high risk people

Systematic reviews have found that diuretics versus placebo significantly decrease the risk of fatal and non-fatal stroke, cardiac events, and total mortality. The biggest benefit is seen in people with the highest baseline risk. Systematic reviews have found no significant difference in mortality or morbidity with diuretics versus β blockers.

LIKELY TO BE BENEFICIAL

Dietary salt restriction

We found no RCTs of the effects of salt restriction on morbidity or mortality. One systematic review has found that a low salt diet versus a usual diet may lead to modest reductions in blood pressure, with more benefit in people older than 45 years than in younger people❶.

Fish oil supplementation

We found no RCTs examining the effects of fish oil supplementation on morbidity or mortality. One systematic review has found that fish oil supplementation in large doses of 3 g daily modestly lowers blood pressure.

Low fat, high fruit and vegetable diet

We found no systematic review and no RCTs examining the effects of low fat, high fruit and vegetable diet on morbidity or mortality of people with raised blood pressure. One RCT found that a low fat, high fruit and vegetable diet versus control diet modestly reduced blood pressure.

Physical activity

We found no RCTs examining the effects of exercise on morbidity or mortality. One systematic review has found that aerobic exercise versus no exercise reduces blood pressure.

Potassium supplementation

We found no RCTs examining the effects of potassium supplementation on morbidity or mortality. One systematic review has found that a daily potassium supplementation of about 60 mmol (2 g, which is about the amount contained in 5 bananas) reduces blood pressure by small amounts.

Reduced alcohol consumption

We found no RCTs examining the effects of reducing alcohol consumption on morbidity or mortality. One systematic review in moderate drinkers (25–50 drinks/week) found inconclusive evidence regarding effects of alcohol reduction on blood pressure.

Smoking cessation

Observational studies have found that smoking is a significant risk factor for cardiovascular disease. We found no direct evidence specifically in people with hypertension that stopping smoking decreases blood pressure.

Weight loss

We found no RCTs examining the effects of weight loss on morbidity and mortality. One systematic review and additional RCTs have found that modest weight reduction in obese people with hypertension may lead to modest reductions in blood pressure.

UNKNOWN EFFECTIVENESS

Calcium supplementation

We found no RCTs examining the effects of calcium supplementation on morbidity or mortality. We found insufficient evidence on the effects of calcium supplementation specifically in people with hypertension. One systematic review in people with and without hypertension found that calcium supplementation may reduce systolic blood pressure by small amounts.

Magnesium supplementation

We found no RCTs examining the effects of magnesium supplementation on morbidity or mortality. We found limited and conflicting evidence on the effect of magnesium supplementation on blood pressure in people with hypertension and normal magnesium concentrations.

What are the effects of interventions aimed at lowering cholesterol?

LIKELY TO BE BENEFICIAL

Cholesterol reduction in high risk people

Systematic reviews have found that reducing cholesterol concentration in asymptomatic people lowers the rate of cardiovascular events. RCTs have found that the magnitude of the benefit is related to an individual's baseline risk of cardiovascular events, and to the degree of cholesterol lowering, rather than to the individual's cholesterol concentration.

Low fat diet

Systematic reviews and RCTs have found that combined use of cholesterol lowering diet and lipid lowering drugs reduces cholesterol concentration more than lifestyle interventions alone.

DEFINITION Primary prevention in this context is the long term management of people at increased risk but with no evidence of cardiovascular disease. Clinically overt ischaemic vascular disease includes acute myocardial infarction, angina, stroke, and peripheral vascular disease. Many adults have no symptoms or obvious signs of vascular disease, even though they have atheroma and are at increased risk of ischaemic vascular events because of one or more risk factors (see aetiology below).

Primary prevention

AETIOLOGY/ RISK FACTORS According to the World Health Report 1999, ischaemic heart disease was the leading single cause for death in the world, the leading single cause for death in high income countries and second to lower respiratory tract infections in low and middle income countries. In 1998 it was still the leading cause for death, with nearly 7.4 million estimated deaths a year in member states of the World Health Organization. This condition had the eighth highest burden of disease in the low and middle income countries (30.7 million disability adjusted life years).[1]

AETIOLOGY/ RISK FACTORS Identified major risk factors for ischaemic vascular disease include increasing age, male sex, raised low density lipoprotein cholesterol, reduced high density lipoprotein cholesterol, raised blood pressure, smoking, diabetes, family history of cardiovascular disease, obesity, and sedentary lifestyle. For many of these risk factors, observational studies show a continuous gradient of increasing risk of cardiovascular disease with increasing levels of the risk factor, with no obvious threshold level. Although by definition event rates are higher in high risk people, of all ischaemic vascular events that occur in the population, most occur in people with intermediate levels of absolute risk because there are many more of them than there are people at high risk; see Appendix 1.[2]

PROGNOSIS A study carried out in Scotland found that about half of people who suffer an acute myocardial infarction die within 28 days, and two thirds of acute myocardial infarctions occur before the person reaches hospital.[3] The benefits of intervention in unselected people with no evidence of cardiovascular disease (primary prevention) are small because in such people the baseline risk is small. However, absolute risk of ischaemic vascular events varies dramatically, even among people with similar levels of blood pressure or cholesterol. Estimates of absolute risk can be based on simple risk equations or tables; see Appendix 1.[4,5]

Please refer to CD-ROM for full text and references.

Secondary prevention of ischaemic cardiac events

Search date March 2002

Cathie Sudlow, Eva Lonn, Michael Pignone, Andrew Ness, and Chararyit Rihal

What are the effects of treatments?

BENEFICIAL

Angiotensin converting enzyme inhibitors in people with left ventricular dysfunction

One systematic review has found that in people who have had a myocardial infarction and have left ventricular dysfunction, angiotensin converting enzyme inhibitors versus placebo significantly reduce mortality, admission to hospital for congestive heart failure, and recurrent non-fatal myocardial infarction after 2 years' treatment.

Angiotensin converting enzyme inhibitors in high risk people without left ventricular dysfunction

One large RCT in people without left ventricular dysfunction found that ramipril versus placebo significantly reduced the combined outcome of cardiovascular death, stroke, and myocardial infarction after about 5 years.

Amiodarone in selected high risk people

Two systematic reviews have found that amiodarone versus placebo significantly reduces the risk of sudden cardiac death, and reduces mortality at 1 year in people at high risk of death after myocardial infarction.

Anticoagulants in the absence of antiplatelet treatment

One systematic review has found that high or moderate intensity oral anticoagulants given alone significantly reduce the risk of serious vascular events in people with coronary artery disease, but are associated with substantial risk of haemorrhage.

Any oral antiplatelet treatment

One systematic review has found that prolonged antiplatelet treatment versus placebo or no antiplatelet treatment reduces the risk of serious vascular events in people at high risk of ischaemic cardiac events.

Aspirin

One systematic review has found that, for prolonged use, aspirin 75–150 mg daily is as effective as higher doses, but found insufficient evidence that doses below 75 mg daily are as effective.

β Blockers

Systematic reviews in people after myocardial infarction have found that long term β blockers reduce all cause mortality, coronary mortality, recurrent non-fatal myocardial infarction, and sudden death. One RCT found that about 25% of people suffer adverse effects.

Cardiac rehabilitation

One systematic review has found that cardiac rehabilitation including exercise reduces the risk of major cardiac events.

Cholesterol lowering drugs

Systematic reviews and large subsequent RCTs have found that lowering cholesterol in people at high risk of ischaemic coronary events substantially reduces the ▶

risk of overall mortality, cardiovascular mortality, and non-fatal cardiovascular events. One systematic review of primary and secondary prevention trials found that statins, in people also given dietary advice, were the only non-surgical treatment for cholesterol reduction to significantly reduce mortality. One systematic review found that the absolute benefits increase as baseline risk increases, but are not additionally influenced by the person's absolute cholesterol concentration.

Coronary artery bypass grafting versus medical treatment alone

One systematic review found that coronary artery bypass grafting reduced the risk of death from coronary artery disease at 5 and 10 years compared with medical treatment alone. Greater benefit occurred in people with poor left ventricular function. One subsequent RCT in people with asymptomatic disease found that revascularisation with coronary artery bypass grafting or coronary percutaneous transluminal angioplasty versus medical treatment alone reduced mortality at 2 years.

Coronary percutaneous transluminal angioplasty versus medical treatment alone

One systematic review found that coronary percutaneous transluminal angioplasty versus medical treatment alone improved angina, but was associated with a higher rate of coronary artery bypass grafting. The review found higher mortality and rates of myocardial infarction with percutaneous transluminal angioplasty versus medical treatment but the difference was not significant. RCTs have found that percutaneous transluminal angioplasty is associated with increased risk of emergency coronary artery bypass grafting and myocardial infarction during and soon after the procedure. One RCT found that percutaneous transluminal angioplasty reduced cardiac events and improved angina severity compared with medical treatment alone in people over the age of 75 years.

Exercise without cardiac rehabilitation

One systematic review has found that exercise alone versus usual care significantly reduces mortality.

Intracoronary stents (better than coronary percutaneous transluminal angioplasty alone)

One systematic review found that intracoronary stents versus coronary percutaneous transluminal angioplasty alone significantly reduced the need for repeat vascularisation. It found no significant difference in mortality or myocardial infarction, but crossover rates from percutaneous transluminal angioplasty alone to stent were high. RCTs found that intracoronary stents improved outcomes after 4–9 months compared with percutaneous transluminal angioplasty alone in people with previous coronary artery bypass grafting, chronic total occlusions, and for treatment of restenosis after initial percutaneous transluminal angioplasty.

Percutaneous revascularisation in people with stable coronary artery disease

One systematic review found that coronary percutaneous transluminal angioplasty versus medical treatment alone improved angina, but was associated with a higher rate of coronary artery bypass grafting. The review found higher mortality and rates of myocardial infarction with percutaneous transluminal angioplasty versus medical treatment but the difference was not significant. RCTs have found that percutaneous transluminal angioplasty is associated with increased risk of emergency coronary artery bypass grafting and myocardial infarction during and soon after the procedure. One RCT found that percutaneous transluminal angioplasty reduced cardiac events and improved angina severity compared with medical treatment alone in people over the age of 75 years.

LIKELY TO BE BENEFICIAL

Blood pressure lowering in people at high risk of ischaemic coronary events

We found no direct evidence of the effects of blood pressure lowering in people with established coronary heart disease. Observational studies, and extrapolation of primary prevention trials of blood pressure reduction, support the lowering of blood pressure in those at high risk of ischaemic coronary events. The evidence for benefit is strongest for β blockers, although not specifically in people with hypertension. The target blood pressure in these people is not clear. Angiotensin converting enzyme inhibitors, calcium channel blockers, and β blockers are discussed separately.

Coronary artery bypass grafting versus percutaneous revascularisation for multi vessel disease (less need for repeat procedures)

One systematic review has found that coronary artery bypass grafting versus percutaneous transluminal angioplasty has no significant effect on death, myocardial infarction, or quality of life. Percutaneous transluminal angioplasty is less invasive but increased the number of repeat procedures.

Eating more fish (particularly oily fish)

One RCT has found that advising people with coronary heart disease to eat more fish (particularly oily fish) significantly reduces mortality at 2 years. A second RCT found that fish oil capsules significantly reduced mortality at 3.5 years.

Mediterranean diet

One RCT has found that advising people with coronary artery disease to eat more bread, fruit, vegetables, and fish, and less meat, and to replace butter and cream with rapeseed margarine significantly reduces mortality at 27 months.

Psychosocial treatment

One systematic review of mainly poor quality RCTs found that psychological treatments versus usual treatment may decrease rates of myocardial infarction or cardiac death in people with coronary heart disease.

Smoking cessation

We found no RCTs of the effects of smoking cessation on cardiovascular events in people with coronary heart disease. Moderate evidence from epidemiological studies indicates that people with coronary heart disease who stop smoking rapidly reduce their risk of recurrent coronary events or death. Treatment with nicotine patches seems safe in people with coronary heart disease.

Stress management

One systematic review of mainly poor quality RCTs found that stress management may decrease rates of myocardial infarction or cardiac death in people with coronary heart disease.

Thienopyridines

One systematic review has found that clopidogrel is at least as safe and effective as aspirin in people at high risk of vascular events.

Secondary prevention of ischaemic cardiac events

UNLIKELY TO BE BENEFICIAL

Advice to eat less fat
RCTs found no strong evidence that low fat diets reduced mortality at 2 years.

Hormone replacement therapy
One large RCT found no evidence that hormone replacement therapy versus placebo reduces major cardiovascular events in postmenopausal women with established coronary artery disease.

Oral glycoprotein IIb/IIIa receptor inhibitors
One systematic review in people with acute coronary syndromes or undergoing percutaneous coronary interventions has found that the oral glycoprotein IIb/IIIa receptor inhibitors versus placebo increase risk of mortality and bleeding.

Vitamin C
Pooled analysis of three small RCTs found no evidence that vitamin C versus placebo provided any substantial benefit.

Vitamin E
Pooled analysis of four large RCTs found no evidence that vitamin E versus placebo given for 1.3–4.5 years altered cardiovascular events and all cause mortality.

Sotalol
One RCT found limited evidence that sotalol versus placebo significantly increased mortality within 1 year.

LIKELY TO BE INEFFECTIVE OR HARMFUL

Adding anticoagulants to antiplatelet treatment
One systematic review and one subsequent RCT found no evidence that addition to aspirin of oral anticoagulation at low (INR*G* < 1.5) or moderate (INR 1.5–3) intensity reduced risk of death or recurrent cardiac events, but found an increased risk of major haemorrhage.

β Carotene
Large RCTs found no evidence of benefit with β carotene, and one RCT found evidence of a significant increase in mortality. Four large RCTs of β carotene supplementation in primary prevention found no cardiovascular benefits, and two of the RCTs raised concerns about increased mortality.

Calcium channel blockers (dihydropyridines)
One systematic review found non-significantly higher mortality with dihydropyridines compared with placebo.

Calcium channel blockers (diltiazem and verapamil)
One systematic review found no benefit from calcium channel blockers in people after myocardial infarction or with chronic coronary heart disease. Diltiazem and verapamil may reduce rates of reinfarction and refractory angina in people after myocardial infarction who do not have heart failure.

Class I antiarrhythmic agents
One systematic review has found that class I antiarrhythmic agents versus placebo given after myocardial infarction significantly increase the risk of cardiovascular mortality and sudden death.

DEFINITION Secondary prevention in this context is the long term management of people with a prior acute myocardial infarction, and of people at high risk of ischaemic cardiac events for other reasons, such as a history of angina or coronary surgical procedures.

Secondary prevention of ischaemic cardiac events

INCIDENCE/ PREVALENCE Coronary artery disease is the leading cause of mortality in developed countries and is becoming a major cause of mortality and morbidity in developing countries. There are pronounced international, regional, and temporal differences in death rates. In the USA, the prevalence of overt coronary artery disease approaches 4%.[1]

AETIOLOGY/ RISK FACTORS Most ischaemic cardiac events are associated with atheromatous plaques that can cause acute obstruction of coronary vessels. Atheroma is more likely in elderly people, in those with established coronary artery disease, and in those with risk factors (such as smoking, hypertension, high cholesterol, diabetes mellitus).

PROGNOSIS Almost 50% of those who suffer an acute myocardial infarction die before they reach hospital. Of those hospitalised, 7–15% die in hospital and another 7–15% die during the following year. People who survive the acute stage of myocardial infarction fall into three prognostic groups, based on their baseline risk❶:[2–4] high (20% of all survivors), moderate (55%), and low (25%) risk. Long term prognosis depends on the degree of left ventricular dysfunction, the presence of residual ischaemia, and the extent of any electrical instability. Further risk stratification procedures include evaluation of left ventricular function (by echocardiography or nuclear ventriculography) and of myocardial ischaemia (by non-invasive stress testing).[4–8] Those with low left ventricular ejection fraction, ischaemia, or poor functional status may be evaluated further by cardiac catheterisation.[9]

Please refer to CD-ROM for full text and references.

Stroke management

Search date September 2002

Gord Gubitz, Peter Sandercock, and Elizabeth Warburton

What are the effects of medical treatments for acute ischaemic stroke?

BENEFICIAL

Aspirin

One systematic review in people with ischaemic stroke confirmed by computerised tomography scan has found that aspirin versus placebo within 48 hours of stroke onset significantly reduces death or dependency at 6 months and significantly increases the number of people making a complete recovery. One prospective combined analysis of two large RCTs found indirect evidence that aspirin should not be delayed if a computerised tomography scan is not available within 48 hours and ischaemic stroke is suspected. Subgroup analysis of results from the two large RCTs found no significant difference in further stroke or death with aspirin versus placebo in people who were subsequently found to have haemorrhagic rather than ischaemic stroke.

Specialised care

One systematic review has found that specialist stroke rehabilitation units versus conventional (less specialised) care significantly reduces death or dependency after a median follow up of 1 year.

TRADE OFF BETWEEN BENEFITS AND HARMS

Thrombolysis

One systematic review in people with ischaemic stroke (without cerebral haemorrhage) which was excluded by computerised tomography scan) has found that thrombolysis versus placebo significantly reduces the risk of the composite outcome of death or dependency after 1–6 months, but significantly increases the risk of death from intracranial haemorrhage measured in the first 7–10 days.

UNLIKELY TO BE BENEFICIAL

Neuroprotective agents (calcium channel antagonists, γ-aminobutyric acid agonists, lubeluzole, glycine antagonists, tirilazad, N-methyl-D-aspartate antagonists)

RCTs found no evidence that, compared with placebo, calcium channel antagonists, tirilazad, lubeluzole, γ-aminobutyric acid agonists, glycine antagonists, or N-methyl-D-aspartate antagonists❻ significantly improve clinical outcomes. One systematic review found that lubeluzole versus placebo was associated with a significant increase in the risk of having Q-T prolongation to more than 450 ms on electrocardiography.

LIKELY TO BE INEFFECTIVE OR HARMFUL

Acute reduction in blood pressure

One systematic review in people with acute stroke found insufficient evidence about the effects of lowering blood pressure versus placebo on clinical outcome, but RCTs have suggested that people treated with antihypertensive agents may have a worse clinical outcome and increased mortality.

◀ **Immediate systemic anticoagulation**

One systematic review comparing systemic anticoagulants (unfractionated heparin, low molecular weight heparin, heparinoids, oral anticoagulants, or specific thrombin inhibitors) versus usual care without systemic anticoagulants found no significant difference in death or dependence after 3–6 months. One systematic review has found that immediate systemic anticoagulation significantly reduces the risk of deep venous thrombosis and symptomatic pulmonary embolus, but increases the risk of intracranial haemorrhage or extracranial haemorrhage. One RCT in people with acute ischaemic stroke and atrial fibrillation found no significant difference with low molecular weight heparin versus aspirin in recurrent ischaemic stroke within 14 days. One RCT in people within 48 hours of stroke onset found no significant difference with high or low dose tinzaparin versus aspirin in people achieving functional independence at 6 months.

What are the effects of surgical treatments for intracerebral haematomas?

UNKNOWN EFFECTIVENESS

Evacuation

We found that the balance between benefits and harms has not been clearly established for the evacuation of supratentorial haematomas. We found no evidence from RCTs on the role of evacuation or ventricular shunting in people with infratentorial haematoma whose consciousness level is declining.

DEFINITION Stroke is characterised by rapidly developing clinical symptoms and signs of focal, and at times global, loss of cerebral function lasting more than 24 hours or leading to death, with no apparent cause other than that of vascular origin.[1] Ischaemic stroke is stroke caused by vascular insufficiency (such as cerebrovascular thromboembolism) rather than haemorrhage.

INCIDENCE/ PREVALENCE Stroke is the third most common cause of death in most developed countries.[2] It is a worldwide problem; about 4.5 million people die from stroke each year. Stroke can occur at any age, but half of all strokes occur in people over 70 years old.[3]

AETIOLOGY/ RISK FACTORS About 80% of all acute strokes are caused by cerebral infarction, usually resulting from thrombotic or embolic occlusion of a cerebral artery.[4] The remainder are caused either by intracerebral or subarachnoid haemorrhage.

PROGNOSIS About 10% of all people with acute ischaemic strokes will die within 30 days of stroke onset.[5] Of those who survive the acute event, about 50% will experience some level of disability after 6 months.[6]

Please refer to CD-ROM for full text and references.

Stroke prevention

Search date May 2002

Gord Gubitz, Gregory Lip, Cathie Sudlow, and Peter Sandercock

---

What are the effects of preventive interventions in people with prior stroke or transient ischaemic attack?

BENEFICIAL

Antiplatelet treatment

One systematic review has found that antiplatelet treatment reduces the risk of serious vascular events in people with prior stroke or transient ischaemic attack compared with placebo or no antiplatelet treatment.

Blood pressure reduction

One systematic review and one subsequent RCT found that antihypertensive treatment reduced stroke among people with a prior stroke or transient ischaemic attack, whether they were hypertensive or not.

Carotid endarterectomy in people with moderate or severe symptomatic carotid artery stenosis

One systematic review in people with a recent carotid territory transient ischaemic event or non-disabling ischaemic stroke has found that carotid endarterectomy versus control treatment significantly reduces the risk of major stroke or death.

Cholesterol reduction

One large RCT has found that simvastatin versus placebo reduced major vascular events, including stroke, in people with prior stroke or transient ischaemic attack over about 5 years. RCTs have found no evidence that non-statin treatments versus placebo or no treatment reduced stroke.

UNKNOWN EFFECTIVENESS

Carotid angioplasty

RCTs found insufficient evidence about the effects of carotid angioplasty versus best "medical treatment".

Carotid endarterectomy in people with severe asymptomatic carotid artery stenosis

Systematic reviews in people with no carotid territory transient ischaemic event or minor stroke within the past few months found limited evidence suggesting that carotid endarterectomy**G** versus medical treatment may significantly reduce the risk of perioperative stroke or death or subsequent ipsilateral stroke over 3 years. However, as the risk of death without surgery in asymptomatic people is relatively low, the balance of benefits and harms from surgery remains unclear.

Different blood pressure lowering regimens

Systematic reviews found no clear evidence of a difference in effectiveness between different antihypertensive drugs. One systematic review found that more intensive treatment reduced stroke and major cardiovascular events but not mortality, compared with less intensive treatment.

UNLIKELY TO BE BENEFICIAL

Alternative antiplatelet agents to aspirin

Systematic reviews have found no good evidence that any antiplatelet treatment is superior to aspirin for long term secondary prevention of serious vascular events. ▶

Clin Evid Concise 2003;9:32–34.

◀ **High dose versus low dose aspirin (no additional benefit but may increase harms)**

One systematic review and one subsequent RCT have found that low dose aspirin (75–150 mg) daily is as effective as higher doses in the prevention of serious vascular events. There was insufficient evidence that doses lower than 75 mg daily are as effective. One systematic review found no association between the dose of aspirin and risk of major extracranial haemorrhage in either direct or indirect comparisons. Another systematic review found no association between the dose of aspirin and risk of gastrointestinal bleeding in an indirect comparison. RCTs directly comparing different doses of aspirin found an increased risk of upper gastrointestinal upset with high (500–1500 mg daily) versus medium (75–325 mg daily) doses. One systematic review of observational studies found an increased risk of gastrointestinal complications with doses of aspirin greater than 300 mg daily. One systematic review found no association between dose of aspirin and risk of intracranial haemorrhage.

LIKELY TO BE INEFFECTIVE OR HARMFUL

Oral anticoagulation in people with prior cerebrovascular ischaemia and normal sinus rhythm

One systematic review in people with prior cerebral ischaemia and in normal sinus rhythm found no significant difference with anticoagulation versus placebo for death or dependency, mortality, or recurrent stroke at about 2 years, but found a significantly increased risk of fatal intracranial haemorrhage (NNH 49, 95% CI 27 to 240). One systematic review has found no significant difference between high intensity (international normalised ratio**G** 3.0–4.5) or low intensity (international normalised ratio 2.5–3.5) anticoagulation versus antiplatelet treatment for preventing recurrent stroke in people with recent cerebral ischaemia of presumed arterial (non-cardiac) origin. High intensity anticoagulation increased the risk of major bleeding compared with antiplatelet treatment.

What are the effects of preventive interventions in people with atrial fibrillation and prior stroke or transient ischaemic attack?

BENEFICIAL

Aspirin in people with contraindications to anticoagulants

Systematic reviews have found that aspirin versus placebo reduces the risk of stroke, but found that aspirin is less effective than anticoagulants. These findings support the use of aspirin in people with atrial fibrillation and contraindications to anticoagulants.

Oral anticoagulates

Systematic reviews have found that adjusted dose warfarin versus placebo significantly reduces the risk of stroke. Systematic reviews have also found that warfarin versus aspirin significantly reduces the risk of stroke in people with previous stroke or transient ischaemic attack. ▶

What are the effects of preventive interventions in people with atrial fibrillation but no other major risk factors for stroke?

LIKELY TO BE BENEFICIAL

Aspirin in people with contraindications to anticoagulants

One systematic review found that aspirin versus placebo significantly reduced the risk of stroke, but another review found no significant difference. These findings support the use of aspirin in people with atrial fibrillation and contraindications to anticoagulants.

Oral anticoagulation

One systematic review has found that warfarin versus placebo significantly reduces fatal and non-fatal ischaemic stroke, provided there is a low risk of bleeding and careful monitoring. The people in the review had a mean age of 69 years. One overview in people less than 65 years old has found no significant difference in the annual stroke rate with warfarin versus placebo.

DEFINITION Prevention in this context is the long term management of people with a prior stroke or transient ischaemic attack, and of people at high risk of stroke Ⓖ for other reasons such as atrial fibrillation. **Stroke:** See definition under stroke management, p 31. **Transient ischaemic attack:** Similar to a mild ischaemic stroke except that symptoms last for less than 24 hours.[1]

INCIDENCE/ PREVALENCE See incidence/prevalence under stroke management, p 31.

AETIOLOGY/ RISK FACTORS See aetiology under stroke management, p 31. Risk factors for stroke include prior stroke or transient ischaemic attack, increasing age, hypertension, diabetes, cigarette smoking, and emboli associated with atrial fibrillation, artificial heart valves, or myocardial infarction. The relation with cholesterol is less clear; an overview of prospective studies among healthy middle aged individuals found no association between total cholesterol and overall stroke risk.[2] However, one review of prospective observational studies in eastern Asian people found that cholesterol was positively associated with ischaemic stroke but negatively associated with haemorrhagic stroke.[3]

PROGNOSIS People with a history of stroke or transient ischaemic attack are at high risk of all vascular events, such as myocardial infarction, but are at particular risk of subsequent stroke (about 10% in the first year and about 5% each year thereafter) Ⓕ[5,6] People with intermittent atrial fibrillation treated with aspirin should be considered at similar risk of stroke, compared to people with sustained atrial fibrillation treated with aspirin (rate of ischaemic stroke/year: 3.2% with intermittent v 3.3% with sustained).[7]

Please refer to CD-ROM for full text and references.

Thromboembolism

Search date March 2002

David Fitzmaurice, FD Richard Hobbs, and Richard McManus

What are the effects of treatments for proximal deep vein thrombosis?

TRADE OFF BETWEEN BENEFITS AND HARMS

Oral anticoagulants

One RCT found that combined acenocoumarol plus intravenous unfractionated heparin versus acenocoumarol alone for initial treatment reduced recurrence of proximal deep vein thrombosis within 6 months. Systematic reviews have found that longer versus shorter duration of anticoagulation is associated with significantly fewer deep vein thrombosis recurrences or thromboembolic complications. One non-systematic review found limited evidence that longer versus shorter duration of warfarin treatment was associated with a significantly increased risk Ⓖ, but another non-systematic review found no significantly increased. The absolute risk of recurrent venous thromboembolism decreases with time, but the relative risk reduction with treatment remains constant. Harms of treatment, including major haemorrhage, continue during prolonged treatment. Individual people have different risk profiles. It is likely that the optimal duration of anticoagulation will vary between people.

Unfractionated and low molecular weight heparin

One systematic review has found no significant difference with long term low molecular weight heparin Ⓖ versus oral anticoagulation in recurrent thromboembolism, major haemorrhage or mortality. Systematic reviews have found that low molecular weight heparin is at least as effective as unfractionated heparin in reducing the incidence of recurrent thromboembolic disease, and have found that short term low molecular weight heparin versus unfractionated heparin is associated with a significantly decreased risk of major haemorrhage.

What are the effects of treatments for isolated calf vein thrombosis?

TRADE OFF BETWEEN BENEFITS AND HARMS

Warfarin plus heparin

One RCT found that warfarin plus intravenous unfractionated heparin versus heparin alone (international normalised ratio Ⓖ 2.5–4.2) reduced the rate of proximal extension. One unblinded RCT found no significant difference in recurrent thromboembolism with 6 versus 12 weeks of anticoagulation.

What are the effects of treatments for pulmonary embolism?

TRADE OFF BETWEEN BENEFITS AND HARMS

Oral anticoagulants

We found no direct evidence about the optimum intensity and duration of anticoagulation in people with pulmonary embolism. The best available evidence requires extrapolation of results from studies of people with proximal deep vein thrombosis.

Clin Evid Concise 2003;9:35–37.

▶

Unfractionated and low molecular weight heparin

One small RCT found that heparin plus warfarin versus no anticoagulation significantly reduced mortality in people with pulmonary embolism at 1 year. One RCT in people with symptomatic pulmonary embolism who did not receive thrombolysis or embolectomy found no significant difference with low molecular weight heparin**G** versus unfractionated heparin in mortality or new episodes of thromboembolism. Another RCT in people with proximal deep vein thrombosis without clinical signs or symptoms of pulmonary embolism but with high probability lung scan findings found that fixed dose low molecular weight heparin versus intravenous heparin significantly reduced the proportion of people with new episodes of venous thromboembolism.

UNLIKELY TO BE BENEFICIAL

Thrombolysis

One systematic review in people with pulmonary embolism has found no significant difference in mortality with thrombolysis plus heparin versus heparin alone, and found that thrombolysis may increase the incidence of intracranial haemorrhage. One small RCT identified by the review found limited evidence that thrombolysis may reduce mortality in people with shock due to massive pulmonary embolism.

What are the effects of computerised decision support on oral anticoagulation management?

UNKNOWN EFFECTIVENESS

Computerised decision support in oral anticoagulation management

We found no RCTs of computerised decision support versus usual management of oral anticoagulation that used clinically important outcomes (major haemorrhage**G** or death).

One systematic review and three subsequent RCTs have found that computerised decision support in oral anticoagulation significantly increases time spent in the target international normalised ratio**G** range. Another subsequent RCT found no significant difference with computerised decision support versus standard manual support in the time spent in the target international normalised ratio range. A subsequent RCT of initiation of warfarin found no significant difference between computerised decision support versus usual care in the time taken to reach therapeutic levels of anticoagulation.

DEFINITION **Venous thromboembolism** is any thromboembolic event occurring within the venous system, including deep vein thrombosis and pulmonary embolism. **Deep vein thrombosis** is a radiologically confirmed partial or total thrombotic occlusion of the deep venous system of the legs sufficient to produce symptoms of pain or swelling. **Proximal deep vein thrombosis** affects the veins above the knee (popliteal, superficial femoral, common femoral, and iliac veins). **Isolated calf vein thrombosis** is confined to the deep veins of the calf and does not affect the veins above the knee. **Pulmonary embolism** is radiologically confirmed partial or total thromboembolic occlusion of pulmonary arteries, sufficient to cause symptoms of breathlessness, chest pain, or both. **Post-thrombotic syndrome** is oedema, ulceration, and impaired viability of the subcutaneous tissues of the leg occurring after deep vein thrombosis. **Recurrence** refers to symptomatic deterioration because of a further (radiologically confirmed) thrombosis, after a previously confirmed thromboembolic event, where there had been an initial, partial, or total symptomatic improvement. **Extension** refers to a radiologically confirmed new, constant, symptomatic intraluminal filling defect extending from an existing thrombosis.

INCIDENCE/ PREVALENCE We found no reliable study of the incidence/prevalence of deep vein thrombosis or pulmonary embolism in the UK. A prospective Scandinavian study found an annual incidence of 1.6–1.8/1000 people in the general population.[1,2] One postmortem study estimated that 600 000 people develop pulmonary embolism each year in the USA, of whom 60 000 die as a result.[3]

AETIOLOGY/ RISK FACTORS Risk factors for deep vein thrombosis include immobility, surgery (particularly orthopaedic), malignancy, smoking, pregnancy, older age, and inherited or acquired prothrombotic clotting disorders.[4] Evidence for these factors is mainly observational. The oral contraceptive pill is associated with death due to venous thromboembolism (ARI with any combined oral contraception: 1–3/million women per year).[5] The principal cause of pulmonary embolism is a deep vein thrombosis.[4]

PROGNOSIS The annual recurrence rate of symptomatic calf vein thrombosis in people without recent surgery is over 25%.[6,7] Proximal extension develops in 40–50% of people with symptomatic calf vein thrombosis.[8] Proximal deep vein thrombosis may cause fatal or non-fatal pulmonary embolism, recurrent venous thrombosis, and the post-thrombotic syndrome. One observational study published in 1946 found 20% mortality from pulmonary emboli in people in hospital with untreated deep vein thrombosis.[9] One non-systematic review of observational studies found that, in people after recent surgery who have an asymptomatic calf vein deep vein thrombosis, the rate of fatal pulmonary embolism was 13–15%.[10] The incidence of other complications without treatment is not known. The risk of recurrent venous thrombosis and complications is increased by thrombotic risk factors.[11]

Please refer to CD-ROM for full text and references.

Varicose veins

Search date November 2002

Clinical Evidence freelance writers

What are effects of treatments in adults with varicose veins? New

LIKELY TO BE BENEFICIAL

Surgery (*v* injection sclerotherapy)

We found no RCTs comparing surgery versus no treatment or compression stockings. One RCT found that surgery significantly improved cure of varicose veins compared with injection sclerotherapy at 5 years in people with varicose veins from saphenofemoral, saphenopopliteal, and perforator incompetence. The RCT did not report separately on effects of surgery for each site of venous incompetence.

UNKNOWN EFFECTIVENESS

Compression stockings

One crossover RCT found no significant difference in symptoms between compression stockings for 4 weeks versus no treatment in people with varicose veins. However, the study may have lacked power to exclude clinically important effects.

Injection sclerotherapy

One systematic review has found no RCTs comparing injection sclerotherapy versus no treatment or compression stockings in people with varicose veins. One RCT has found no significant difference between injection sclerotherapy with polidocanol versus sodium tetradecyl sulphate for improving appearance of varicose veins not due to saphenofemoral or saphenopopliteal incompetence at 16 weeks.

DEFINITION Although we found no consistent definition of varicose veins,[1] the term is commonly taken to mean veins that are distended and tortuous. Any vein may become varicose, but the term "varicose veins" conventionally applies to varices of the superficial leg veins. The condition is caused by poorly functioning valves within the lumen of the veins. Blood flows from the deep to the superficial venous systems through these incompetent valves, causing persistent superficial venous hypertension, which leads to varicosity of the superficial veins. Common sites of valvular incompetence include the saphenofemoral and saphenopopliteal junctions and perforating veins connecting the deep and superficial venous systems along the length of the leg. Sites of venous incompetence are determined by clinical examination or, more reliably, by Doppler ultrasound. Symptoms of varicose veins include distress about cosmetic appearance, pain, itch, limb heaviness, and cramps. This review focuses on uncomplicated, symptomatic varicose veins. We have excluded treatments for chronic venous ulceration and other complications. We have also excluded studies that solely examine treatments for small, dilated veins in the skin of the leg, known as thread veins, spider veins, or superficial telangiectasia.

INCIDENCE/ PREVALENCE One large US cohort study found the annual incidence of varicose veins to be 2.6% in women and 1.9% in men.[2] Incidence was constant over the age of 40 years. The prevalence of varicose veins in Western populations is about 25–30% among women and 10–20% in men.[3]

AETIOLOGY/ RISK FACTORS One large case control study found that women with two or more pregnancies were at increased risk of varicose veins compared with women with fewer than two pregnancies (RR about 1.2–1.3 after adjustment for age, height, and weight).[2] It found that obesity was also a risk factor, although only among women (RR about 1.3). One narrative systematic review found insufficient evidence about effects of other suggested risk factors, including genetic predisposition; prolonged sitting or standing; tight undergarments; low fibre diet; constipation; deep vein thrombosis; and smoking.[3]

PROGNOSIS We found no reliable data about prognosis, nor about the frequency of complications, which include chronic inflammation of affected veins (phlebitis), venous ulceration, and rupture of varices.

Please refer to CD-ROM for full text and references.

Absence seizures

Search date May 2002

Ewa Posner

What are the effects of treatments for typical absence seizures in children?

TRADE OFF BETWEEN BENEFITS AND HARMS

Ethosuximide

We found no systematic review or RCTs comparing ethosuximide versus placebo. There is consensus that ethosuximide is beneficial. Ethosuximide is associated with rare but serious adverse effects, including aplastic anaemia, skin reactions, and renal and hepatic impairment. We found no RCTs comparing ethosuximide versus other anticonvulsants (except valproate) in children with typical absence seizures.

Lamotrigine

One RCT found that lamotrigine versus placebo significantly increased the number of children who remained seizure free, but lamotrigine is associated with serious skin reactions. We found no RCTs comparing lamotrigine versus other anticonvulsants in children with typical absence seizures.

Valproate

We found no RCTs comparing valproate versus placebo. There is consensus that valproate is beneficial. Valproate is associated with rare but serious adverse effects, including behavioural and cognitive abnormalites, liver necrosis, and pancreatitis. Three small RCTs found no significant difference between valproate and ethosuximide. We found no RCTs comparing valproate versus other anticonvulsants (except ethosuximide) in children with typical absence seizures.

UNKNOWN EFFECTIVENESS

Gabapentin

One brief RCT found no significant difference between gabapentin versus placebo in the frequency of typical absence seizures.

DEFINITION Absence seizures are sudden, short (seconds) episodes of unconsciousness. Depending on electroencephalogram findings they are divided into typical and atypical seizures. Typical absence seizures are associated with an electroencephalogram showing regular symmetrical three cycles a second generalised spike and wave complexes. Absence seizures may be the only type of seizures experienced by a child and this then constitutes an epileptic syndrome(G) called childhood absence epilepsy. In many children, typical absence seizures coexist with other types of seizures. Atypical absence seizures do not show the characteristic (for typical absence seizures) electroencephalogram pattern, are usually one of many types of seizures in a child with a background of learning disability and severe epilepsy and tend to be less defined in time.[1] This differentiation into typical versus atypical seizures is important as the natural history and response to treatment varies in the two groups. Interventions for atypical absence seizures are not included in this topic.

INCIDENCE/ PREVALENCE About 10% of seizures in children with epilepsy are typical absence seizures.[1]

AETIOLOGY/ RISK FACTORS The cause is presumed to be genetic.

PROGNOSIS In childhood absence epilepsy where typical absence seizures are the only type of seizures suffered by the child the prognosis is excellent, the seizures cease spontaneously after a few years. In other epileptic syndromes (where absence seizures may coexist with other types of seizures) prognosis is varied, depending on the syndrome. Absence seizures have significant impact on quality of life. The episode of unconsciousness may occur at any time. Absence seizures usually occur without warning. Affected children need to take precaution to prevent injury during absences. Often school staff are the first to notice the recurrent episodes of absences and the treatment is necessitated by the impact on learning.

Please refer to CD-ROM for full text and references.

Acute otitis media

Search date October 2002

Paddy O'Neill and Tony Roberts

What are the effects of treatments?

LIKELY TO BE BENEFICIAL

Ibuprofen

One RCT in children aged 1–6 years receiving antibiotic treatment found that ibuprofen versus placebo significantly reduced earache as assessed by parental observation after 2 days.

Paracetamol

One RCT in children aged 1–6 years receiving antibiotic treatment found that paracetamol versus placebo significantly reduced earache as assessed by parental observation after 2 days.

TRADE OFF BETWEEN BENEFITS AND HARMS

Antibiotics versus placebo

We found four systematic reviews comparing antibiotics versus placebo in acute otitis media (AOM) but using different inclusion criteria and outcome measures. One review in children aged 4 months to 18 years found a significant reduction in symptoms with a range of antibiotics (cephalosporins, erythromycin, penicillins, trimethoprim–sulfamethoxazole [co-trimoxazole]) versus placebo after 7–14 days of treatment. Another review in children aged less than 2 years found no significant difference in clinical improvement with antibiotics (penicillins, sulphonamides, co-trimoxazole) versus placebo alone or versus placebo with myringotomy**G**. A third review in children aged 4 weeks to 18 years found that antibiotics (ampicillin, amoxicillin) versus placebo or observational treatment significantly reduced clinical failure rate within 2–7 days. The final review in children aged 6 months to 15 years found that early use of antibiotics (erythromycin, penicillins) versus placebo significantly reduced the proportion of children still in pain 2–7 days after presentation and reduced the risk of developing contralateral AOM. This review also found that antibiotics increased the risk of vomiting, diarrhoea, or rashes.

Choice of antibiotic regimen

One systematic review in children aged 4 months to 18 years found no significant difference between a range of antibiotics in rate of treatment success at 7–14 days or of middle ear effusion at 30 days. Another systematic review in children aged 4 weeks to 18 years found no significant difference between antibiotics in clinical failure rates within 7–14 days. The second review also found that adverse effects, primarily gastrointestinal, were more common with cefixime versus amoxicillin or ampicillin, and were more common with amoxicillin/clavulanate (original formulation) versus azithromycin.

Immediate versus delayed antibiotic treatment

One RCT in children aged 6 months to 10 years found that immediate versus delayed antibiotic treatment significantly reduced the number of days of earache, ear discharge, and amount of daily paracetamol used after the first 24 hours of illness but found no difference in daily pain scores. It also found a significant increase in diarrhoea with immediate versus delayed antibiotic treatment. ▶

Short versus longer courses of antibiotics

One systematic review and two subsequent RCTs have found that 10 day versus 5 day courses of antibiotics significantly reduce treatment failure, relapse, and reinfection at 8–19 days, but found no significant difference at 20–30 days.

LIKELY TO BE BENEFICIAL

Myringotomy *New*

One RCT in infants aged 3 months to 1 year found no significant difference in resolution of clinical symptoms with myringotomy only versus antibiotic only or myringotomy plus antibiotic but found higher rates of persistent infection with myringotomy only. A second RCT in children aged 2–12 years found no significant difference in reduction of pain at 24 hours or 7 days with myringotomy versus no treatment. A third RCT in children aged 7 months to 12 years found significantly higher rates of initial treatment failure (resolution of symptoms within 12 hours) for severe episodes of AOM treated by myringotomy and placebo versus antibiotic.

What are the effects of interventions to prevent recurrence?

LIKELY TO BE BENEFICIAL

Xylitol chewing gum or syrup

One RCT found that xylitol syrup or chewing gum versus control significantly reduced the incidence of AOM over 3 months. It found no significant difference with xylitol lozenges versus control gum. More children taking xylitol versus control withdrew because of abdominal pain or other unspecified reasons.

TRADE OFF BETWEEN BENEFITS AND HARMS

Long term antibiotic prophylaxis

One systematic review in children and adults has found that long term antibiotic prophylaxis versus placebo significantly reduces recurrence of acute otitis media after 1 month. However, one subsequent RCT in children aged 3 months to 6 years found no significant difference between antibiotic prophylaxis and placebo in preventing recurrence. We found insufficient evidence on which antibiotic to use, for how long, and how many previous episodes of AOM justify starting preventive treatment.

LIKELY TO BE INEFFECTIVE OR HARMFUL

Tympanostomy (ventilation tubes) *New*

One small RCT found that tympanostomy**G** tube insertion versus myringotomy alone or no surgery significantly reduced the mean number of AOM episodes during the first 6-month period after treatment but not during the subsequent 18 months. It also found a trend for more recurrent infections and worse hearing, after tube extrusion, in those treated with tympanostomy.

DEFINITION Otitis media is an inflammation in the middle ear. Subcategories include AOM, recurrent AOM, and chronic suppurative otitis media. AOM is the presence of middle ear effusion in conjunction with rapid onset of one or more signs or symptoms of inflammation of the middle ear. Uncomplicated AOM is limited to the middle ear cleft.[1] AOM presents with systemic and local signs, and has a rapid onset. The persistence of an effusion beyond 3 months without signs of infection defines otitis media with effusion (also known as "glue ear"). Chronic suppurative otitis media is characterised by continuing inflammation in the middle ear causing discharge (otorrhoea) through a perforated tympanic membrane.

Acute otitis media

INCIDENCE/ PREVALENCE AOM is common and has a high morbidity and low mortality in otherwise healthy children. In the UK, about 30% of children under 3 years old visit their general practitioner with AOM each year and 97% receive antimicrobial treatment.[2] By 3 months of age, 10% of children have had an episode of AOM. It is the most common reason for outpatient antimicrobial treatment in the USA.[3]

AETIOLOGY/ RISK FACTORS The most common bacterial causes for AOM in the USA and UK are *Streptococcus pneumoniae*, *Haemophilus influenzae*, and *Moraxella catarrhalis*.[2] Similar pathogens are found in Colombia.[4] The incidence of penicillin resistant *S pneumoniae* has risen, but rates differ between countries. The most important risk factors for AOM are young age and attendance at daycare centres, such as nursery schools. Other risk factors include being white; male sex; a history of enlarged adenoids, tonsillitis, or asthma; multiple previous episodes; bottle feeding; a history of ear infections in parents or siblings; and use of a soother or pacifier. The evidence for an effect of environmental tobacco smoke is controversial.[2]

PROGNOSIS In about 80% of children the condition resolves in about 3 days without antibiotic treatment. Serious complications are rare in otherwise healthy children but include hearing loss, mastoiditisⒼ, meningitis, and recurrent attacks.[2] The World Health Organization estimates that each year 51 000 children under the age of 5 years die from complications of otitis media in developing countries.[5]

Please refer to CD-ROM for full text and references.

Asthma and other wheezing disorders of childhood

Search date October 2002

Duncan Keeley and Michael McKean

What are the effects of treatments for acute asthma in children?

BENEFICIAL

Oxygen

An RCT of oxygen versus no oxygen treatment in acute severe asthma would be considered unethical. One prospective cohort study and clinical experience support the need for oxygen in acute asthma.

High dose inhaled corticosteroids

We found one systematic review that identified four RCTs comparing high dose inhaled versus oral corticosteroids in children. Three RCTs found no significant difference in hospital admission with nebulised budesonide or dexamethasone versus oral prednisolone in children with mild to moderate asthma. One RCT in children with moderate to severe asthma found that oral prednisolone versus inhaled fluticasone significantly reduced hospital admission and improved lung function at 4 hours. A subsequent RCT in children aged 4–16 years found that nebulised fluticasone versus oral prednisolone significantly improved lung function over 7 days. Another RCT in children aged 5–16 years admitted to hospital with severe asthma found no significant difference with nebulised budesonide versus oral prednisolone in lung function at 24 hours or 24 days after admission.

Inhaled ipratropium bromide added to β_2 agonists (in emergency room)

One systematic review has found that in children aged 18 months to 17 years multiple doses of inhaled ipratropium bromide plus an inhaled β_2 agonist (fenoterol or salbutamol❸) versus the β_2 agonist alone reduce hospital admissions and improve lung function in children with severe asthma exacerbations. In children with mild to moderate asthma exacerbations, a single dose of inhaled ipratropium bromide plus a β_2 agonist (fenoterol, salbutamol, or terbutaline) versus a β_2 agonist alone significantly improves lung function for up to 2 hours, but does not significantly reduce hospital admissions.

Metered dose inhaler plus spacer devices for delivery of β_2 agonists (as effective as nebulisers)

One systematic review in children with acute but not life threatening asthma who were old enough to use a spacer has found no significant difference in hospital admission rates with a metered dose inhaler plus a spacer versus nebulisation for delivering β_2 agonists (fenoterol, salbutamol, or terbutaline) or β agonist (orciprenaline❸). Children using metered dose inhaler with spacer may have shorter stays in emergency departments, less hypoxia, and lower pulse rates compared with children receiving β_2 agonist by nebulisation.

Oral corticosteroids

One systematic review has found that oral corticosteroids (prednisone or prednisolone) versus placebo within 45 minutes of an acute asthma attack significantly reduce hospital admission.

▶

Clin Evid Concise 2003;9:45–50.

LIKELY TO BE BENEFICIAL

Intravenous theophylline

One systematic review found that in children aged 1–19 years admitted to hospital with severe asthma, intravenous theophylline versus placebo significantly improved lung function and symptom scores 6–8 hours after treatment but found no significant difference in number of bronchodilator treatments required or length of hospital stay. A subsequent RCT found that in children aged 1–17 years admitted to intensive care unit with severe asthma, intravenous theophylline versus control significantly decreased the time to reach clinical asthma score G of 3 or less but found no significant difference in length of stay in intensive care unit.

UNKNOWN EFFECTIVENESS

Inhaled ipratropium bromide added to β_2 agonists (after initial stabilisation) New

One RCT in children admitted to hospital with initially stabilised severe asthma found no significant difference in clinical asthma scores during the first 36 hours with nebulised ipratropium bromide versus placebo added to salbutamol and corticosteroid (hydrocortisone or prednisone).

What are the effects of single agent prophylaxis in childhood asthma?

BENEFICIAL

Inhaled corticosteroids

One systematic review has found that inhaled corticosteroids (betamethasone, beclometasone, budesonide, flunisolide, or fluticasone) versus placebo improve symptoms and lung function in children with asthma. Two systematic reviews of studies with long term follow up and a subsequent long term RCT have found no evidence of growth retardation in children with asthma treated with inhaled corticosteroids. Some shorter term studies found reduced growth velocity.

One RCT in children aged 6–16 years found no significant difference in improvement of asthma symptoms with inhaled beclometasone versus theophylline, but found less use of bronchodilators and oral corticosteroids with inhaled beclometasone.

Small RCTs have found inhaled corticosteroids to be more effective than sodium cromoglicate in improving symptoms and lung function.

RCTs in children aged 5–16 years have found that inhaled corticosteroids (beclometasone, budesonide, or fluticasone) versus inhaled long acting β_2 agonists (salmeterol) or inhaled nedocromil improve symptoms and lung function in children with asthma.

Inhaled nedocromil New

Two RCTs in children aged 6–17 years found that inhaled nedocromil versus placebo significantly reduces asthma symptom scores, asthma severity, bronchodilator use, and lung function. One large RCT in children aged 5–12 years with mild to moderate asthma found no significant difference with nedocromil versus budesonide versus placebo in lung function, hospital admission rate, or the symptom score on diary cards, but found that budesonide was superior to nedocromil, and that nedocromil was superior to placebo in several measures of asthma symptoms and morbidity.

◀ **Oral montelukast** *New*

One RCT in children aged 6–14 years found that oral montelukast versus placebo significantly increased (from baseline) the mean morning forced expiratory volume in 1 second and significantly reduced the total daily β_2 agonist use but found no significant difference in daytime asthma symptom score or in nocturnal awakenings with asthma. Another RCT in children aged 2–5 years found that oral montelukast versus placebo significantly improved average daytime symptom scores and reduced the need for rescue oral steroid courses but found no significant difference in average overnight asthma symptom scores. We found no RCTs directly comparing oral montelukast versus inhaled corticosteroids.

LIKELY TO BE BENEFICIAL

Inhaled sodium cromoglicate *New*

One systematic review found insufficient evidence for prophylactic treatment with sodium cromoglicate in children aged less than 1 year to 18 years. Several small comparative RCTs have found sodium cromoglicate to be less effective than inhaled corticosteroids in improving symptoms and lung function.

TRADE OFF BETWEEN BENEFITS AND HARMS

Inhaled salmeterol *New*

Two RCTs in children aged 4–14 years found that inhaled salmeterol versus placebo significantly improved lung function but found conflicting evidence about a reduced salbutamol use. One RCT comparing inhaled salmeterol versus beclometasone found that salmeterol was associated with a significant deterioration in bronchial reactivity.

Oral theophylline *New*

One small RCT in children aged 6–15 years found that oral theophylline versus placebo significantly increased mean morning peak expiratory flow rate and significantly reduced the mean number of acute night time attacks and doses of bronchodilator used. Another RCT in children aged 6–16 years found no significant difference in improvement of asthma symptoms with oral theophylline versus inhaled beclometasone, but found greater use of bronchodilators and oral corticosteroids with theophylline over 1 year. Theophylline has serious adverse effects (cardiac arrhythmia, convulsions) if therapeutic blood concentrations are exceeded.

What are the effects of additional treatments in childhood asthma inadequately controlled by standard dose inhaled corticosteroids?

UNKNOWN EFFECTIVENESS

Increased dose of inhaled corticosteroid

One RCT in children aged 6–16 years taking inhaled beclometasone comparing the addition of a second dose of inhaled corticosteroid (beclometasone) versus placebo found no significant difference in lung function, symptom scores, exacerbation rates, or bronchial reactivity but found significant reduction of growth velocity at 1 year.

Long acting β_2 agonists

One RCT in children aged 6–16 years found that addition of a long acting β_2 agonist (salmeterol) increased peak expiratory flow rates in the first few months of treatment but found no increase after 1 year. A second short term RCT in children ▶

aged 4–16 years also found increased morning peak expiratory flow rates and more symptom free days at 3 months with addition of a long acting β_2 agonist (salmeterol).

Oral leukotriene receptor antagonists New

One crossover RCT in children aged 6–14 years with persistent asthma who had been taking inhaled budesonide for at least 6 weeks found that the addition of oral montelukast versus placebo significantly improved lung function and decreased the proportion of days with asthma exacerbations over 4 weeks. These differences were statistically significant but modest in clinical terms.

Oral theophylline

One small RCT found that addition of theophylline versus placebo to previous treatment significantly increased the proportion of symptom free days and significantly reduced the use of additional β agonist (orciprenaline) and additional corticosteroid (beclometasone or prednisolone) over 4 weeks.

What are the effects of treatments for acute wheezing in infants?

UNKNOWN EFFECTIVENESS

Addition of ipratropium bromide to long acting β_2 agonist New

One RCT identified by a systematic review in infants aged 3–24 months found that addition of ipratropium bromide to fenoterol versus fenoterol alone significantly reduced the proportion of infants receiving further treatment 45 minutes after initial treatment.

High dose inhaled corticosteroids New

One systematic review found that high dose inhaled corticosteroids versus placebo reduced the requirement for oral corticosteroids but the difference was not statistically significant. The review also found a clear preference for the inhaled corticosteroids by the children's parents over placebo. The clinical importance of these results is unclear.

Inhaled ipratropium bromide

We found no RCTs comparing inhaled ipratropium bromide versus placebo for treating acute wheeze.

Oral corticosteroids

One small RCT found no significant difference in daily symptom scores with oral prednisolone versus placebo.

Short acting β_2 agonists New

One RCT in infants aged 3 months to 2 years found that nebulised salbutamol versus placebo significantly improved respiratory rate but found no significant difference in hospital admission. Another RCT that included infants aged less than 18 months to 36 months found no significant difference in change from baseline in clinical symptom scores with nebulised salbutamol versus placebo.

Short acting β_2 agonists delivered by metered dose inhaler/spacer versus nebuliser

Two RCTs in children aged up to 5 years found no significant difference in hospital admission with delivery of salbutamol through a metered dose inhaler plus spacer versus nebulised salbutamol. Another RCT in infants aged 1–24 months found no significant difference in improvement of symptoms with delivery of terbutaline through a metered dose inhaler plus spacer versus nebulised terbutaline. Nebulised β_2 agonists may cause tachycardia, tremor, and hypokalaemia.

What are the effects of prophylaxis in wheezing infants?

LIKELY TO BE BENEFICIAL

Oral short acting β_2 agonist *New*
One RCT identified by a systematic review in infants aged 3–14 months found that oral salbutamol versus placebo significantly reduced treatment failures.

TRADE OFF BETWEEN BENEFITS AND HARMS

Higher dose inhaled corticosteroids *New*
One RCT in infants aged 6–30 months found that higher prophylactic doses of inhaled corticosteroids (budesonide) versus placebo significantly reduced symptoms and the proportion of children with acute wheezing episodes during a 12 week period but found no significant reduction in the proportion of wheezing episodes per infant. Another RCT in infants aged 11–36 months found that higher prophylactic doses of inhaled corticosteroid (budesonide) significantly reduced the proportion of days requiring oral prednisolone and symptoms of wheezing and sleep disturbance but found no significant improvement for cough. Higher doses of inhaled corticosteroids have the potential for adverse effects.

UNKNOWN EFFECTIVENESS

Inhaled ipratropium bromide *New*
One small RCT identified by a systematic review found no significant difference in relief of symptoms with nebulised ipratropium bromide versus placebo. The study may have lacked power to exclude a clinically important difference between treatments.

Inhaled short acting β_2 agonist *New*
Two RCTs identified by a systematic review in infants aged up to 2 years found no significant improvement in symptoms with inhaled salbutamol versus placebo.

Lower dose inhaled corticosteroids *New*
Three RCTs found no clear evidence of effectiveness with lower prophylactic doses of inhaled corticosteroids (budesonide) in children aged 1 week to 6 years with recurrent wheeze.

UNLIKELY TO BE BENEFICIAL

Addition of inhaled corticosteroid to short acting β_2 agonist *New*
One RCT found no significant improvement in symptoms with addition of inhaled beclometasone versus placebo to inhaled salbutamol.

DEFINITION **Childhood asthma** is characterised by chronic or recurrent cough and wheeze. The diagnosis is confirmed by demonstrating reversible airway obstruction in children old enough to perform peak flow measurements or spirometry. Diagnosing asthma in children requires exclusion of other causes of recurrent respiratory symptoms. **Wheezing in infants** is characterised by a high pitched purring or whistling sound produced predominantly during breathing out and is commonly associated with an acute viral infection such as bronchiolitis (see bronchiolitis, p 53) or asthma. These are not easy to distinguish clinically.

INCIDENCE/ PREVALENCE **Childhood asthma:** Surveys have found increasing prevalence in children diagnosed with asthma. The increase is more than can be explained by an increased readiness to diagnose asthma. One questionnaire study from Aberdeen, Scotland, surveyed 2510 children aged 8–13 years in 1964 and 3403 children in 1989. Over the 25 years, diagnosis of asthma rose from 4% to 10%.[1] The increase in prevalence of childhood asthma from the 1960s to

1980s was accompanied by an increase in hospitals admissions over the same period. In England and Wales this was a sixfold increase.[2] **Wheezing in infants** is common and seems to be increasing though the magnitude of any increase is not clear. One Scottish cross-sectional study (2510 children aged 8–13 years in 1964 and 3403 children in 1989) found that prevalence of wheeze rose from 10% in 1964 to 20% in 1989 and episodes of shortness of breath rose from 5% to 10% over the same period.[1] Difficulties in defining clear groups (phenotypes) and the transient nature of the symptoms, which often resolve spontaneously, have confounded many studies.

AETIOLOGY/ RISK FACTORS **Childhood asthma:** Asthma is more common in children with a personal or family history of atopy; severity and frequency of wheezing episodes and presence of variable airway obstruction or bronchial hyperresponsiveness. Precipitating factors for symptoms and acute episodes include infection, house dust mites, allergens from pet animals, exposure to tobacco smoke, and anxiety. **Wheezing in infants:** Most wheezing episodes in infancy are precipitated by viral respiratory infections.

PROGNOSIS **Childhood asthma:** A British longitudinal study of children born in 1970 found that 29% of 5 year olds wheezing in the past year were still wheezing at the age of 10 years.[3] Another study followed a group of children in Melbourne, Australia from age 7 years (in 1964) into adulthood. The study found a large proportion (73%) of 14 year olds with infrequent symptoms had little or no symptoms by the age of 28 years, whereas two thirds of those 14 year olds with frequent wheezing still had recurrent attacks at the age of 28 years.[4] **Wheezing in infants:** The results of one cohort study (826 infants followed from birth to 6 years) suggests that there may be at least three different prognostic categories for wheezing in infants.[5] The study found one group (14% of total, with risk factors for atopic asthma such as elevated immunoglobulin E levels and maternal history of asthma) were "persistent wheezers" who initially suffered wheeze during viral infections, but the wheezing persisted into school age.[5] A second group (20% of total, with reduced lung function as infants but no early markers of atopy) were "transient wheezers" who also suffered wheeze during viral infections but stopped wheezing after the first 3 years of life. A third group (15% of total) were "late onset wheezers" who did not wheeze when aged under 3 years but had developed wheeze by school age.[5] Another retrospective cohort study found that 14% of children with one attack and 23% of children with four or more attacks in the first year of life had experienced at least one wheezing illness in their past year at age 10 years.[3] Administering inhaled treatments to young children can be difficult. Inconsistencies in results could reflect the effects of the differences in the drugs used, delivery devices used, dosages used, and the differences in the pattern of wheezing illnesses and treatment responses among young children.

Please refer to CD-ROM for full text and references.

Attention deficit hyperactivity disorder

Search date April 2002

Carol Joughin, Paul Ramchandani, and Morris Zwi

What are the effects of treatments?

LIKELY TO BE BENEFICIAL

Dexamfetamine

Limited evidence from two systematic reviews suggests that dexamfetamine versus placebo significantly improves some behavioural outcomes but increases anorexia and appetite disturbance. The second systematic review could not draw firm conclusions about the effects of dexamfetamine versus methylphenidate.

Methylphenidate

A systematic review has found that methylphenidate versus placebo significantly reduces core symptoms in children aged 5–18 years, but may disturb sleep and appetite. The review could not draw firm conclusions about the effects of methylphenidate versus dexamfetamine or versus tricyclic antidepressants. The review also found that methylphenidate versus psychological/behavioural treatment improves symptoms in the medium term, but the clinical importance of these findings is unclear.

Methylphenidate plus behavioural treatment

One systematic review found inconsistent results for combination treatments (medication plus psychological/behavioural treatment) versus placebo. A second systematic review has found that combination treatments versus psychological/behavioural treatments alone significantly improve attention deficit hyperactivity disorder symptoms.

UNKNOWN EFFECTIVENESS

Clonidine

Limited evidence from one systematic review suggests that clonidine versus placebo for 4 –12 weeks reduces core symptoms, but the clinical importance of these findings is unclear.

Psychological/behavioural treatment

One systematic review of two small RCTs found insufficient evidence about the effects of psychological/behavioural treatment versus standard care. One large subsequent RCT found no significant difference between psychological/behavioural treatment versus standard care in behaviour rating scales.

DEFINITION Attention deficit hyperactivity disorder is "a persistent pattern of inattention and/or hyperactivity and impulsivity that is more frequent and severe than is typically observed in individuals at a comparable level of development" (DSM-IV).[1] Inattention, hyperactivity, and impulsivity are commonly known as the core symptoms**G** of attention deficit hyperactivity disorder. Symptoms must be present for at least 6 months, observed before the age of 7 years, and "clinically significant impairment in social, academic, or occupational functioning" must be evident in more than one setting. The symptoms must not be better explained by another disorder such as an anxiety disorder**G**, mood disorder, psychosis, or autistic disorder.[1,] The World Health Organization's *International statistical classification of diseases and related health problems* (ICD-10)[2] uses the term "hyperkinetic disorder" for a more restricted diagnosis. It differs from the DSM-IV classification[3] as all three problems of attention, hyperactivity, and impulsiveness must be present, more stringent criteria for "pervasiveness" across situations must be met, and the presence of another disorder is an exclusion criterion. ▶

Attention deficit hyperactivity disorder

INCIDENCE/ PREVALENCE Prevalence estimates of attention deficit hyperactivity disorder vary according to the diagnostic criteria used and the population sampled. DSM-IV prevalence estimates among school children range from 3–5%,[1] but other estimates vary from 1.7–16%.[4,5] No objective test exists to confirm the diagnosis of attention deficit hyperactivity disorder, which remains a clinical diagnosis. Other conditions frequently coexist with attention deficit hyperactivity disorder. Oppositional defiant disorder**G** is present in 35% (95% CI 27% to 44%) of children with attention deficit hyperactivity disorder, conduct disorder**G** in 26% (95% CI 13% to 41%), anxiety disorder in 26% (95% CI 18% to 35%), and depressive disorder**G** in 18% (95% CI 11% to 27%).[6]

AETIOLOGY/ RISK FACTORS The underlying causes of attention deficit hyperactivity disorder are not known.[6] There is limited evidence that it has a genetic component.[7–9] Risk factors also include psychosocial factors.[10] There is increased risk in boys compared to girls, with ratios varying from 3 : 1[6] to 4 : 1.[3]

PROGNOSIS More than 70% of hyperactive children may continue to meet criteria for attention deficit hyperactivity disorder in adolescence, and up to 65% of adolescents may continue to meet criteria for attention deficit hyperactivity disorder in adulthood.[5] Changes in diagnostic criteria cause difficulty with interpretation of the few outcome studies. One cohort of boys followed up for an average of 16 years found a ninefold increase in antisocial personality disorder and a fourfold increase in substance misuse disorder.[7]

Please refer to CD-ROM for full text and references.

Bronchiolitis

Search date October 2001

Juan M Lozano and Elaine Wang

What are the effects of preventive interventions?

BENEFICIAL

Respiratory syncytial virus immunoglobulins or palivizumab (monoclonal antibody) in children at high risk

One systematic review has found that, in children born prematurely, in children with bronchopulmonary dysplasia, and in children with a combination of risk factors, prophylactic respiratory syncytial virus immunoglobulin or palivizumab (monoclonal antibody) versus placebo or no prophylaxis reduces admission rates to hospital and intensive care units.

UNKNOWN EFFECTIVENESS

Nursing interventions (cohort segregation⊖, handwashing, gowns, masks, gloves, and goggles) in children admitted to hospital

We found no RCTs about the effects of these interventions.

What are the effects of treatments?

UNKNOWN EFFECTIVENESS

Antibiotics (routine)

We found no evidence about children with bronchiolitis alone. One unblinded RCT in children with bronchiolitis and uncomplicated pneumonia (crackles on auscultation, or consolidation on a chest radiograph) found no significant difference in clinical scores with routine use of antibiotics (ampicillin, penicillin, or erythromycin) versus placebo, but it may not have been sufficiently powered to exclude a clinically important effect.

Bronchodilators

Systematic reviews have found that inhaled bronchodilators versus placebo significantly improve overall clinical scores in the short term in children treated in hospital, emergency departments and outpatient clinics, but have found no evidence that bronchodilators reduce admission rates or produce a clinically important improvement in oxygen saturation.

Corticosteroids

One systematic review and eight additional RCTs found limited and conflicting evidence on the effects of corticosteroids versus placebo.

Respiratory syncytial virus immunoglobulins, pooled immunoglobulins, or palivizumab (monoclonal antibody)

RCTs found insufficient evidence about the effects of immunoglobulin treatment versus placebo in children admitted to hospital with bronchiolitis.

Ribavirin

One systematic review in children admitted to hospital with respiratory syncytial virus bronchiolitis found no significant difference in mortality, the risk of respiratory deterioration, or length of hospital stay with ribavarin (tribvarin) versus no treatment, but found that ribavirin significantly reduced the duration of ventilation. One small subsequent RCT found no significant difference with ribavarin versus placebo in hospital stay, oxygen needs, recurrence of disease, or admission rates, but it may have been too small to exclude a clinically important difference.

Bronchiolitis

DEFINITION Bronchiolitis is a virally induced acute bronchiolar inflammation that is associated with signs and symptoms of airway obstruction. Diagnosis is based on clinical findings. Clinical manifestations include fever, rhinitis (inflammation of the nasal mucosa), tachypnoea, expiratory wheezing, cough, rales, use of accessory muscles, apnoea (absence of breathing), dyspnoea (difficulty in breathing), alar flaring (flaring of the nostrils), and retractions (in-drawing of the intercostal soft tissues on inspiration). The disease severity**Ⓖ** of bronchiolitis may be classified clinically as mild, moderate, or severe.

INCIDENCE/ PREVALENCE Bronchiolitis is the most common lower respiratory tract infection in infants, occurring in a seasonal pattern with highest incidence in the winter in temperate climates,[1] and in the rainy season in warmer countries. Each year in the USA, about 21% of infants have lower respiratory tract disease and 6–10/1000 infants are admitted to hospital for bronchiolitis (1–2% of children < 12 months of age).[2] The peak rate of admission occurs in infants aged between 2 and 6 months.[3]

AETIOLOGY/ RISK FACTORS Respiratory syncytial virus is responsible for bronchiolitis in 70% of cases. This figure reaches 80–100% in the winter months. However, in early spring parainfluenza virus type 3 is often responsible.[1]

PROGNOSIS **Morbidity and mortality:** Disease severity is related to the size of the infant, and proximity and to the frequency of contact with infective infants. Children at increased risk of morbidity and mortality are those with congenital heart disease, chronic lung disease, history of premature birth, hypoxia, and age less than 6 weeks.[4] Other factors associated with a prolonged or complicated hospital stay include a history of apnoea or respiratory arrest, pulmonary consolidation, as shown on a chest radiograph, and (in North America) native American or Inuit race.[5] The risk of death within 2 weeks is high for children with congenital heart disease (3.4%) or chronic lung disease (3.5%) compared with other groups combined (0.1%).[4] Rates of admission to intensive care units (range 31–36%) and need for mechanical ventilation (range 11–19%) are similar among all high risk groups.[4] The percentage of these children needing oxygen supplementation is also high (range 63–80%).[4] In contrast, mortality in children with bronchiolitis but without these risk factors is less than 1%, and rates of ICU admission and ventilation in such children are markedly lower (15% and 8%).[6] **Long term prognosis:** Information on long term prognosis varies among studies. One small prospective study of two matched cohorts (25 children with bronchiolitis; 25 children without) found no evidence that bronchiolitis requiring outpatient treatment is associated with an increased risk of asthma in the long term.[7] Possible confounding factors include variation in illness severity, smoke exposure, and crowding.[8] We found one prospective study in 50 randomly selected infants admitted with bronchiolitis, followed up by questionnaire for 5 years and a visit in the fifth year. It found a doubling of asthma incidence compared with the general population, although there was large (30%) loss to follow up and no matched control group.[9]

Please refer to CD-ROM for full text and references.

Cardiorespiratory arrest in children

Search date October 2002

Kate Ackerman and David Creery

What are the effects of treatments for non-submersion out of hospital cardiorespiratory arrest?

LIKELY TO BE BENEFICIAL

Bag–mask ventilation

We found no RCTs. One controlled clinical trial in children requiring airway management in the community found no significant difference between endotracheal intubation and bag–mask ventilation in survival or neurological outcome.

Bystander cardiopulmonary resuscitation

It is widely accepted that cardiopulmonary resuscitation should be undertaken in children who have arrested. Placebo controlled trials would be considered unethical. One systematic review of observational studies found that children who received bystander cardiopulmonary resuscitation versus no bystander cardiopulmonary resuscitation were more likely to survive to hospital discharge.

Intubation

See bag–mask ventilation.

Airway management and ventilation; direct current cardiac shock (for ventricular fibrillation or pulseless ventricular tachycardia G); standard dose intravenous adrenaline (epinephrine)

Although we found no direct evidence to support their use, widespread consensus based on indirect evidence and extrapolation from adult data holds that these interventions should be universally applied to children who have arrested. Placebo controlled trials would be considered unethical.

UNKNOWN EFFECTIVENESS

High dose intravenous adrenaline (epinephrine); intravenous bicarbonate; intravenous calcium; training parents to perform cardiopulmonary resuscitation

We found no RCTs or prospective cohort studies on the effects of these interventions in children who have arrested in the community.

DEFINITION Non-submersion out of hospital cardiorespiratory arrest in children is a state of pulselessness and apnoea occurring outside of a medical facility and not caused by submersion in water.[1]

INCIDENCE/ PREVALENCE We found 12 studies (3 prospective, 9 retrospective) reporting the incidence of non-submersion out of hospital cardiorespiratory arrest in children T.[2–13] Eleven studies reported the incidence in both adults and children, and eight reported the incidence in children.[2–9,11–13] Incidence of arrests in the general population ranged from 2.2–5.7/100 000 people a year (mean 3.1, 95% CI 2.1 to 4.1). Incidence of arrests in children ranged from 6.9–18.0/100 000 children a year (mean 10.6, 95% CI 7.1 to 14.1).[8] One prospective study (300 children) found that about 50% of out of hospital cardiorespiratory arrests occurred in children under 12 months, and about two thirds occurred in children under 18 months.[11]

AETIOLOGY/ RISK FACTORS We found 26 studies reporting the causes of non-submersion pulseless arrests G in a total of 1574 children. The commonest causes of arrest were undetermined causes as in sudden infant death syndrome G (39%), trauma (18%), chronic disease (7%), and pneumonia (4%) T.[1,3–12,14–28]

Cardiorespiratory arrest in children

PROGNOSIS We found no systematic review that investigated non-submersion arrests alone. We found 27 studies (5 prospective, 22 retrospective; total of 1754 children) that reported out of hospital arrest.[1–12,14–28] The overall survival rate following out of hospital arrest was 5% (87 children). Nineteen of these studies (1140 children) found that of the 48 surviving children, 12 (25%) had no or mild neurological disability and 36 (75%) had moderate or severe neurological disability. We found one systematic review (search date 1997), which reported outcomes after cardiopulmonary resuscitation for both in hospital and out of hospital arrests in children of any cause, including submersion.[29] Studies were excluded if they did not report survival. The review found evidence from prospective and retrospective observational studies that out of hospital arrest of any cause in children carries a poorer prognosis than arrest within hospital (132/1568 children [8%] survived to hospital discharge after out of hospital arrest *v* 129/544 children [24%] after in hospital arrests). About half of the survivors were involved in studies that reported neurological outcome. Of these, survival with "good neurological outcome" (i.e. normal or mild neurological deficit) was higher in children who arrested in hospital compared with those who arrested elsewhere (60/77 surviving children [78%] in hospital *v* 28/68 [41%] elsewhere).[29]

Please refer to CD-ROM for full text and references.

Constipation in children

Search date April 2002

Gregory Rubin

What are the effects of treatments?

LIKELY TO BE BENEFICIAL

Biofeedback training (short term benefit only)

Three RCTs found that biofeedback plus conventional treatment (laxatives alone or laxatives plus dietary advice and toilet training) versus conventional treatment alone significantly improved defaecation dynamics and reduced rates of soiling after 3–7 months. Two of the RCTs found no significant difference after 1 year.

Medical treatment plus toilet training

One small RCT in children with encopresis (see definition below) found short term benefit from the addition of toilet training to medical treatment (enemas and osmotic or stimulant laxatives).

Osmotic laxatives

One RCT in children aged 8 months to 16 years found no significant difference with lactitol versus lactulose in stool frequency and consistency of stools, but found that lactulose significantly increased the proportion of children with abdominal pain and flatulence. Another RCT in children aged 11 months to 13 years found that lactitol versus lactulose significantly increased stool frequency and consistency after 15 days' treatment. A third RCT in infants aged 0–6 months found that lactulose significantly improved ease of evacuation and consistency of stools from baseline after 14 days' treatment. However, the benefits shown in these three RCTs are comparisons of outcomes before and after treatment, and were not necessarily because of the treatments.

TRADE OFF BETWEEN BENEFITS AND HARMS

Cisapride

RCTs in an outpatient setting in people aged 2–18 years found that cisapride versus placebo significantly improved stool frequency and symptoms of constipation after 8–12 weeks of treatment. We found no evidence in primary care settings. Cisapride has been withdrawn in several countries because of suspected adverse cardiac effects, and is not widely licensed for use in children. See comments on cisapride under gastro-oesophageal reflux in children, p 64.

UNKNOWN EFFECTIVENESS

Increased dietary fibre

We found no RCTs in children on the effects of increasing dietary fibre.

Stimulant laxatives

We found no RCTs in children on the effects of stimulant laxatives versus placebo or alternative treatments. One small RCT in children with encopresis found short term benefit from the addition of toilet training or biofeedback to stimulant or osmotic laxatives.

DEFINITION Constipation is characterised by infrequent bowel evacuations, hard, small faeces, or difficult or painful defaecation. The frequency of bowel evacuation varies from person to person.[1] Encopresis is defined as involuntary bowel movements in inappropriate places at least once a month for 3 months or more, in children aged 4 years and older.[2]

Constipation in children

INCIDENCE/ PREVALENCE Constipation with or without encopresis is common in children. It accounts for 3% of consultations to paediatric outpatient clinics and 25% of paediatric gastroenterology consultations in the USA.[3] Encopresis has been reported in 1.5% of children at school entry. The peak incidence is at 2–4 years of age.

AETIOLOGY/ RISK FACTORS No cause is discovered in 90–95% of children with constipation. Low fibre intake and a family history of constipation may be associated factors.[4] Psychosocial factors are often suspected, although most children with constipation are developmentally normal.[3] Chronic constipation can lead to progressive faecal retention, distension of the rectum, and loss of sensory and motor function. Organic causes for constipation are uncommon, but include Hirschsprung's disease (1/5000 births; male : female 4 : 1; constipation invariably present from birth), cystic fibrosis, anorectal physiological abnormalities, anal fissures, constipating drugs, dehydrating metabolic conditions, and other forms of malabsorption.[3]

PROGNOSIS Childhood constipation can be difficult to treat and often requires prolonged support, explanation, and medical treatment. In one long term follow up study of children presenting under the age of 5 years, 50% recovered within 1 year and 65–70% recovered within 2 years; the remainder required laxatives for daily bowel movements or continued to soil for years.[3] It is not known what proportion continue to have problems into adult life, although adults presenting with megarectum or megacolon often have a history of bowel problems from childhood.

Please refer to CD-ROM for full text and references.

Depression in children and adolescents

Search date September 2002

Philip Hazell

What are the effects of treatments?

BENEFICIAL

Cognitive therapy (in mild to moderate depression)

One systematic review in children and adolescents with mild to moderate depression has found that cognitive behavioural therapy**G** significantly improves symptoms compared with non-specific support.

LIKELY TO BE BENEFICIAL

Interpersonal therapy in adolescents (in mild to moderate depression)

Two RCTs found that interpersonal therapy**G** versus clinical monitoring or waiting list control significantly increased recovery rate over 12 weeks in adolescents with mild to moderate depression.

TRADE OFF BETWEEN BENEFITS AND HARMS

Selective serotonin reuptake inhibitors

One RCT found no significant difference, one RCT found equivocal results (statistically significant differences on some depression measures but not others), and one RCT found a significant improvement in depressive symptoms with fluoxetine versus placebo after 8–9 weeks. One RCT found that, in adolescents with major depression, paroxetine versus placebo significantly improved remission after 8 weeks. We found no RCTs on other selective serotonin reuptake inhibitors. Selective serotonin reuptake inhibitors are frequently associated with dizziness, lightheadedness, drowsiness, poor concentration, nausea, headache, and fatigue if treatment is reduced or stopped.

UNKNOWN EFFECTIVENESS

Cognitive therapy (depressed adolescents with depressed parent)

One RCT in depressed adolescents with depressed parents found no significant difference in recovery from depression with cognitive behavioural therapy plus usual care versus usual care alone over 2 years.

Electroconvulsive therapy

We found no RCTs on electroconvulsive therapy in children and adolescents with depression.

Intravenous clomipramine (adolescents)

One small RCT found that in non-suicidal adolescents, intravenous clomipramine versus placebo significantly reduced depression scores at 6 days. However, the trial was too small and brief for us to draw reliable conclusions.

Lithium

One RCT found no significant difference with lithium versus placebo in global assessment or depression scores after 6 weeks in children with depression and family history of bipolar affective disorder. Lithium was associated with adverse effects.

Long term effects of treatments

We found no systematic review or RCTs examining long term outcomes of interventions for depression in children and adolescents.

▶

Monoamine oxidase inhibitors

One RCT found insufficient evidence to compare moclobemide versus placebo in children aged 9–15 years with major depression. We found no RCTs on non-reversible monoamine oxidase inhibitors in children or adolescents.

St John's Wort

We found no RCTs on St John's Wort (*Hypericum perforatum*) in children or adolescents with depression.

Venlafaxine

One RCT found no significant difference with venlafaxine versus placebo in improvement of depressive symptoms in children and adolescents with major depression after 6 weeks.

Family therapy; group treatments other than cognitive behavioural therapy

We found insufficient evidence in children and adolescents about the effects of these interventions.

UNLIKELY TO BE BENEFICIAL

Oral tricyclic antidepressants (adolescents)

One systematic review found no significant difference with oral tricyclic antidepressants (amitriptyline, desipramine, imipramine, nortriptyline) versus placebo in depression scores in adolescents and children with depression. Subgroup analyses found that oral tricyclic antidepressants versus placebo significantly reduced symptoms in adolescents but not in children. The review also found that oral tricyclic antidepressants were associated with adverse effects.

LIKELY TO BE INEFFECTIVE OR HARMFUL

Oral tricyclic antidepressants (children)

Subgroup analyses in one systematic review found no significant difference with oral tricyclic antidepressants (amitriptyline, desipramine, imipramine, nortriptyline) versus placebo in children with depression. The review also found that oral tricyclic antidepressants were associated with adverse effects.

DEFINITION Compared with adult depression, depression in children (6–12 years) and adolescents (13–18 years) may have a more insidious onset, may be characterised more by irritability than sadness, and occurs more often in association with other conditions such as anxiety, conduct disorder, hyperkinesis, and learning problems.[1]

INCIDENCE/ PREVALENCE Estimates of prevalence of depression among children and adolescents in the community range from 2–6%.[2,3] Prevalence tends to increase with age, with a sharp rise around onset of puberty. Pre-adolescent boys and girls are affected equally by the condition, but depression is seen more frequently among adolescent girls than boys.[4]

AETIOLOGY/ RISK FACTORS The aetiology is uncertain, but may include genetic vulnerability,[5] childhood events and current psychosocial adversity.[4]

PROGNOSIS In children and adolescents, the recurrence rate following a first depressive episodes in childhood or adolescence is 70% by 5 years, which is similar to the recurrence rate in adults. It is not clear if this is related to severity of depression.[4] Young people experiencing a moderate to severe depressive episode may be more likely than adults to have a manic episode within the next few years.[4,6] Trials of treatment for child and adolescent depression have found high rates of spontaneous remission (as much as two thirds of people in some inpatient studies).

Please refer to CD-ROM for full text and references.

Gastroenteritis in children

Search date June 2002

Jacqueline Dalby-Payne and Elizabeth Elliott

What are the effects of treatments?

BENEFICIAL

Intravenous fluids (as effective as oral rehydration solutions)

One systematic review in children with mild to moderate dehydration found no significant difference with intravenous fluids versus oral rehydration solutions in duration of diarrhoea, time spent in hospital, or weight gain at discharge. One RCT in children with severe dehydration found that intravenous fluids versus oral rehydration solutions significantly increased the duration of diarrhoea and reduced weight gain at discharge, and were associated with more adverse effects.

Oral rehydration solutions (as effective as intravenous fluids)

See intravenous fluids above.

LIKELY TO BE BENEFICIAL

Lactose-free feeds (for duration of diarrhoea)

One systematic review has found that lactose-free feeds versus lactose-containing feeds reduce the duration of diarrhoea in children with mild to severe dehydration. Subsequent RCTs found conflicting results.

Loperamide (reduces duration of diarrhoea, but adverse effects are unclear)

Two RCTs found that, in children with mild to moderate dehydration, loperamide versus placebo significantly reduces the duration of diarrhoea. Another RCT found no significant difference with loperamide versus placebo in the duration of diarrhoea. We found insufficient evidence about adverse effects.

UNKNOWN EFFECTIVENESS

Clear fluids for rehydration (other than oral rehydration solutions)

We found no systematic review or RCTs on "clear fluids" (water, carbonated drinks, and translucent fruit juices) versus oral rehydration solutions for treatment of mild to moderate dehydration caused by acute gastroenteritis.

DEFINITION Acute gastroenteritis is characterised by rapid onset of diarrhoea with or without vomiting, nausea, fever, and abdominal pain.[1] In children, the symptoms and signs can be non-specific.[2] Diarrhoea is defined as the frequent passage of unformed liquid stools.[3]

INCIDENCE/ PREVALENCE Worldwide, about 3–5 billion cases of acute gastroenteritis occur in children under 5 years of age each year.[4] In the UK, acute gastroenteritis accounts for 204/1000 general practitioner consultations in children under 5 years of age each year.[5] Gastroenteritis leads to hospital admission in 7/1000 children under 5 years of age per year in the UK[5] and 13/1000 in the USA.[6] In Australia, gastroenteritis accounts for 6% of all hospital admissions in children under 15 years of age.[7]

AETIOLOGY/ RISK FACTORS In developed countries, acute gastroenteritis is predominantly caused by viruses (87%), of which rotavirus is most common;[8–11] bacteria cause most of the remaining cases, predominantly Campylobacter, Salmonella, Shigella, and *Escherichia coli*. In developing countries, bacterial pathogens are more frequent, although rotavirus is also a major cause of gastroenteritis.

PROGNOSIS Acute gastroenteritis is usually self limiting but if untreated can result in morbidity and mortality secondary to water and electrolyte losses. Acute diarrhoea causes 4 million deaths per year in children under 5 years of age in Asia (excluding China), Africa, and Latin America, and over 80% of deaths occur in children under 2 years of age.[12] Although death is uncommon in developed countries, dehydration secondary to gastroenteritis is a significant cause of morbidity and need for hospital admission.[6,7,13]

Please refer to CD-ROM for full text and references.

Gastro-oesophageal reflux in children

Search date May 2002

Yadlapalli Kumar and Rajini Sarvananthan

What are the effects of treatments?

UNKNOWN EFFECTIVENESS

Domeperidone

One small RCT in children aged 5 months to 11 years found insufficient evidence about the effects of domperidone versus placebo.

Feed thickeners

We found no clear evidence about the effects of feed thickeners. One small RCT in infants aged 1–16 weeks found no significant difference in regurgitation reported by parents with carob flour thickened feeds versus placebo thickened feeds. Another small RCT in infants aged 5–11 months found that carob flour versus traditional formula thickened with rice flour significantly reduced gastro-oesophageal reflux symptoms and episodes of vomiting.

H_2 antagonists

One small RCT in children aged 1 month to 14 years found that cimetidine (an H_2 antagonist) versus placebo significantly improved clinical or endoscopic features of gastro-oesophageal reflux complicated by oesophagitis over 12 weeks.

Metoclopramide

Three small RCTs found insufficient evidence about the effects of metoclopramide versus placebo. One small RCT found insufficient evidence about the effects of metoclopramide versus sodium alginate or versus placebo.

Positioning (left lateral or prone)

Small crossover RCTs in children aged under 6 months found limited evidence that prone or left lateral positioning versus supine positioning improved oesophageal pH variables, but both positions may be associated with sudden infant death syndrome.

Sodium alginate

One small RCT in childrea aged under 2 years found that sodium alginate versus placebo for 8 days significantly reduced episodes of regurgitation reported by parents. One small RCT in children aged 4 months to 17 years found insufficient evidence about the effects of sodium alginate versus metoclopramide or versus placebo.

Proton pump inhibitors; surgery (fundoplication)

We found no RCTs about the effects of these interventions.

LIKELY TO BE INEFFECTIVE OR HARMFUL

Cisapride

One systematic review found no significant difference with cisapride versus placebo in clinical symptoms. Cisapride is not widely licensed for use in children and has been withdrawn or its use restricted in several countries because of an association with heart rhythm abnormalities.

Gastro-oesophageal reflux in children

DEFINITION Gastro-oesophageal reflux disease is the passive transfer of gastric contents into the oesophagus due to transient or chronic relaxation of the lower oesophageal sphincter.[1] A survey of 69 children (median age 16 months) with gastro-oesophageal reflux disease attending a tertiary referral centre found that presenting symptoms were recurrent vomiting (72%), epigastric and abdominal pain (36%), feeding difficulties (29%), failure to thrive (28%), and irritability (19%).[2] Over 90% of children with gastro-oesophageal reflux disease have vomiting before 6 weeks of age.[1]

INCIDENCE/ PREVALENCE Gastro-oesophageal regurgitation is considered a problem if it is frequent, persistent, and associated with other symptoms such as increased crying, discomfort with regurgitation and frequent back arching.[1,3] A cross-sectional survey of parents of 948 infants attending 19 primary care paediatric practices found that regurgitation of at least one episode a day was reported in 51% of infants aged 0–3 months. "Problematic" regurgitation occurred in significantly fewer infants (14% *v* 51%; P < 0.001).[3] Peak regurgitation reported as "problematic" was reported in 23% of infants aged six months.[3]

AETIOLOGY/ RISK FACTORS Risk factors for gastro-oesophageal reflux disease include immaturity of the lower oesophageal sphincter, chronic relaxation of the sphincter, increased abdominal pressure, gastric distension, hiatus hernia, and oesophageal dysmotility.[1] Premature infants and children with severe neurodevelopmental problems or congenital oesophageal anomalies are particularly at risk.[1]

PROGNOSIS Regurgitation is considered benign, and most cases resolve spontaneously by 12–18 months of age.[4] In a cross-sectional survey of 948 parents, the peak age for reporting four or more episodes of regurgitation was at 5 months of age (23%), which decreased to 7% at 7 months (P < 0.001). The prevalence of "problematic" regurgitation also reduced from 23% in infants aged 6 months to 3.25% in infants aged 10–12 months.[3] Rare complications of gastro-oesophageal reflux disease include oesophagitis with haematemesis and anaemia, respiratory problems (such as cough, apnoea, and recurrent wheeze), and failure to thrive.[1] A small comparative study (40 children) suggested that, when compared with healthy children, infants with gastro-oesophageal reflux disease had slower development of feeding skills and had problems affecting behaviour, swallowing, food intake, and mother–child interaction.[5]

Please refer to CD-ROM for full text and references.

Infantile colic

Search date May 2002

Teresa Kilgour and Sally Wade

What are the effects of treatments?

LIKELY TO BE BENEFICIAL

Whey hydrolysate milk

One RCT found limited evidence that replacing cows' milk formula with whey hydrolysate formula🅖 significantly reduced crying recorded in a parental diary.

TRADE OFF BETWEEN BENEFITS AND HARMS

Dicycloverine

One systematic review found limited evidence that dicycloverine (dicyclomine)🅖 versus placebo reduced crying in infants with colic. One RCT found that dicycloverine versus placebo significantly reduced the proportion of infants with colic. RCTs found that dicycloverine versus placebo increased drowsiness, constipation, and loose stools, but the difference did not reach significance. Case reports of harms in infants have included breathing difficulties, seizures, syncope, asphyxia, muscular hypotonia, and coma.

UNKNOWN EFFECTIVENESS

Car ride stimulation

One RCT found no evidence that car ride stimulation reduced maternal anxiety and hours of infant crying over 2 weeks more than reassurance🅖 and support alone.

Casein hydrolysate milk

RCTs found insufficient evidence about the effects of replacing cows' milk formula with casein hydrolysate hypoallergenic formula.

Cranial osteopathy

We found no RCTs about the effects of cranial osteopathy🅖 in infants with colic.

Herbal tea

One small RCT found that herbal tea (containing extracts of camomile, vervain, liquorice, fennel, and balm mint in a sucrose solution) versus sucrose solution significantly improved symptoms of colic rated by parents at 7 days.

Focused counselling

One RCT found no evidence that counselling mothers about specific management techniques (responding to crying with gentle soothing motion, avoiding over stimulation, using a pacifier, and prophylactic carrying) reduced maternal anxiety and hours of infant crying over 2 weeks more than reassurance and support alone. Another small RCT found that focused counselling versus substitution of soya or cows' milk with casein hydrolysate formula significantly decreased duration and extent of crying.

Infant massage

One RCT found no significant difference with massage versus a crib vibrator in colic related crying or parental rating of symptoms of infantile colic, but it may have lacked power to detect a clinically important difference.

Low lactose (lactase treated) milk

RCTs found no significant difference in duration of crying with low lactose treated milk versus untreated milk.

Reduction of stimulation of the infant
One RCT found limited evidence that advice to reduce stimulation (by not patting, lifting, or jiggling the baby, or by reducing auditory stimulation) versus an empathetic interview significantly reduced crying after 7 days in infants under 12 weeks.

Soya based infant feeds
One small RCT found that soya based infant feeds Ⓖ versus standard cows' milk formula significantly reduced the duration of crying.

Spinal manipulation
Two RCTs found inconclusive results about the effects of spinal manipulation Ⓖ.

Sucrose solution
One small crossover RCT found limited evidence that sucrose solution versus placebo significantly improved symptoms of colic as rated by parents after 12 days.

UNLIKELY TO BE BENEFICIAL

Increased carrying
One RCT found no significant difference in daily crying time with carrying the infant, even when not crying, for at least an additional 3 hours a day versus a general advice group (to carry, check baby's nappy, feed, offer pacifier, place baby near mother, or use background stimulation such as music). The "advice to carry" group carried their babies for 4.5 hours daily compared with 2.6 hours daily in the general advice group.

Simethicone (activated dimeticone)
One RCT found no significant difference with simethicone (activated dimeticone) Ⓖ versus placebo in the presence of colic when rated by carers. Another RCT found no significant difference with simethicone versus placebo in improvement as rated by parental interview, 24 hour diary, or behavioural observation. Another poor quality RCT found that simethicone versus placebo significantly reduced the number of crying attacks on days 4–7 of treatment.

DEFINITION Infantile colic is defined as excessive crying in an otherwise healthy baby. The crying typically starts in the first few weeks of life and ends by 4–5 months. Excessive crying is defined as crying that lasts at least 3 hours a day, for 3 days a week, for at least 3 weeks.[1]

INCIDENCE/ PREVALENCE Infantile colic causes 1/6 families to consult a health professional. One systematic review of fifteen community based studies found a wide variation in prevalence, which depended on study design and method of recording.[2] The two best prospective studies identified by the review yielded prevalence rates of 5% and 19%.[2] One RCT (89 breast and formula fed infants) found that, at 2 weeks of age, the prevalence of crying more than 3 hours a day was 43% among formula fed infants and 16% among breastfed infants. The prevalence at 6 weeks was 12% (formula fed) and 31% (breast fed).[3]

AETIOLOGY/ RISK FACTORS The cause of infantile colic is unclear and, despite its name, might not have an abdominal cause. It may reflect part of the normal distribution of infantile crying. Other possible explanations are painful gut contractions, lactose intolerance, gas, or parental misinterpretation of normal crying.[1]

PROGNOSIS Infantile colic improves with time. One study found that 29% of infants aged 1–3 months cried for more than 3 hours a day, but by 4–6 months of age the prevalence had fallen to 7–11%.[4]

Please refer to CD-ROM for full text and references.

Measles

Search date December 2002

Clinical Evidence freelance writers

What are the effects of preventive interventions?

BENEFICIAL

Live combined measles, mumps, and rubella (MMR) vaccine; live monovalent measles vaccine

Large cohort studies, large time series, and population surveillance data from different countries have all found that combined MMR**G** and live monovalent measles vaccination programmes reduce the risk of measles infection to near zero, especially in populations in which vaccine coverage**G** is high.

We found no RCTs comparing the effects of MMR versus no vaccination or placebo on measles infection rates. Such trials are likely to be considered unethical because of the large body of whole-population evidence finding benefit from vaccination.

Unlike live monovalent measles vaccine**G**, MMR additionally protects against mumps and rubella, which themselves cause serious complications (mumps causes orchitis, pancreatitis, infertility, meningoencephalitis, deafness, and congenital fetal abnormalities; rubella causes deafness, blindness, heart defects, liver, spleen and brain damage, and stillbirth).

One systematic review, one RCT, one large population based survey, and one population based study found no evidence that MMR was associated with acute developmental regression**G**. Large time series studies have consistently found no evidence that MMR or live monovalent measles vaccine was associated with autism.

One large, long term population surveillance study and one population based case control study found no evidence that either MMR or monovalent measles vaccine was associated with inflammatory bowel disease. One large cohort study and two population based case control studies found no association between monovalent measles vaccine and inflammatory bowel disease.

One systematic review and one additional RCT found that MMR and monovalent measles vaccine were associated with a small and similar risk of self limiting fever within 3 weeks of vaccination compared with 100% risk of acute fever in people with measles.

DEFINITION Measles is an infectious disease caused by a ribonucleic acid paramyxomavirus. The illness is characterised by an incubation period of 10–12 days; a prodromal period of 2–4 days with upper respiratory tract symptoms; Koplik's spots on mucosal membranes and high fever; followed by further fever, and a widespread maculopapular rash that persists for 5–6 days.[1]

INCIDENCE/ PREVALENCE Measles incidence varies widely according to vaccination coverage. Worldwide, there are an estimated 30 million cases of measles each year,[2] but an incidence of only 0–10/100 000 people in countries with widespread vaccination programmes, such as the USA, UK, Mexico, India, China, Brazil, and Australia.[3] In the USA, before licensing of effective vaccines, more than 90% of people were infected by the age of 15 years. After licensing in 1963, incidence fell by about 98%.[1] Mean annual incidence in Finland was 366/100 000 in 1970,[4] but declined to about zero by the late 1990s.[5] Similarly, annual incidence declined to about zero in Chile, the English speaking Caribbean, and Cuba during the 1990s when vaccination programmes were introduced.[6,7]

AETIOLOGY/ RISK FACTORS Measles is highly contagious. The virus is spread through airborne droplets that persist for up to 2 hours in closed areas following the presence of an infected person. Measles is highly contagious. As with other infectious diseases, risk factors include overcrowding, low herd immunity**G**, and immunosuppression. People with immunosuppression, children younger than 5 years of age, and adults older than 20 years of age have a higher risk of severe complications and death, although these also occur in healthy people (see prognosis below).[1] Newborn babies have a lower risk of measles than older infants, owing to the persistence of protective maternal antibodies, although in recent US outbreaks, maternal antibody protection was lower than expected.[1]

PROGNOSIS The World Health Organization estimated that in the year 2000, measles caused 777 000 deaths and 27.5 million disability adjusted life years.[8] **Disease in healthy people:** In developed countries, most prognostic data come from the pre-vaccination era and from subsequent outbreaks in non-vaccinated populations. In the USA, about 30% of reported measles cases involve complications of the disease. From 1989–1991 in the USA, measles resurgence among young children (< 5 years) who had not been immunised led to 55 622 cases with more than 11 000 hospital admissions and 125 deaths.[1] Measles complications include diarrhoea (8%), otitis media (7%), pneumonia (6%), death (0.1–0.2%), acute encephalitis (about 0.1% followed by death in 15% and permanent neurological damage in about 25%), seizures (with or without fever in 0.6–0.7%), idiopathic thrombocytopenia (1/6000 reported cases), and subacute scerlosing panencephalitis causing degeneration of the central nervous system and death 7 years after measles infection (range 1 month to 27 years; 0.5–1.0/100 000 reported cases).[1,9] Measles during pregnancy results in higher risk of premature labour, spontaneous abortion, and low birth weight infants. An association with birth defects remains uncertain.[1] **Disease in malnourished or immunocompromised people:** In malnourished or immunocompromised people, particularly those with vitamin A deficiency, measles case fatality can be as high as 25%. Worldwide, measles is a major cause of blindness and causes 5% of deaths in young children (< 5 years).[1,10]

Please refer to CD-ROM for full text and references.

Nocturnal enuresis

Search date June 2002

Sara Bosson and Natalie Lyth

What are the effects of interventions for short term relief of symptoms?

BENEFICIAL

Desmopressin (intranasal)

One systematic review has found that intranasal desmopressin versus placebo significantly reduces bedwetting by at least one night a week, and increases the chance of attaining 14 consecutive dry nights.

Dry bed training

One systematic review has found that a significantly greater proportion of children achieved 14 consecutive dry nights with dry bed training versus no treatment.

Enuresis alarm

One systematic review has found that significantly greater proportion of children achieved 14 consecutive dry nights with enuresis alarms versus no treatment.

LIKELY TO BE BENEFICIAL

Desmopressin (oral)

One RCT in children aged 6–16 years found that oral desmopressin (0.2–0.6 mg) versus placebo significantly increased the proportion of children achieving 50% or greater reduction in number of wet nights for 14 days.

Laser acupuncture

One RCT found no significant difference in the number of wet nights in children aged over 5 years with laser acupuncture versus intranasal desmopressin.

Standard home alarm clock

One RCT found that a significantly higher proportion of children achieved 14 consecutive dry nights with standard home alarm clock versus waking after 3 hours' sleep.

TRADE OFF BETWEEN BENEFITS AND HARMS

Tricyclic drugs (imipramine, desipramine)

One systematic review has found that tricyclic drugs (imipramine, desipramine) versus placebo significantly increase the chance of attaining 14 consecutive dry nights. It found no significant difference with imipramine versus an alarm during the treatment period but found that children using an enuresis alarm had fewer wet nights per week after the treatment had stopped. The review found that tricyclic drugs versus placebo increased adverse effects such as anorexia, anxiety reaction, constipation, depression, diarrhoea, dizziness, drowsiness, dry mouth, headache, irritability, lethargy, sleep disturbance, upset stomach, and vomiting.

What are the effects of interventions for long term relief of symptoms?

BENEFICIAL

Enuresis alarm

One systematic review has found that significantly greater proportion of children achieve 14 consecutive dry nights with enuresis alarms versus no treatment, and ▶

that 31–61% of children were still dry at 3 months. The review found that children using an alarm were 9 times less likely to relapse than children taking desmopressin. One RCT found that a significantly higher proportion of children achieved 4 weeks of dryness with alarm plus intranasal desmopressin (40 μg) versus alarm alone.

UNKNOWN EFFECTIVENESS

Dry bed training

One systematic review found no significant difference in the proportion of dry nights in the long term with dry bed training versus no treatment.

Standard home alarm clock

One RCT found that a significantly higher proportion of children achieved 14 consecutive dry nights with standard home alarm clock versus waking after 3 hours' sleep, but found no significant difference in the proportion of dry nights at 3 months.

Ultrasound

We found no RCTs on use of ultrasound. One small controlled trial in children aged 6–14 years found that ultrasound versus control significantly increased the proportion of dry nights for up to 12 months.

UNLIKELY TO BE BENEFICIAL

Adding intranasal desmopressin to alarm

Two RCTs found no significant difference with addition of intranasal desmopressin (40 μg) versus placebo to an alarm in long term relief from bed wetting

DEFINITION Nocturnal enuresis is the involuntary discharge of urine at night in the absence of congenital or acquired defects of the central nervous system or urinary tract in a child aged 5 years or older.[1] Disorders that have bedwetting as a symptom (termed "nocturnal incontinence") can be excluded by a thorough history, examination, and urinalysis. "Monosymptomatic" nocturnal enuresis is characterised by night time symptoms only and accounts for 85% of cases. Nocturnal enuresis is defined as primary if the child has never been dry for a period of more than 6 months, and secondary if such a period of dryness preceded the onset of wetting.

INCIDENCE/ PREVALENCE Between 15% and 20% of 5 year olds, 7% of 7 year olds, 5% of 10 year olds, 2–3% of 12–14 year olds, and 1–2% of people aged 15 years and over wet the bed twice a week on average.[2]

AETIOLOGY/ RISK FACTORS Nocturnal enuresis is associated with several factors, including small functional bladder capacity, nocturnal polyuria, and arousal dysfunction. Linkage studies have identified associated genetic loci on chromosomes 8q, 12q, 13q, and 22q11.[3–6]

PROGNOSIS Nocturnal enuresis has widely differing outcomes, from spontaneous resolution to complete resistance to all current treatments. About 1% of adults remain enuretic. Without treatment, about 15% of children with enuresis become dry each year.[7] We found no RCTs on the best age to start treatment in children with nocturnal enuresis. Anecdotal experience suggests that reassurance is sufficient below the age of 7 years. Behavioural treatments, such as alarms, require motivation and commitment from the child and a parent. Anecdotal experience suggests that children under the age of 7 years may not exhibit the commitment needed.

Please refer to CD-ROM for full text and references.

Nosebleeds in children

Search date October 2002

Gerald McGarry

What are the effects of treatments?

LIKELY TO BE BENEFICIAL

Antiseptic cream

One RCT found that chlorhexidine/neomycin cream versus no treatment significantly reduced nosebleeds at 8 weeks.

UNKNOWN EFFECTIVENESS

Antiseptic cream versus cautery

One small RCT comparing chlorhexidine/neomycin cream versus silver nitrate cautery found no significant difference in nose bleeds at 8 weeks. Some children found the smell and taste of the antiseptic cream unpleasant. All children found cautery painful, despite the use of local anaesthesia.

Cautery plus antiseptic cream

One small RCT found insufficient evidence about the effects of silver nitrate cautery plus chlorhexidine/neomycin cream versus chlorhexidine/neomycin cream alone.

Cautery versus no treatment

We found no RCTs about the effects of this intervention.

DEFINITION Recurrent idiopathic epistaxis is recurrent, self limiting, nasal bleeding in children for which no specific cause is identified. There is no consensus on the frequency or severity of recurrences.

INCIDENCE/ PREVALENCE A cross sectional study of 1218 children (aged 11–14 years) found that 9% had frequent episodes of epistaxis.[1] It is likely that only the most severe episodes are considered for treatment.

AETIOLOGY/ RISK FACTORS In children, most epistaxis occurs from the anterior part of the septum in the region of Little's area.[2] Initiating factors include local inflammation, mucosal drying, and local trauma (including nose picking).[2] Epistaxis caused by other specific local (e.g. tumours) or systemic factors (e.g. clotting disorders) is not considered here.

PROGNOSIS Recurrent epistaxis is less common in adolescents over 14 years and many children "grow out" of this problem.

Please refer to CD-ROM for full text and references.

Reducing pain during blood sampling in infants

Search date September 2002

Linda Franck and Ruth Gilbert

What are the effects of blood sampling method?

BENEFICIAL

Venepuncture versus heel puncture

RCTs in term infants have found that venepuncture versus heel puncture significantly reduces pain responses (particularly crying) during blood sampling, and reduces the need for repeat punctures.

Automated devices versus manual lancets

RCTs in preterm and term infants have found that automated devices versus manual lancets for heel puncture are less painful, cause less bruising, and reduce the time needed to obtain a sample.

What are the effects of interventions to reduce pain related distress during heel puncture?

BENEFICIAL

Oral sucrose

Systematic reviews and additional RCTs have found that oral sucrose versus water or no treatment significantly reduces pain responses (particularly the duration of crying). One RCT found that sucrose did not appear to increase the benefit of holding. One RCT in preterm infants found no significant difference in pain score between a pacifier**G** dipped in sucrose versus a pacifier alone. One RCT found insufficient evidence about the effects of oral sucrose versus lidocaine–prilocaine emulsion (EMLA®) in term infants undergoing heel puncture.

LIKELY TO BE BENEFICIAL

Holding (skin to skin) in term infants

RCTs found that crying was reduced in infants held during heel puncture.

Oral glucose

RCTs have found that oral glucose versus water or versus no treatment significantly reduces pain responses (particularly the duration of crying).

Other sweeteners

RCTs have found that other sweeteners (hydrogenated glucose**G** or an artificial sweetener, 10 parts cyclamate and 1 part saccharin) versus water significantly reduce pain scores and the percentage of time spent crying.

Pacifiers

RCTs in term and preterm infants have found that pacifiers given before heel puncture versus no treatment reduce pain responses.

Positioning (tucking arms and legs) in preterm infants

RCTs found limited evidence that pain responses were reduced by tucking the arms and legs into a mid-line flexed position during heel puncture.

Clin Evid Concise 2003;9:73–75.

Rocking

One RCT found limited evidence that rocking by the examiner versus no intervention reduced pain in neonates undergoing heel puncture. Another RCT found no significant difference in pain response with simulated rocking by a mechanical device versus water given before heel puncture.

UNKNOWN EFFECTIVENESS

Multiple doses of sweet solution

One small RCT found no significant difference with multiple versus single doses of sucrose in pain scores for heel puncture.

Swaddling

RCTs found no significant difference in pain responses from swaddling or positioning.

UNLIKELY TO BE BENEFICIAL

Breast milk

RCTs found no evidence that breast milk or breast feeding versus water reduced pain responses or crying in neonates.

Prone position

One RCT found no significant difference in pain score with prone position versus side or supine position during heel puncture. One RCT found that handling (as if being prepared for a lumbar puncture) versus no handling significantly increased pain and crying for up to 2 minutes after heel puncture.

Topical anaesthetics

Systematic reviews and additional RCTs found no evidence of reduced pain responses, particularly crying, following heel puncture with topical anaesthetic (lidocaine, lidocaine–prilocaine emulsion, or tetracaine [amethocaine]) compared with placebo.

Warming

One RCT in term infants found no benefit of warming prior to heel puncture.

What are the effects of interventions to reduce pain related distress during venepuncture?

LIKELY TO BE BENEFICIAL

Oral glucose

RCTs have found that oral glucose versus water or versus no treatment significantly reduces pain responses (particularly the duration of crying). One RCT found no significant difference in pain scores between sucrose and glucose for venepuncture. We found no RCTs about the effects of oral glucose versus topical anaesthesia.

Oral sucrose

RCTs have found that oral sucrose versus water or no treatment significantly reduces pain responses (particularly the duration of crying). One RCT found no significant difference in pain scores between sucrose and glucose for venepuncture. One RCT in preterm infants found no significant difference in pain score between a pacifier dipped in sucrose versus a pacifier alone.

Pacifiers

One RCT in term infants undergoing venepuncture found that pacifiers versus water or versus no treatment significantly reduced pain responses.

Topical anaesthetics

RCTs found limited evidence that lidocaine–prilocaine emulsion versus placebo reduced pain responses to venepuncture. RCTs found that tetracaine (amethocaine) versus placebo reduced pain scores and the number of infants who cried during venepuncture. We found no RCTs about the effects of oral glucose versus topical anaesthesia.

UNKNOWN EFFECTIVENESS

Breast milk

We found no RCTs on the effects of breast milk during venepuncture.

Other sweeteners

We found no RCTs of other sweeteners for venepuncture.

DEFINITION Methods of sampling blood in infants include heel puncture, venepuncture, and arterial puncture. Heel puncture involves lancing of the lateral aspect of the infant's heel, squeezing the heel, and collecting the pooled capillary blood. Venepuncture involves aspirating blood through a needle in a peripheral vein. Arterial blood sampling is not discussed in this review.

INCIDENCE/ PREVALENCE Almost every infant in the developed world undergoes heel puncture to screen for metabolic disorders (e.g. phenylketonuria). Many infants have repeated heel punctures or venepunctures to monitor blood glucose or haemoglobin. Preterm or ill neonates receiving intensive care may have 1–21 painful procedures a day.[1–3] Heel punctures comprise 61–87% and venepuncture comprise 8–13% of the invasive procedures performed on ill infants. Analgesics are rarely given specifically for blood sampling procedures, but 5–19% of infants receive analgesia for other indications.[2,3] In one study, comfort measures were provided during 63% of venepunctures and 75% of heel punctures.[3]

AETIOLOGY/ RISK FACTORS Blood sampling in infants can be difficult to perform, particularly in preterm or ill infants. Young infants may have increased sensitivity and more prolonged responses to pain than older age groups.[4] Factors that may affect the infant's pain responses include postconceptional age, previous pain experience, and procedural technique.

PROGNOSIS Pain caused by blood sampling is associated with acute behavioural and physiological deterioration.[4] Experience of pain during heel puncture appears to heighten pain responses during subsequent blood sampling.[5] Other adverse effects of blood sampling include bleeding, bruising, haematoma, and infection. Extremely rarely, heel puncture can result in cellulitis, osteomyelitis, calcaneal spurs, calcified cysts, and necrotising chondritis.[6–9]

Please refer to CD-ROM for full text and references.

Sudden infant death syndrome

Search date July 2002

David Creery and Angelo Mikrogianakis

What are the effects of interventions to reduce the risk of sudden infant death syndrome?

BENEFICIAL

Advice to avoid prone sleeping

One non-systematic review of observational studies and 11 additional observational studies found that campaigns involving advice to encourage non-prone sleeping positions were followed by a reduced incidence of sudden infant death syndrome. RCTs are unlikely to be conducted.

LIKELY TO BE BENEFICIAL

Advice to avoid tobacco smoke exposure

One non-systematic review of observational studies and three additional observational studies found that campaigns to reduce several sudden infant death syndrome risk factors, which included tobacco smoke exposure, were followed by a reduced incidence of sudden infant death syndrome. RCTs are unlikely to be conducted.

UNKNOWN EFFECTIVENESS

Advice to avoid bed sharing

One observational study found that a campaign to reduce several sudden infant death syndrome risk factors, which included advice to avoid bed sharing, was followed by a reduced incidence of sudden infant death syndrome. RCTs are unlikely to be conducted.

Advice to avoid over heating or over wrapping

One non-systematic review of observational studies and one additional observational study found that campaigns to reduce several sudden infant death syndrome risk factors, which included over wrapping, were followed by a reduced incidence of sudden infant death syndrome. RCTs are unlikely to be conducted.

Advice to breast feed

One non-systematic review of observational studies and two additional observational studies found that campaigns to reduce several sudden infant death syndrome risk factors, which included advice to breast feed, were followed by a reduced incidence of sudden infant death syndrome. RCTs are unlikely to be conducted.

Advice to avoid soft sleeping surfaces; advice to promote soother use

We found no evidence on the effects of these interventions in the prevention of sudden infant death syndrome.

DEFINITION Sudden infant death syndrome (SIDS) is the sudden death of an infant aged under 1 year that remains unexplained after review of the clinical history, examination of the scene of death, and postmortem.

INCIDENCE/ PREVALENCE The incidence of SIDS has varied over time and among nations (incidence per 1000 live births of SIDS in 1996: Netherlands 0.3; Japan 0.4; Canada 0.5; England and Wales 0.7; USA 0.8; and Australia 0.9).[1]

Clin Evid Concise 2003;9:76–77.

Sudden infant death syndrome

AETIOLOGY/ RISK FACTORS By definition, the cause of SIDS is not known. Observational studies have found an association between SIDS and several risk factors, including prone sleeping**G** position,[2,3] prenatal or postnatal exposure to tobacco smoke,[4] soft sleeping surfaces,[5,6] hyperthermia/over wrapping**T**,[7,8] bed sharing (particularly with mothers who smoke),[9,10] lack of breast feeding,[11,12] and soother**G** use.[7,13]

PROGNOSIS Although by definition prognosis is not applicable for an affected infant, the incidence of SIDS is increased in the siblings of that infant.[14,15]

Please refer to CD-ROM for full text and references.

Urinary tract infection in children

Search date January 2002

James Larcombe

What are the effects of treatment of acute infection?

BENEFICIAL

Longer versus short courses of oral antibiotics

One systematic review identified two RCTs that found a significantly higher cure rate (eradication of causative organism on follow up culture) with longer (10 days) versus shorter (single dose/1 day) courses of oral antibiotics (amoxicillin, cefadroxil) in children with urinary tract infections. Another systematic review in children and adolescents aged < 18 years with uncomplicated cystitis found that conventional (≥ 5 days) versus short courses (≤ 4 days) significantly increased cure rate, but the significant difference disappeared when single dose studies were excluded. The difference in cure rate between short and conventional courses remained significant for amoxicillin but not co-trimoxazole.

LIKELY TO BE BENEFICIAL

Co-trimoxazole (3 day course)

One systematic review found no significant difference in cure rate between a 3 day and a conventional (7–10 day) course of co-trimoxazole.

Oral versus initial intravenous antibiotics

One RCT found no significant difference with oral versus initial intravenous antibiotics (cephalosporins) in duration of fever, reinfection, renal scarring, or extent of scarring in children aged 2 years or younger with first confirmed urinary tract infection. The RCT found weak evidence from a post hoc subgroup analysis in children with grades III–IV reflux**G** that renal scarring at 6 months may be more common with oral versus initial intravenous treatment.

UNKNOWN EFFECTIVENESS

Immediate empirical versus delayed antibiotic treatment

We found no RCTs on the effects of giving early empirical treatment versus awaiting the results of microscopy or culture in acute urinary tract infection in children. One RCT found no significant difference in risk of renal scarring with antibiotic (cephalosporins) treatment within 24 hours versus 24 hours after the onset of fever in children under 2 years with urinary tract infections.

UNLIKELY TO BE BENEFICIAL

Longer versus short courses of initial intravenous antibiotics

Two RCTs found no significant difference with long (7–10 days) versus short (3 days) course of initial intravenous antibiotic (ceftriaxone) treatment on development of renal scarring in children with acute pyelonephritis**G**.

LIKELY TO BE INEFFECTIVE OR HARMFUL

Prolonged delay in treatment (> 7 days)

Five retrospective studies found that medium to long term delays (4 days to 7 years) in treatment may be associated with an increase of renal scarring.

Single dose amoxicillin

One systematic review found a significant difference in cure rate between a conventional (10 day) versus a single dose of amoxicillin.

Which children with a first urinary tract infection benefit from diagnostic imaging?

UNLIKELY TO BE BENEFICIAL

Routine diagnostic imaging in all children with first urinary tract infection

We found no RCTs. One systematic review of descriptive studies found no evidence of benefit from routine diagnostic imaging of all children with a first urinary tract infection. We found indirect evidence suggesting that children at increased risk of morbidity may benefit from investigation.

What are the effects of preventive interventions?

LIKELY TO BE BENEFICIAL

Immunotherapy

One systematic review in premature and in low birth weight neonates has found that intravenous immunoglobulinsⒼ versus placebo significantly reduce the occurrence of serious infections, including urinary tract infections. One RCT found that pidotimod (an immunotherapeutic agent) versus placebo significantly reduces urinary tract infection recurrence in children.

Prophylactic antibiotics

One systematic review and an additional RCT found limited evidence that prophylactic antibiotics (co-trimoxazole, nitrofurantoin) versus placebo or no treatment reduced urinary tract infection recurrence in children. One RCT found that nitrofurantoin versus trimethoprim significantly reduced recurrence of urinary tract infection over 6 months but also found that significantly more children discontinued treatment with nitrofurantoin versus trimethoprim because of adverse effects. We found no RCTs evaluating the optimum duration of prophylactic antibiotics.

UNKNOWN EFFECTIVENESS

Surgical correction of moderate to severe bilateral vesicouretic reflux (grades III–IV) with bilateral nephropathy

One small RCT found a steady, but not significant, decline in glomerular filtration rate over 10 years with medical treatment versus surgery in children with moderate to severe bilateral vesicoureteric reflux.

UNLIKELY TO BE BENEFICIAL

Surgical correction of minor functional anomalies

We found no RCTs. One observational study suggested that children with minor anomalies do not develop renal scarring and therefore may not benefit from surgery.

Surgical correction of moderate to severe vesicoureteric reflux with adequate glomerular filtration rate (similar benefits to medical management)

One systematic review and one subsequent RCT found that, although surgery abolished reflux, there was no significant difference between surgical versus medical management (prophylactic antibiotic treatment) in preventing recurrence or complications from urinary tract infection after 6 months to 5 years in children with moderate to severe vesicoureteric reflux.

Urinary tract infection in children

DEFINITION Urinary tract infection (UTI) is defined by the presence of a pure growth of more than 10^5 colony forming units of bacteria per mL. Lower counts of bacteria may be clinically important, especially in boys and in specimens obtained by urinary catheter. Any growth of typical urinary pathogens is considered clinically important if obtained by suprapubic aspiration. In practice, three age ranges are usually considered on the basis of differential risk and different approaches to management: children under 1 year; young children (1–4, 5, or 7 years, depending on the information source); and older children (up to 12–16 years). Recurrent UTI is defined as a further infection by a new organism. Relapsing UTI is defined as a further infection with the same organism.

INCIDENCE/ PREVALENCE Boys are more susceptible before the age of 3 months; thereafter the incidence is substantially higher in girls. Estimates of the true incidence of UTI depend on rates of diagnosis and investigation. At least 8% of girls and 2% of boys will have a UTI in childhood.[1]

AETIOLOGY/ RISK FACTORS The normal urinary tract is sterile. Contamination by bowel flora may result in urinary infection if a virulent organism is involved or if the child is immunosuppressed. In neonates, infection may originate from other sources. *Escherichia coli* accounts for about three quarters of all pathogens. *Proteus* is more common in boys (about 30% of infections). Obstructive anomalies are found in 0–4% and vesicoureteric reflux in 8–40% of children being investigated for their first UTI.[2] Although vesicoureteric reflux is a major risk factor for adverse outcome, other as yet unidentified triggers may also need to be present.

PROGNOSIS After first infection, about half of girls have a further infection in the first year and three quarters within 2 years.[3] We found no figures for boys, but a review suggests that recurrences are common under 1 year of age but rare subsequently.[4] Renal scarring occurs in 5–15% of children within 1–2 years of their first UTI, although 32–70% of these scars are noted at the time of initial assessment.[2] The incidence of renal scarring rises with each episode of infection in childhood.[5] An RCT comparing oral versus intravenous antibiotics found retrospectively that new renal scarring after a first urinary tract infection was more common in children with vesicoureteric reflux than in children without reflux (logistic regression model: AR of scarring 16/107 [15%] with reflux *v* 10/165 [6%] without reflux; RR 2.47, 95% CI 1.17 to 5.24).[6] A study (287 children with severe vesicoureteral reflux treated either medically or surgically for any UTI) evaluated the risk of renal scarring with serial DMSA**G** scintigraphy over 5 years. It found that younger children (< 2 years) were at greater risk of renal scarring than older children regardless of treatment allocation for the infection (AR for deterioration in DMSA scan over 5 years 21/86 [24%] for younger children *v* 27/201 [13%] for older children; RR 1.82, 95% CI 1.09 to 3.03).[7] Renal scarring is associated with future complications: poor renal growth; recurrent adult pyelonephritis; impaired glomerular function; early hypertension; and end stage renal failure.[8–11] A combination of recurrent urinary infection, severe vesicoureteric reflux, and the presence of renal scarring at first presentation is associated with the worst prognosis.

Please refer to CD-ROM for full text and references.

Anal fissure

Search date September 2002

Marion Jonas and John Scholefield

What are the effects of treatments for chronic anal fissure?

BENEFICIAL

Internal anal sphincterotomy

One systematic review found no significant difference with internal anal sphincterotomy**G** versus anal stretch in persistence of fissures, and that both procedures healed 70–95% of fissures. It found no significant difference with open versus closed internal sphincterotomy in persistence of fissures. Three RCTs have found that sphincterotomy significantly improved fissure healing compared with topical glyceryl trinitrate (GTN) after 6 weeks to 1 year.

LIKELY TO BE BENEFICIAL

Anal advancement flap (as effective as internal anal sphincterotomy)

One RCT found no significant difference with lateral internal anal sphincterotomy versus anal advancement flap**G** in patient satisfaction or fissure healing.

Botulinum A toxin-haemagglutinin complex (botulinum A toxin-hc)

One small RCT found that botulinum A toxin-hc**G** versus placebo increased fissure healing after 2 months. One small RCT found that botulinum A toxin-hc versus topical GTN 0.2% significantly increased fissure healing rates after 2 months. Two RCTs found no significant difference with high dose versus low dose botulinum A toxin-hc in healing rates after 2–3 months.

Topical glyceral trinitrate (GTN)

Two RCTs found that topical GTN**G** versus placebo significantly increased fissure healing after 8 weeks. Two further RCTs found no significant difference in fissure healing after 4 weeks of treatment, although they may have lacked power to detect a clinically important benefit. Three RCTs have found that sphincterotomy significantly improved fissure healing compared with topical GTN after 6 weeks to 1 year. One systematic review found that botulinum A toxin-hc versus GTN significantly increased fissure healing after 2 months. One RCT found no significant difference with glyceryl trinitrate ointment versus a glyceryl trinitrate patch in fissure healing after 8 weeks. One RCT found no significant difference between topical GTN versus topical diltiazem in healing at 8 weeks.

TRADE OFF BETWEEN BENEFITS AND HARMS

Anal stretch

One systematic review found no significant difference with internal anal sphincterotomy versus anal stretch**G** in persistence of fissures, and that both procedures healed 70–95% of fissures. Anal stretch versus internal anal sphincterotomy significantly increased rates of flatus incontinence.

UNKNOWN EFFECTIVENESS

Botulinum A toxin-haemagglutinin complex (botulinum A toxin-hc) plus nitrates *New*

We found no RCTs comparing botulinum toxin A-hc plus nitrates versus placebo. One small RCT in people with anal fissures that had failed to heal with topical nitrates found that botulinum A toxin-hc plus topical isosorbide dinitrate three times daily versus botulinum A toxin-hc alone significantly increased fissure healing at 6 weeks but found no significant difference at 8 or 12 weeks.

Diltiazem

We found no placebo controlled RCTs. One small RCT found no significant difference with oral diltiazem versus topical diltiazem in fissure healing after 8 weeks. One small RCT found no significant difference in healing rate between topical diltiazem versus topical GTN at 8 weeks.

Indoramin

One RCT found no significant difference with oral indoramin versus placebo in fissure healing after 6 weeks, but may have been too smal to detect a clinically important difference.

DEFINITION Anal fissure is a split or tear in the lining of the distal anal canal. It is a very painful condition often associated with fresh blood loss from the anus and perianal itching. **Acute anal fissures** have sharply demarcated, fresh mucosal edges, and often with granulation tissue at the base. **Chronic anal fissures** margins are indurated, there is less granulation tissue, and muscle fibres of the internal anal sphincter may be seen at the base. Fissures persisting for longer than 6 weeks are generally defined as chronic.

INCIDENCE/ PREVALENCE Anal fissures are common in all age groups, but we found no evidence to quantify the incidence.

AETIOLOGY/ RISK FACTORS Low intake of dietary fibre may be a risk factor for the development of acute anal fissures.[1] People with anal fissure often have raised resting anal canal pressures with anal spasm.[2,3] Men and women are equally affected by anal fissures, and up to 11% of women develop anal fissures after childbirth.[4]

PROGNOSIS Placebo controlled studies found that 70–90% of untreated "chronic" fissures did not heal during the study.[5,6]

Please refer to CD-ROM for full text and references.

Appendicitis

Search date June 2002

John Simpson and William Speake

What are the effects of treatments?

BENEFICIAL

Adjuvant antibiotics

One systematic review and one subsequent RCT in children and adults with simple or complicated appendicitis**G** undergoing appendicectomy have found that prophylactic antibiotics versus no antibiotics significantly reduce wound infections and intra-abdominal abscesses.

LIKELY TO BE BENEFICIAL

Adjuvant antibiotics (in children with complicated appendicitis)

Subgroup analysis from one systematic review has found that antibiotics versus no antibiotics significantly reduce the number of wound infections in children with complicated appendicitis.

Laparoscopic surgery versus open surgery (in children)

One systematic review has found that laparoscopic surgery versus open surgery significantly reduces the number of wound infections and the length of hospital stay, but found no significant difference in postoperative pain, time to mobilisation, or proportion of intra-abdominal abscesses.

TRADE OFF BETWEEN BENEFITS AND HARMS

Antibiotics versus surgery

One RCT in adults with suspected appendicitis found that conservative treatment with antibiotics versus appendicectomy significantly reduced pain and morphine consumption during the period of 12 hours to 10 days after starting treatment. However, the RCT found that 35% of people following conservative management were readmitted within 1 year with acute appendicitis and subsequently had an appendicectomy.

Laparoscopic surgery versus open surgery (in adults)

One systematic review has found that laparoscopic surgery versus open surgery significantly reduces the number of wound infections, pain on the first postoperative day, the duration of hospital stay, and the time taken to return to work, but significantly increases the proportion of postoperative intra-abdominal abscesses.

UNKNOWN EFFECTIVENESS

Adjuvant antibiotics (in children with simple appendicitis)

Subgroup analysis from one systematic review has found no significant difference in the number of wound infections with antibiotics versus no antibiotics in children with simple appendicitis. One subsequent RCT in children with simple appendicitis found no significant difference with antibiotic prophylaxis versus no antibiotic prophylaxis in wound infections, but the RCT may have been too small to exclude a clinically important difference.

Open surgery versus no treatment

We found no RCTs of surgery versus no surgery.

▶

Stump inversion at open appendicectomy *New*

One RCT found no significance difference with double invagination versus simple ligation in wound infection, length of hospital stay, or intra-abdominal abscesses. Another RCT found a significantly higher incidence of wound infection with double invagination versus simple ligation but found no significant difference between groups for intra-abdominal abscesses or length of hospital stay.

DEFINITION Acute appendicitis is acute inflammation of the vermiform appendix.

INCIDENCE/PREVALENCE The incidence of acute appendicitis is falling, although the reason for this is unclear. The reported lifetime risk of appendicitis in the USA is 8.7% in males and 6.7% in females,[1] and there are about 60 000 cases reported annually in England and Wales. Appendicitis is the most common surgical emergency requiring operation.

AETIOLOGY/RISK FACTORS The aetiology of appendicitis is uncertain although various theories exist. Most relate to luminal obstruction, which prevents escape of secretions and inevitably leads to a rise in intraluminal pressure within the appendix. This can lead to subsequent mucosal ischaemia, and the stasis provides an ideal environment for bacterial overgrowth. Potential causes of the obstruction are faecoliths, often due to constipation, lymphoid hyperplasia, or caecal carcinoma.[2]

PROGNOSIS The prognosis of untreated appendicitis is unknown, although spontaneous resolution has been reported in at least 1/13 (8%) episodes.[3] The recurrence of appendicitis after conservative management,[3,4] and recurrent abdominal symptoms in certain patients,[5] suggests that chronic appendicitis and recurrent acute or subacute appendicitis may also exist.[6] The standard treatment for acute appendicitis is appendicectomy. The mortality from acute appendicitis is less than 0.3%, rising to 1.7% after perforation.[7] The most common complication of appendicectomy is wound infection occurring in between 5 and 33% of cases.[8] Intra-abdominal abscess formation occurs less frequently in 2% of appendicectomies.[9] A perforated appendix in childhood does not appear to have subsequent negative consequences on female fertility.[10]

Please refer to CD-ROM for full text and references.

Colonic diverticular disease

Search date October 2002

John Simpson and Robin Spiller

What are the effects of treatments for uncomplicated diverticular disease?

LIKELY TO BE BENEFICIAL

Rifaximin (plus glucomannan v glucomannan alone)

One RCT found that oral rifaximin**G** plus glucomannan versus glucomannan plus placebo significantly increases the proportion of people with uncomplicated diverticular disease**G** who are symptom free after 12 months of treatment.

UNKNOWN EFFECTIVENESS

Bran and ispaghula husk

Two small RCTs found no consistent effect of bran or ispaghula husk versus placebo on symptom relief after 12–16 weeks.

Elective surgery

We found no RCTs of elective open or laparoscopic colonic resection.

Lactulose

One RCT found no significant difference with lactulose versus a high fibre diet in the number of people who considered themselves to be "much improved" after 12 weeks.

Methylcellulose

One small RCT found no significant difference with methylcellulose versus placebo in mean symptom score after 3 months.

What are the effects of treatments to prevent complications of diverticular disease?

UNKNOWN EFFECTIVENESS

Increased fibre intake

We found no RCTs of advice to consume a high fibre diet or of dietary fibre supplementation.

TRADE OFF BETWEEN BENEFITS AND HARMS

Mesalazine (after an attack of acute diverticulitis) *New*

One RCT found that mesalazine reduced symptomatic recurrence compared with no treatment in people previously treated for an episode of acute diverticulitis**G**, but associated with abdominal pain.

What are the effects of treatments for acute diverticulitis?

UNKNOWN EFFECTIVENESS

Medical treatment

We found no RCTs of medical treatment versus placebo. One RCT comparing intravenous cefoxitin versus intravenous gentamicin plus intravenous clindamycin found no significant difference in rates of clinical cure. Observational studies in people with acute diverticulitis have found low mortality rates with medical treatment, but found that recurrence rates may be high.

Clin Evid Concise 2003;9:85–86.

Colonic diverticular disease

Surgery (for diverticulitis complicated by generalised peritonitis)

We found no RCTs of surgery versus no surgery or versus medical treatment. One RCT comparing acute resection versus no acute resection (involving a transverse colostomy) of the sigmoid colon found no significant difference in mortality. A second RCT comparing primary versus secondary sigmoid colonic resection found no significant difference in mortality, but found that primary resection significantly reduced rates of postoperative peritonitis and emergency reoperation.

DEFINITION Colonic diverticula are mucosal out pouchings through the large bowel wall. They are often accompanied by structural changes (elastosis of the taenia coli, muscular thickening, and mucosal folding). They are usually multiple and occur most frequently in the sigmoid colon.

INCIDENCE/ PREVALENCE In the UK, the incidence of diverticulosis🅖 increases with age; about 5% of people are affected in their fifth decade of life and about 50% by their ninth decade.[1] Diverticulosis is common in developed countries, although there is a lower prevalence of diverticulosis in Western vegetarians consuming a diet high in roughage.[2] Diverticulosis is almost unknown in rural Africa and Asia.[3]

AETIOLOGY/ RISK FACTORS There is an association between low fibre diets and diverticulosis of the colon.[3] Prospective observational studies have found that both physical activity and a high fibre diet are associated with a lower risk of developing diverticular disease.[4,5] One case control study found an association between the ingestion of non-steroidal anti-inflammatory drugs and the development of severe diverticula complications, including pericolic abscess, generalised peritonitis, bleeding, and fistula formation.[6] People in Japan, Singapore, and Thailand develop diverticula that mainly affect the right side of the colon.[7]

PROGNOSIS Symptoms will develop in 10–25% of people with diverticula at some point in their lives.[1] It is unclear why some people develop symptoms and some do not. Even after successful medical treatment of acute diverticulitis almost two thirds of people suffer recurrent pain in the lower abdomen.[8] Recurrent diverticulitis is observed in 7–42% of people with diverticular disease, and after recovery from the initial attack the calculated yearly risk of suffering a further episode is 3%.[9] About half of recurrences occur within 1 year of the initial episode and 90% occur within 5 years.[10] Complications of diverticular disease (perforation, obstruction, haemorrhage, and fistula formation) are each seen in about 5% of people with colonic diverticula when followed up for 10–30 years.[11] Intra-abdominal abscess formation may also occur.

Please refer to CD-ROM for full text and references.

Colorectal cancer

Search date April 2002

Charles Maxwell-Armstrong and John Scholefield

What are the effects of treatments?

BENEFICIAL

Adjuvant chemotherapy

Three systematic reviews and one subsequent RCT have found that adjuvant chemotherapy significantly reduces mortality compared with surgery alone in people with Dukes' A, B, and C colorectal cancer**G**. One RCT found that adding levamisole to adjuvant fluoruracil did not reduce mortality or recurrence rate compared with adjuvant fluorouracil alone in people with Dukes' A, B, and C colorectal cancer. One RCT found mortality or recurrence rates were similar with adjuvant fluorouracil plus high or low dose folinic acid in people with Dukes' A, B, and C colorectal cancer.

TRADE OFF BETWEEN BENEFITS AND HARMS

Preoperative radiotherapy

One systematic review found that preoperative radiotherapy reduced mortality and local recurrence compared with no radiotherapy, but a second systematic review and two subsequent RCTs found no significant difference with preoperative versus no radiotherapy. One RCT found that preoperative versus postoperative radiotherapy did not reduce mortality but preoperative radiotherapy significantly reduced local tumour recurrence. One systematic review has found that preoperative radiotherapy significantly increases postoperative morbidity.

UNKNOWN EFFECTIVENESS

Routine follow up

One systematic review and one additional RCT have found conflicting evidence on the effects of routine follow up.

Total mesorectal excision

We found no RCTs of total mesorectal excision**G** in people with rectal cancer. Observational studies suggest that total mesorectal excision may reduce the rate of local recurrence compared with conventional surgery.

DEFINITION Colorectal cancer is a malignant neoplasm arising from the lining (mucosa) of the large intestine (colon and rectum). Nearly two thirds of colorectal cancers occur in the rectum or sigmoid colon. Colorectal cancer may be categorised as Dukes' A, B, or C.

INCIDENCE/ PREVALENCE Colorectal cancer is the third most common malignancy in the developed world. It accounts for about 20 000 deaths each year in the UK and 60 000 deaths each year in the USA. Although the incidence of, and mortality from, colorectal cancer has changed little over the past 40 years, the incidence of the disease has fallen recently in both the UK and the USA.[1,2] In the UK, about a quarter of people with colorectal cancer present as emergencies with either intestinal obstruction or perforation.[3,4]

AETIOLOGY/ RISK FACTORS Colon cancer affects almost equal proportions of men and women, most commonly between the ages of 60 and 80 years. Rectal cancer is more common in men.[1] The pathogenesis of colorectal cancer involves genetic and environmental factors. The most important environmental factor is probably diet.[5]

Clin Evid Concise 2003;9:87–88.

Colorectal cancer

PROGNOSIS Overall 5 year survival is about 50% and has not changed over the past 40 years. Disease specific mortality in both USA and UK cancer registries is decreasing but the reasons for this are unclear.[1,2] Surgery is undertaken with curative intent in over 80% of people, but about half suffer recurrence.

Please refer to CD-ROM for full text and references.

Gastro-oesophageal reflux disease

Search date November 2002

Paul Moayyedi, Brendan Delaney, and David Foreman

What are the effects of interventions in the initial treatment of gastro-oesophageal reflux disease (GORD) associated with oesophagitis?

BENEFICIAL

H_2 receptor antagonists

One systematic review in people with oesophagitis found that H_2 receptor antagonists significantly increased healing compared with placebo, but reduced healing compared with proton pump inhibitors.

Proton pump inhibitors

One systematic review has found that proton pump inhibitors increased incidence of healing compared with placebo or H_2 receptor antagonists. One systematic review found that esomeprazole significantly increased healing at 4 weeks compared with omeprazole. RCTs have found no significant difference in clinical benefit among other proton pump inhibitors.

UNKNOWN EFFECTIVENESS

Antacids/alginates

Two RCTs found limited evidence that antacids versus placebo reduced symptom scores at 4–8 weeks, but found no significant difference in endoscopic healing. We found limited evidence on the effects of antacids versus H_2 receptor antagonists in people with oesophagitis. The first RCT found no significant difference between antacids versus cimetidine on endoscopic healing at 8 weeks. The second RCT found that antacids were significantly less effective for healing compared with ranitidine at 12 weeks.

Lifestyle advice

RCTs found insufficient evidence on the effects of lifestyle measures for the treatment of reflux oesophagitis.

LIKELY TO BE INEFFECTIVE OR HARMFUL

Motility stimulants

One RCT found that cisapride significantly increased endoscopic healing compared with placebo at 12 weeks. The use of cisapride has been restricted in some countries because of concerns about heart rhythm abnormalities. We found no RCTs of domperidone or metoclopramide.

What are the effects of interventions in the maintenance treatment of GORD associated with oasophagitis?

BENEFICIAL

Proton pump inhibitors

RCTs have found that proton pump inhibitors compared with placebo or H_2 receptor antagonists increase remission rates in people with healed reflux oesophagitis at 6–18 months. RCTs have found that proton pump inhibitors compared with placebo or H_2 receptor antagonists increase remission rates in people with healed reflux oesophagitis at 6–18 months. One systematic review has found that ▶

standard dose lansoprazole (30 mg/day) was as effective as omeprazole (20 mg/day) for maintaining healing at 12 months. However, it found that lower dose lansoprazole (15 mg/day) was less effective than higher dose lansoprazole (30 mg/day), omeprazole, or esomeprazole for maintaining healing for up to 12 months.

TRADE OFF BETWEEN BENEFITS AND HARMS

Laparoscopic surgery

One systematic review found no fully published RCTs comparing laparoscopic surgery versus medical treatment for maintenance treatment in people with GORD and oesophagitis. Two RCTs found no significant difference between open and laparasopic fundoplication for remission at 3 months to 2 years. One RCT found that complication rates were lower with laparoscopic versus open surgery.

Open surgery

RCTs have found that open Nissen fundoplication compared with medical treatment improved the endoscopic grade of oesophagitis in people with chronic GORD and oesophagitis at between 3 and 38 months. However, longer term follow up from one of those RCTs found no significant difference in endoscopic appearance between surgery and medical treatment at 10 years. Two RCTs found no significant difference between open and laparascopic fundoplication for remission at 3 months to 2 years. One RCT found that mortality was higher with open surgery compared with medical treatment. One RCT found that complication rates were higher with open versus laparoscopic surgery.

UNKNOWN EFFECTIVENESS

Antacids/alginates

We found no RCTs on the effects of antacids/alginates on long term management of reflux oesophagitis.

H_2 receptor antagonists

One RCT found no significant difference between ranitidine versus placebo for relapse of oesophagitis at 6 months in people with previously healed reflux oesophagitis. RCTs have found that H_2 receptor antagonists are less effective than proton pump inhibitors for maintaining remission up to 12 months.

Lifestyle advice

We found no RCTs on the effects of lifestyle advice on long term management of reflux oesophagitis.

LIKELY TO BE INEFFECTIVE OR HARMFUL

Motility stimulants

We found limited evidence on the effects of cisapride compared with placebo. Three RCTs found that cisapride compared with placebo improved maintenance of healing at 6–12 months. Two further RCTs found no evidence of a difference. However, they might have lacked power to detect a clinically important effect. We found no RCTs comparing other prokinetics versus placebo or each other in people with GORD and oesophagitis. The use of cisapride has been restricted in some countries because of concerns about effects on heart rhythms.

DEFINITION GORD is defined as reflux of gastroduodenal contents into the oesophagus causing symptoms that are sufficient to interfere with quality of life.[1] People with GORD often have symptoms of heartburn and acid regurgitation.[2] GORD can be classified according to results of upper gastrointestinal endoscopy. An endoscopy showing mucosal breaks in the distal oesophagus indicate the presence of oesophagitis, which is graded in severity from grade A (mucosal breaks of < 5 mm in the oesophagus) to grade D (circumferential breaks in the oesophageal mucosa).[1,3] Alternatively, severity may be graded according to the Savary–Miller classification (grade I: linear, non-confluent erosions to grade IV: severe ulceration or stricture).

INCIDENCE/ PREVALENCE Surveys from Europe and the USA suggest that 20–25% of the population have symptoms of GORD, and 7% have heartburn daily.[4,5] In primary care settings, about 25–40% of people with GORD have oesophagitis on endoscopy, but most have endoscopy negative reflux disease.[6]

AETIOLOGY/ RISK FACTORS We found no evidence of clear predictive factors for GORD. Obesity is reported to be a risk factor for GORD but epidemiological data are conflicting.[7,8] Smoking and alcohol are also thought to predispose to GORD, but observational data are limited.[8,9] It has been suggested that some foods, such as coffee, mints, dietary fat, onions, citrus fruits, or tomatoes, may predispose to GORD.[10] However, we found insufficient data on the role of these factors. We found limited evidence that drugs that relax the lower oesophageal sphincter, such as calcium channel blockers, may promote GORD.[11] Twin studies suggest that there may be a genetic predisposition to GORD.[9]

PROGNOSIS GORD is a chronic condition, with about 80% of people relapsing once medication is discontinued.[12] Many people therefore require long term medical treatment or surgery. Endoscopy negative reflux disease remains stable, with a minority of people developing oesophagitis over time.[13] However, people with severe oesophagitis may develop complications such as oesophageal stricture and Barrett's oesophagus.[1]

Please refer to CD-ROM for full text and references.

Helicobacter pylori infection

Search date April 2002

Brendan Delaney, Paul Moayyedi, and David Forman

What are the effects of treatments?

BENEFICIAL

H pylori eradication for healing and preventing recurrence of duodenal ulcer

Systematic reviews and one subsequent RCT have found that *H pylori* eradication versus acid suppression or antisecretory treatment increases the proportion of ulcers healed at 6 weeks and reduces 1 year recurrence. One systematic review has found that *H pylori* eradication versus ulcer healing alone or versus ulcer treatment plus subsequent acid suppression maintenance treatment significantly reduced the risk of rebleeding.

H pylori eradication for healing and preventing recurrence of gastric ulcer

One systematic review has found that *H pylori* eradication treatment versus antisecretory treatment significantly reduces recurrent ulcers at 1 year. Observational evidence identified by the review found that eradication treatment heals 83% of gastric ulcers within 6 weeks of starting treatment. We found no RCTs of *H pylori* eradication treatment on preventing complications of gastric ulcers.

LIKELY TO BE BENEFICIAL

H pylori eradication for non-ulcer dyspepsia

One systematic review in people with non-ulcer dyspepsia has found that *H pylori* eradication versus placebo significantly reduces dyspeptic symptoms at 3–12 months.

H pylori eradication rather than empirical acid suppression for uninvestigated dyspepsia

One RCT found that *H pylori* eradication versus placebo significantly increased relief from dyspeptic symptoms after 1 year.

H pylori eradication rather than endoscopy in people with uninvestigated dyspepsia not at risk of malignancy

One systematic review and one subsequent RCT have found no significant difference between *H pylori* testing plus eradication versus management based on initial endoscopy in dyspepsia after 1 year.

Three day quadruple regimen (*v* 1 week triple regimen)

One RCT comparing a 3 day quadruple regimen versus a 1 week triple regimen found no significant difference in *H pylori* eradication at 6 weeks, but found that people taking the 3 day quadruple regimen experienced significantly fewer days of adverse effects.

Triple regimen (*v* dual regimen)

We found no systematic review or RCTs of the effects of dual regimen**G** versus triple regimens**G** on dyspeptic symptom scores, proportion of subjects with symptoms, quality of life, or mortality. One systematic review has found that dual versus triple regimens eradicate *H pylori* from fewer people.

Two week triple regimen (*v* 1 wk triple regimen)

One systematic review found that 14 days versus 7 days treatment with proton pump inhibitor based triple regimens significantly increased *H pylori* cure rates. ▶

UNKNOWN EFFECTIVENESS

H pylori eradication for gastric B cell lymphoma

We found no RCTs of *H pylori* eradication treatment in people with B cell gastric lymphomaⒼ. Observational studies found limited evidence that 60–93% of people with localised, low grade B cell lymphoma respond to *H pylori* eradication treatment, avoiding the need for radical surgery, radiotherapy, or chemotherapy.

H pylori eradication for prevention of gastric cancer (adenocarcinoma)

We found no RCTs of *H pylori* eradication in people at risk of gastric cancer. One RCT in people with gastric atrophy or intestinal metaplasia found that *H pylori* eradication versus no eradication increased the regression of high risk lesions. We found consistent evidence from observational studies of an association between *H pylori* infection and increased risk of distal gastric adenocarcinoma of the stomach.

One triple regimen versus another

We found no systematic review or RCTs of the effects of different triple regimensⒼ on dyspeptic symptom scores, proportion of subjects with symptoms, quality of life, or mortality. One systematic review has found that clarithromycin 500 mg twice daily versus clarithromycin 250 mg twice daily plus a proton pump inhibitorⒼ plus amoxicillin significantly increases *H pylori* eradication, but found no significant difference between clarithromycin 500 mg twice daily versus clarithromycin 250 mg twice daily plus a proton pump inhibitor plus metronidazole in *H pylori* eradication rates. Another systematic review has found that a triple regimen containing ranitidine bismuthⒼ plus clarithromycin plus metronidazole versus a triple regimen containing ranitidine bismuth plus clarithromycin plus amoxicillin significantly increases eradication at 5–7 days.

UNLIKELY TO BE BENEFICIAL

H pylori eradication in people with gastro-oesophageal reflux disease

One RCT in people with gastro-oesophageal reflux disease found no significant difference with *H pylori* eradication treatment versus placebo in symptomatic relapse.

DEFINITION *H pylori* is a Gram negative flagellated spiral bacterium found in the stomach. Infection with *H pylori* is predominantly acquired in childhood. The organism is associated with lifelong chronic gastritis and may cause other gastroduodenal disorders.

INCIDENCE/ PREVALENCE *H pylori* prevalence rates vary with birth cohort and social class in the developed world. Prevalence rates in many developed countries tend to be much higher (50–80%) in those born prior to 1950 in comparison to rates (< 20%) in those born more recently. In many developing countries the infection has a high prevalence (80–95%) irrespective of the period of birth.[1] Adult prevalence is believed to represent the persistence of a historically higher rate of infection acquired in childhood, rather than increasing acquisition of infection during life.

AETIOLOGY/ RISK FACTORS Overcrowded conditions associated with childhood poverty lead to increased transmission and higher prevalence rates. Adult reinfection rates are low — less than 1% a year.[1]

Helicobacter pylori infection

PROGNOSIS *H pylori* infection is believed to be causally related to the development of duodenal and gastric ulceration, gastric B cell lymphoma, and distal gastric cancer. About 15% of people infected with *H pylori* will develop a peptic ulcer, and 1% of people will develop gastric cancer during their lifetime.[2] *H pylori* infection is not associated with a specific type of dyspeptic symptom.

Please refer to CD-ROM for full text and references.

Pancreatic cancer

Search date November 2002

Clinical Evidence freelance writers

What are the effects of surgical treatments in people with pancreatic cancer that is considered suitable for complete tumour resection? New

UNKNOWN EFFECTIVENESS

Pylorus-preserving pancreaticoduodenectomy

Four small RCTs found no evidence that pylorus-preserving surgery improved overall quality of life or 5 year survival compared with classical Whipple's procedure**G**. The studies may have lacked power to detect clinically important differences for these outcomes.

Surgery*

We found no RCTs comparing surgery versus non-surgical treatment in people with resectable pancreatic cancer. Observational data provide limited evidence that surgery may reduce mortality compared with non-surgical treatment, although results may be confounded by differences in disease stage.

*RCTs comparing surgery versus no surgery may be considered unethical in people with pancreatic cancer that is considered suitable for complete tumour resection.

What are the effects of adjuvant treatments in people with resected pancreatic cancer? New

LIKELY TO BE BENEFICIAL

Systemic fluorouracil-based chemotherapy after resection

One RCT has found that adjuvant fluorouracil-based chemotherapy improves median survival compared with no adjuvant chemotherapy in people with resected pancreatic cancer. However, it found no evidence that fluorouracil improved 5 year survival directly, although the study may have lacked power to detect a difference. A second RCT did not directly compare chemotherapy alone versus no chemotherapy.

UNKNOWN EFFECTIVENESS

Systemic gemcitabine-based chemotherapy after resection

One systematic review found insufficient evidence about effects of adjuvant gemcitabine compared with no adjuvant chemotherapy in people with resected pancreatic cancer.

DEFINITION Primary adenocarcinoma of the pancreas. Other pancreatic malignancies, such as carcinoid tumour, are not considered in the present review. Pancreatic cancer is staged according to disease spread. Stage I disease is limited to the pancreas, duodenum, bile duct, or peri-pancreatic tissues, with no distant metastases or regional lymph node involvement. Stages II–IV describe disease that has spread more extensively or become metastatic. A pancreatic tumour is considered resectable if surgery aims to completely remove all cancerous tissue. Early stage tumours in the tail or body of the pancreas are more likely to be resectable than the more common, later stage cancers in the head of the pancreas. Other factors that influence resectability include proximity of the tumour to major blood vessels and perceived peri-operative risk. Symptoms include pain, jaundice, nausea, weight loss, loss of appetite, and symptoms of gastrointestinal obstruction and diabetes. ▶

Pancreatic cancer

INCIDENCE/ PREVALENCE Pancreatic cancer is the eighth most frequent cancer in the UK.[1] Annual incidence in England and Wales is about 12/100 000. Prevalence is similar in males and females, with 5–10% presenting with resectable disease.[2] Pancreatic cancer is the fifth most common cause of cancer death in higher income countries, responsible for about 26 000 deaths each year in the US.[3]

AETIOLOGY/ RISK FACTORS Pancreatic cancer is more likely in people who smoke and have high alcohol intake. Dietary factors, such as lack of fruit and vegetables, are also reported risk factors.[4] One meta-analysis of observational studies found that people with diabetes mellitus of more than 5 years' duration are more likely to develop pancreatic cancer compared with the general population.[5] However, estimates of the magnitude of increased risk vary. Additional risk factors include pancreatitis and, in some cases, a family history.[1]

PROGNOSIS Prognosis is poor. One year survival is about 12%, with 5 year survival ranging from less than 1% in those with advanced cancer at presentation to 5% in those with early stage cancer at presentation.[1,6]

Please refer to CD-ROM for full text and references.

Stomach cancer

Search date May 2002

Peter McCulloch

What are the effects of treatments?

LIKELY TO BE BENEFICIAL

Complete surgical resection

RCTs of complete surgical excision are unlikely to be conducted. Observational studies and multivariate analysis of RCTs have found a strong association between survival and complete excision of the primary tumour.

Subtotal gastrectomy (as effective as total gastrectomy) for resectable distal tumours

RCTs in people with primary tumours in the distal stomach have found no significant difference with total(G) versus subtotal(G) gastrectomy in 5 year survival or postoperative mortality.

UNKNOWN EFFECTIVENESS

Adjuvant chemotherapy

Systematic reviews and subsequent RCTs have found limited evidence that adjuvant chemotherapy(G) versus surgery alone significantly increases survival. RCTs in people from Japan have found conflicting results on the effects of adjuvant chemotherapy versus surgery alone on survival. Two RCTs found that adjuvant chemotherapy versus surgery alone significantly increased postoperative complications. The size of any benefit remains uncertain, and many recent adjuvant chemotherapy regimens have not been evaluated fully in RCTs.

Conservative (as effective as radical) lymphadenectomy

Two RCTs comparing conservative versus radical lymphadenectomy found no significant difference in 5 year survival rates. One RCT found that radical versus conservative lymphadenectomy significantly increased perioperative mortality.

LIKELY TO BE INEFFECTIVE OR HARMFUL

Removal of adjacent organs

One RCT found no significant difference with radical gastrectomy plus splenectomy versus radical gastrectomy alone in 5 year survival rates or postoperative mortality. The RCT found that radical gastrectomy plus splenectomy versus radical gastrectomy alone significantly increased the number of postoperative infections. Retrospective analyses of observational studies and RCTs in people with stomach cancer found that removal of additional organs (spleen and distal pancreas) versus no organ removal increased morbidity and mortality.

DEFINITION Stomach cancer is usually an adenocarcinoma arising in the stomach and includes tumours arising at or just below the gastro-oesophageal junction (type II and III junctional tumours). Tumours are staged according to degree of invasion and spread(T).

INCIDENCE/ PREVALENCE The incidence of stomach cancer varies among countries and by sex (incidence per 100 000 population per year in Japanese men is about 80, Japanese women 30, British men 18, British women 10, white American men 11, white American women 7).[1] Incidence has declined dramatically in North America, Australia, and New Zealand since 1930, but the decline in Europe has been slower.[2] In the USA stomach cancer remains relatively common among particular ethnic groups, especially Japanese Americans and some ▶

Hispanic groups. The incidence of cancer of the proximal stomach and gastro-oesophageal junction is rising rapidly in most Western countries; the reasons for this are poorly understood.[3,4]

AETIOLOGY/ RISK FACTORS Distal stomach cancer is strongly associated with lifelong infection with *Helicobacter pylori* and poor dietary intake of antioxidant vitamins (A, C, and E).[5,6] In Western Europe and North America, distal stomach cancer is associated with relative socioeconomic deprivation. Proximal stomach cancer is strongly associated with smoking (OR about 4),[7] and is probably associated with gastro-oesophageal reflux, obesity, high fat intake, and medium to high socioeconomic status.

PROGNOSIS Invasive stomach cancer (stages T2–T4) is fatal without surgery. Mean survival without treatment is less than 6 months from diagnosis.[8,9] Intramucosal or submucosal cancer (stage T1) may progress slowly to invasive cancer over several years.[10] In the USA, over 50% of people recently diagnosed with stomach cancer have regional lymph node metastasis or involvement of adjacent organs. The prognosis after macroscopically and microscopically complete resection (R0) is related strongly to disease stage Ⓖ, particularly penetration of the serosa (stage T3) and lymph node involvement. Five year survival rates range from over 90% in intramucosal cancer to about 20% in people with stage T3N2 disease Ⓣ. In Japan, the 5 year survival rate for people with advanced disease is reported to be about 50%, but the explanation for the difference remains unclear. Comparisons between Japanese and Western practice are confounded by factors such as age, fitness, and disease stage, as well as by tumour location, because many Western series include gastro-oesophageal junction adenocarcinoma with a much lower survival after surgery.

Please refer to CD-ROM for full text and references.

Chronic suppurative otitis media

Search date July 2002

Jose Acuin

What are the effects of treatments in adults?

LIKELY TO BE BENEFICIAL

Topical antibiotics

RCTs found limited evidence that topical quinolone antibiotics versus placebo improved otoscopic appearances. RCTs found insufficient evidence to compare different topical antibiotics or to assess clinical effects of adding topical antibiotics to systemic antibiotics or of preoperative topical antibiotics. RCTs have found few adverse events associated with short term use. One systematic review found that topical antibiotics were significantly more effective than systemic antibiotics for reducing otoscopic features of chronic suppurative otitis media.

UNKNOWN EFFECTIVENESS

Ear cleansing

We found no RCTs of ear cleansing**G** (aural toilet) versus no treatment.

Systemic antibiotics

We found insufficient evidence about the effects of systemic antibiotics versus placebo, no treatment, or topical antiseptics. One systematic review found that systemic antibiotics were significantly less effective than topical antibiotics in reducing otoscopic features of chronic suppurative otitis media. We found no evidence about long term treatment.

Topical antibiotics plus topical steroids

One systematic review found insufficient evidence from three RCTs about effects on symptoms of topical antibiotics plus topical steroids versus placebo or topical steroids alone.

Topical antiseptics

We found no RCTs comparing topical antiseptics versus placebo or no treatment. One RCT compared topical antiseptics plus ear cleansing under microscopic control versus topical antibiotics alone or versus oral antibiotics. It found no significant difference in the rate of persistent activity on otoscopy. However, the RCT was too small to exclude a clinically important difference.

Topical steroids

We found no RCTs comparing topical steroids versus placebo or no treatment.

Tympanoplasty with or without mastoidectomy

We found no RCTs comparing tympanoplasty**G** with or without mastoidectomy**G** versus no surgery for chronic suppurative otitis media without cholesteatoma**G**.

What are the effects of treatments in children?

UNKNOWN EFFECTIVENESS

Ear cleansing

One systematic review found no significant difference in persistent otorrhoea or tympanic perforations with a simple form of ear cleansing versus no ear cleansing. However, a clinically important effect cannot be excluded.

Systemic antibiotics

RCTs found insufficient evidence about the effects of systemic antibiotics in children with chronic suppurative otitis media.

Topical antibiotics

We found no RCTs comparing topical antibiotics versus placebo.

Topical antibiotics plus topical steroids

We found insufficient evidence from small RCTs to compare topical antibiotics plus topical steroids versus cleansing only or topical antiseptics. We found no RCTs comparing topical antibiotics plus topical steroids versus either topical treatment alone.

Topical antiseptics

Two RCTs found no significant reduction in otorrhoea with topical antiseptics versus placebo after 2 weeks. One RCT found no significant difference in otorrhoea with topical antiseptics versus topical antibiotic plus steroid. However, the RCTs were too small to exclude a clinically important effect.

Topical steroids

We found no RCTs comparing topical steroids versus placebo.

Tympanoplasty with or without mastoidectomy

We found no RCTs comparing tympanoplasty with or without mastoidectomy versus no surgery for chronic suppurative otitis media without cholesteatoma.

DEFINITION Chronic suppurative otitis media is a persistent inflammation of the middle ear or mastoid cavity. Synonyms include "chronic otitis media (without effusion)", chronic mastoiditis, and chronic tympanomastoiditis. Chronic suppurative otitis media is characterised by recurrent or persistent ear discharge (otorrhoea) over 2–6 weeks through a perforation of the tympanic membrane. Typical findings also include thickened granular middle ear mucosa, mucosal polyps, and cholesteatoma within the middle ear. Chronic suppurative otitis media is differentiated from chronic otitis media with effusion, in which there is an intact tympanic membrane with fluid in the middle ear but no active infection. Chronic suppurative otitis media does not include chronic perforations of the eardrum that are dry, or only occasionally discharge, and have no signs of active infection.

INCIDENCE/ PREVALENCE The worldwide prevalence of chronic suppurative otitis media is 65–330 million people. Between 39–200 million (60%) suffer from significant hearing impairment. Otitis media has been estimated to cause 28 000 deaths and loss of over 2 million Disability Adjusted Life Years(G) in 2000,[1] 94% of which are in developing countries. Most of these deaths are likely to be due to chronic suppurative otitis media because acute otitis media is a self limiting infection(T).[2–32]

AETIOLOGY/ RISK FACTORS Chronic suppurative otitis media is assumed to be a complication of acute otitis media, but the risk factors for chronic suppurative otitis media are not clear. Frequent upper respiratory tract infections and poor socioeconomic conditions (overcrowded housing,[33] hygiene, and nutrition) may be related to the development of chronic suppurative otitis media.[34,35] Improvement of housing, hygiene, and nutrition in Maori children was associated with a halving of the prevalence of chronic suppurative otitis media between 1978 and 1987.[36] See acute otitis media, p 42.

PROGNOSIS Most children with chronic suppurative otitis media have mild to moderate hearing impairment (about 26–60 dB increase in hearing thresholds) based on surveys among children in Africa, Brazil,[37] India,[38] and Sierra Leone,[39] and among the general population in Thailand.[40] In many developing countries, chronic suppurative otitis media represents the most frequent cause of moderate hearing loss (40–60 dB).[41] Persistent hearing loss during the first 2 years of life may increase learning disabilities and poor scholastic performance.[42] Spread of infection may lead to life threatening complications such as intracranial infections and acute mastoiditis.[43] The frequency of serious complications has fallen 10-fold to about 0.24% in Thailand and 1.8% in Africa. This is believed to be associated with increased use of antibiotic treatment, tympanoplasty, and mastoidectomy.[44–46] Cholesteatoma is another serious complication that has been found in a variable proportion of people with chronic suppurative otitis media (range 0–60%).[47–50] In the West, the incidence of cholesteatoma is low (in 1993 in Finland the age standardised incidence of cholesteatoma was 8 new cases per 100 000 population/year).[51]

Please refer to CD-ROM for full text and references.

Menière's disease

Search date October 2002

Adrian James and Marc Thorp

What are the effects of treatments for acute attacks?

UNKNOWN EFFECTIVENESS

Anticholinergics; benzodiazepines; betahistine

We found no RCTs on the effects of these interventions.

What are the effects of prophylactic interventions?

UNKNOWN EFFECTIVENESS

Betahistine (for vertigo or tinnitus)

Six RCTs found insufficient evidence about the effects of betahistine versus placebo on the frequency and severity of attacks of vertigo, tinnitus, and aural fullness. Two small RCTs in people with definite or possible Menière's disease found no significant difference with betahistine versus trimetazidine in hearing or tinnitus. One of these RCTs found that betahistine versus trimetazidine significantly decreased the proportion of people reporting that the intensity of vertigo was "substantially better or cured". The other RCT found no significant difference with betahistine versus trimetazidine in vertigo intensity.

Diuretics

One small crossover RCT in people with possible Menière's disease found no significant difference with triamterene plus hydrochlorothiazide versus placebo in change in hearing over 17 weeks, and found insufficient evidence on vertigo and tinnitus

Trimetazidine

We found no RCTs comparing trimetazidine versus placebo to prevent attacks of Menière's disease. Two small RCTs in people with definite or possible Menière's disease found no significant difference with trimetazidine versus betahistine in hearing or tinnitus. One of these RCTs found that trimetazidine versus betahistine significantly increased the number of people reporting that the intensity of vertigo was "substantially better or cured". The other RCT found no significant difference with trimetazidine versus betahistine in vertigo intensity.

Dietary modification; psychological support; systemic aminoglycosides; vestibular rehabilitation

We found no RCTs on the effects of these interventions.

UNLIKELY TO BE BENEFICIAL

Betahistine (for hearing loss)

Four RCTs found no change in hearing as assessed by changes in pure tone audiograms with betahistine versus placebo. Two small RCTs in people with definite or possible Menière's disease found no significant difference with betahistine versus trimetazidine in hearing or tinnitus.

Clin Evid Concise 2003;9:102–103.

LIKELY TO BE INEFFECTIVE OR HARMFUL

Lithium

Two small crossover RCTs in people with possible Menière's disease found no difference with lithium versus placebo in vertigo, tinnitus, aural fullness, or hearing, and found that lithium was associated with tremor, thirst, and polyuria in some people.

DEFINITION Menière's disease is characterised by recurrent episodes of spontaneous rotational vertigo and sensorineural hearing loss with tinnitus and a feeling of fullness or pressure in the ear. It may be unilateral or bilateral. Acute episodes may occur in clusters of about 6–11 a year, although remission may last several months.[1] The diagnosis is made clinically.[2] It is important to distinguish Menière's disease from other types of vertigo that might occur independently with hearing loss and tinnitus, and respond differently to treatment (e.g. benign positional vertigo, acute labyrinthitis). Strict diagnostic criteria help. In this review we applied the classification of the American Academy of Otolaryngology–Head and Neck Surgery to indicate the diagnostic rigour used in RCTs**T**.

INCIDENCE/ PREVALENCE Menière's disease is most common between 40–60 years of age, although younger people can be affected.[6,7] In Europe, the incidence is about 50–200/100 000 a year. A survey of general practitioner records of 27 365 people in the UK found an incidence of 43 affected people in a 1 year period (157/100 000).[8] Diagnostic criteria were not defined in this survey. A survey of over 8 million people in Sweden found an incidence of 46/100 000 a year with diagnosis strictly based on the triad of vertigo, hearing loss, and tinnitus.[9] From smaller studies, the incidence appears lower in Uganda[10] and higher in Japan (350/100 000 based on a national survey of hospital attendances during a single wk).[7]

AETIOLOGY/ RISK FACTORS Menière's disease is associated with endolymphatic hydrops (raised endolymph pressure in the membranous labyrinth of the inner ear),[11] but a causal relationship between Menière's disease and endolymphatic hydrops remains unproven.[12] Specific disorders associated with hydrops (such as temporal bone fracture, syphilis, hypothyroidism, Cogan's syndrome**G**, and Mondini dysplasia**G**, can produce similar symptoms to Menière's disease.

PROGNOSIS Menière's disease is progressive, but fluctuates unpredictably. It is difficult to distinguish natural resolution from the effects of treatment. Significant improvement of vertigo is usually seen in the placebo arm of RCTs.[13,14] Acute attacks of vertigo often increase in frequency during the first few years after presentation then decrease in frequency in association with sustained deterioration in hearing.[6] In most people, vertiginous episodes eventually cease completely.[15] In one 20 year cohort study in 34 people, 28 (82%) people had at least moderate hearing loss (mean pure tone hearing loss > 50 dB)[1] and 16 (47%) developed bilateral disease. Symptoms other than hearing loss improve in 60–80% of people irrespective of treatment.[16]

Please refer to CD-ROM for full text and references.

Middle ear pain and trauma during air travel

Search date November 2002

Simon Janvrin

What are the effects of preventive interventions?

LIKELY TO BE BENEFICIAL

Oral decongestants in adults

One RCT in adult passengers with a history of ear pain during air travel found limited evidence that oral pseudoephedrine versus placebo significantly decreased symptoms of barotrauma during air travel. One other RCT in adult passengers with a history of ear pain during air travel found limited evidence that oral pseudoephedrine versus placebo significantly decreased ear pain and hearing loss during air travel.

UNKNOWN EFFECTIVENESS

Oral decongestants in children

One small RCT in children up to the age of 6 years found no significant difference with oral pseudoephedrine versus placebo in ear pain at take off or landing.

Topical nasal decongestants

One small RCT in adults with a history of ear pain during air travel found no significant difference with oxymetazoline nasal spray versus placebo in symptoms of barotrauma.

DEFINITION The effects of air travel on the middle ear can include ear drum pain, vertigo, hearing loss, and ear drum perforation.

INCIDENCE/ PREVALENCE The prevalence of symptoms depends on the altitude, type of aircraft, and characteristics of the passengers. One point prevalence study found that 20% of adult and 40% of child passengers had negative pressure in the middle ear after flight, and that 10% of adults and 22% of children had auroscopic evidence of damage to the ear drum.[1] We found no data on the incidence of perforation, which seems to be extremely rare in commercial passengers.

AETIOLOGY/ RISK FACTORS During aircraft descent, the pressure in the middle ear drops relative to that in the ear canal. A narrow, inflamed, or poorly functioning Eustachian tube impedes the necessary influx of air. As the pressure difference between the middle and outer ear increases, the ear drum is pulled inward.

PROGNOSIS In most people, symptoms resolve spontaneously. Experience in military aviation shows that most ear drum perforations will heal spontaneously.[2]

Please refer to CD-ROM for full text and references.

Otitis media with effusion

Search date March 2002

Ian Williamson

What are the effects of preventive interventions?

UNKNOWN EFFECTIVENESS

Change in modifiable risk factors

We found no RCTs on the effects of avoiding risk factors such as passive smoking and bottle feeding in preventing otitis media with effusion.

What are the effects of treatments?

LIKELY TO BE BENEFICIAL

Autoinflation with nasal balloon (short term benefit)

One systematic review has found that autoinflation with a nasal balloon versus no treatment significantly improves effusion. Some children may find autoinflation difficult.

TRADE OFF BETWEEN BENEFITS AND HARMS

Antimicrobial drugs (possible short term benefit)

One systematic review found limited evidence that antimicrobial drugs versus placebo or no treatment significantly increased resolution of effusion at up to 1 month. A subsequent systematic review found no significant difference with antimicrobial drugs versus placebo, but timing of the outcome was unclear. Adverse effects (mainly nausea, vomiting, and diarrhoea) were reported in 2–32% of children.

UNKNOWN EFFECTIVENESS

Topical steroids

One small RCT found limited evidence that topical steroids plus antibiotics improved short term symptoms as compared with antibiotics alone. It did not report on adverse events.

Grommets with or without adenoidectomy; other autoinflation devices; tonsillectomy

We found insufficient evidence on the effects of these interventions.

UNLIKELY TO BE BENEFICIAL

Mucolytics

One systematic review found no significant difference between 1–3 month courses of carbocisteine versus placebo or no treatment in resolution of effusion. Three small RCTs of bromhexine versus placebo found conflicting results.

LIKELY TO BE INEFFECTIVE OR HARMFUL

Antihistamines plus oral decongestants

One systematic review found no significant difference between antihistamines plus oral decongestants versus placebo in clearance of effusion after 4 weeks.

Oral steroids

One systematic review found no significant difference between oral steroids versus placebo in clearance of effusion after 2 weeks. Oral steroids may cause behavioural changes, increased appetite, and weight gain. ▶

Clin Evid Concise 2003;9:105–106.

Otitis media with effusion

DEFINITION Otitis media with effusion (OME), or "glue ear", is serous or mucoid but not mucopurulent fluid in the middle ear. Children usually present with hearing loss and speech problems. In contrast to those with acute otitis media (see topic, p 42), children with OME do not suffer from acute ear pain, fever, or malaise. Hearing loss is usually mild and often identified when parents express concern regarding their child's behaviour, school performance, or language development.

INCIDENCE/ PREVALENCE One study in the UK found that, at any time, 5% of children aged 2–4 years have persistent (at least 3 months) bilateral hearing loss associated with OME. The prevalence declines considerably beyond age 6 years.[1] About 80% of children aged 10 years have been affected by OME at some time in the past. OME is the most common reason for referral for surgery in children in the UK. Middle ear effusions also occur infrequently in adults after upper respiratory tract infection or after air travel.

AETIOLOGY/ RISK FACTORS Contributory factors include upper respiratory tract infection and narrow upper respiratory airways. Prospective case control studies have identified risk factors, including age 6 years or younger at first onset, daycare centre attendance, high number of siblings, low socioeconomic group, frequent upper respiratory tract infection, bottle feeding, and household smoking.[2,3] Most factors are associated with about twice the risk of developing OME.[4]

PROGNOSIS In 5% of preschool children, OME (identified by tympanometric screening) persists for at least 1 year.[5,6] One large cohort study (534 children) found that middle ear disease increased reported hearing difficulty at age 5 years (OR 1.44, 95% CI 1.18 to 1.76) and was associated with delayed language development in children up to age 10 years.[7]

Please refer to CD-ROM for full text and references.

Seasonal allergic rhinitis

Search date May 2002

Aziz Sheikh, Sukhmeet Panesar, and Sangeeta Dhami

What are the effects of treatments on quality of life? New

BENEFICIAL

Oral fexofenadine

Three RCTs found that fexofenadine versus placebo significantly improved quality of life and rhinitis symptoms.

LIKELY TO BE BENEFICIAL

Oral montelukast plus loratadine

One RCT comparing montelukast plus loratadine versus montelukast alone, loratadine alone, or placebo found that montelukast plus loratadine significantly improved daytime nasal symptoms score compared with other treatments. The RCT found that montelukast plus loratadine significantly improved quality of life compared with placebo.

UNKNOWN EFFECTIVENESS

Intranasal antihistamines; intranasal ipratropium bromide; oral decongestants; oral decongestants plus oral antihistamines; oral leukotriene receptor antagonists; other oral antihistamines

We found no RCTs evaluating these interventions for quality of life.

What are the effects of treatments on rhinitis symptoms? New

BENEFICIAL

Intranasal levocabastine

RCTs have found that intranasal levocabastine versus placebo significantly improves symptoms of seasonal allergic rhinitis.

Oral antihistamines (acrivastine, azatadine, brompheniramine, cetirizine, ebastine, fexofenadine, loratadine, or mizolastine)

Numerous RCTs have found that oral antihistamines (acrivastine, azatadine, brompheniramine, cetirizine, ebastine, loratadine, or mizolastine) versus placebo significantly improved rhinitis symptoms. Drowsiness, sedation, or somnolence were the most commonly reported adverse events.

Oral pseudoephedrine plus oral antihistamines

RCTs have found that pseudoephedrine plus oral antihistamines (fexofenadine, acrivastine, cetirizine, terfenadine, triprolidine, loratadine, azatadine) versus pseudoephedrine or oral antihistamine or placebo alone significantly improved overall symptoms of seasonal allergic rhinitis. The most common adverse events reported with combination treatment were headache and insomnia.

LIKELY TO BE BENEFICIAL

Oral montelukast plus loratadine

One RCT comparing montelukast plus loratadine versus montelukast alone, loratadine alone, or placebo found that montelukast plus loratadine significantly improved daytime nasal symptoms score compared with other treatments. ▶

Seasonal allergic rhinitis

TRADE OFF BETWEEN BENEFITS AND HARMS

Oral astemizole

RCTs have found that astemizole versus placebo significantly improves rhinitis symptoms but astemizole has been associated with prolongation of the QTc interval, and has the potential to induce ventricular arrhythmias.

Oral terfenadine

RCTs have found conflicting results about effectiveness of terfenadine versus placebo on rhinitis symptoms. Terfenadine is associated with risk of fatal cardiac toxicity if used in conjunction with macrolide antibiotics, oral antifungal agents, or grapefruit juice.

UNKNOWN EFFECTIVENESS

Intranasal azelastine

RCTs have found conflicting results on effectiveness of intranasal azelastine versus placebo on symptoms of seasonal allergic rhinitis. Two small RCTs found no significant difference in nasal symptoms between intranasal antihistamines (azelastine, levocabastine) and oral antihistamines (cetirizine, terfenadine)

Intranasal ipratropium bromide

We found no systematic review or published RCTs.

Other oral leukotriene receptor antagonists

We found no RCTs comparing only oral leukotriene receptor antagonists versus placebo.

DEFINITION Seasonal allergic rhinitis or "hay fever" is a symptom complex that may affect several organ systems. Symptoms will typically consist of seasonal sneezing, nasal itching, nasal blockage, and watery nasal discharge.[1] Eye symptoms (red eyes, itchy eyes, and tearing) are common. Other symptoms may include peak seasonal coughing, wheezing, and shortness of breath, oral allergy syndrome (manifesting as an itchy swollen oropharynx on eating stoned fruits), and systemic symptoms such as tiredness, fever, a pressure sensation in the head, and itchiness. Confirming the presence of pollen hypersensitivity using objective allergy tests such as skin prick tests, detection of serum specific IgE, and nasal provocation challenge testing may improve diagnostic accuracy.

INCIDENCE/ PREVALENCE Seasonal allergic rhinitis is found throughout the world. Epidemiological evidence suggests that there is considerable geographical variation its prevalence. Prevalence is found to be highest in socioeconomically developed countries where the condition may affect as much as 25% of the population.[2–4] Prevalence and severity are increasing, possibly resulting from improved living standards and reduced risk of childhood infections, which in turn lead to immune deviation of T helper cells in early life (the so called "hygiene hypothesis").[5,6] Although males and females of all ages may be affected, the peak age of onset is adolescence.[7]

AETIOLOGY/ RISK FACTORS Seasonal allergic rhinitis is an IgE mediated Type-1 hypersensitivity reaction to grass, tree, or weed pollen that is most commonly responsible for inducing clinical symptoms. Allergy to other seasonal aeroallergens such as fungal spores may also provoke symptoms. This will typically manifest as the development in or an exacerbation of symptoms during the relevant pollen season and an increase in symptom intensity when outdoors because pollen exposure is then increased. Risk factors include a personal or family history of atopy or other allergic disorders, male sex, birth order (increased risk being seen in first born), and small family size.[8,9]

PROGNOSIS Seasonal allergic rhinitis may cause considerable impairment in quality of life interfering with work, sleep, and recreational activities.[10] Other allergic problems such as asthma and eczema frequently coexist thus adding to the impact of rhinitis.[11]

Please refer to CD-ROM for full text and references.

Tinnitus

Search date October 2002

Angus Waddell and Richard Canter

What are the effects of treatments for chronic tinnitus?

LIKELY TO BE BENEFICIAL

Tricyclic antidepressants

One small RCT in people with depression and chronic tinnitus found that tricyclic antidepressants (nortriptyline) versus placebo significantly improved tinnitus related disability, audiometric tinnitus loudness matching, and symptoms of depression, but found no significant difference in tinnitus severity at 6 weeks. One small RCT in people with tinnitus but without depression found that a greater proportion of people rated themselves as improved with tricyclic antidepressants (amitriptyline) versus placebo at 6 weeks

UNKNOWN EFFECTIVENESS

Psychotherapy

One systematic review found insufficient evidence about effects of cognitive behavioural treatment, relaxation therapy, counselling, education, hypnosis, biofeedback, or stress management compared with other or no treatment in people with chronic tinnitus.

Acupuncture; antiepileptics; baclofen; benzodiazepines; cinnarizine; electromagnetic stimulation; hyperbaric oxygen; hypnosis; low power laser; nicotinamide; tinnitus masking devices; zinc

We found insufficient evidence about the effects of these interventions.

LIKELY TO BE INEFFECTIVE OR HARMFUL

Ginkgo biloba

One systematic review and one subsequent RCT found no significant difference with ginkgo biloba versus placebo in tinnitus symptoms.

Tocainide

One RCT found no significant difference with tocainide versus placebo in improving symptoms, but found evidence that tocainide caused significantly more adverse effects after 30 days' treatment.

DEFINITION Tinnitus is defined as the perception of sound, which does not arise from the external environment, from within the body (e.g. vascular sounds), or from auditory hallucinations related to mental illness. This review concerns the management of chronic tinnitus, where tinnitus is the only, or the predominant, symptom in an affected person.

INCIDENCE/ PREVALENCE Up to 18% of the general population in industrialised countries are mildly affected by chronic tinnitus, and 0.5% report tinnitus having a severe effect on their ability to lead a normal life.[1]

AETIOLOGY/ RISK FACTORS Tinnitus may occur as an isolated idiopathic symptom or in association with any type of hearing loss. Tinnitus may be a particular feature of presbyacusis, noise induced hearing loss, Menière's disease Ⓖ (see benefits under Menière's disease, p 102), or the presence of an acoustic neuroma. In people with toxicity from aspirin or quinine, tinnitus can occur while hearing thresholds remain normal. Tinnitus is also associated with depression, although it may be unclear whether the tinnitus is a manifestation of the depressive illness or a factor contributing to its development.[2]

PROGNOSIS Tinnitus may have an insidious onset, with a long delay before clinical presentation. It may persist for many years or decades, particularly when associated with a sensorineural hearing loss. In Menière's disease both the presence and intensity of tinnitus can fluctuate. Tinnitus may cause disruption of sleep patterns, an inability to concentrate, and depression.[3]

Please refer to CD-ROM for full text and references.

Tonsillitis

Search date August 2002

William McKerrow

What are the effects of tonsillectomy for severe tonsillitis in children and adults?

TRADE OFF BETWEEN BENEFITS AND HARMS

Tonsillectomy versus antibiotics in children

Two systematic reviews found limited evidence that tonsillectomy may benefit some children with severe tonsillitis, but found insufficient evidence to compare surgical versus medical treatment. One subsequent RCT in less severely affected children found that surgery significantly reduced the frequency of tonsillitis compared with medical treatment over 3 years. The modest benefit may be outweighed by morbidity associated with the generation in populations with low incidence of tonsillitis.

UNKNOWN EFFECTIVENESS

Tonsillectomy versus antibiotics in adults

We found no RCTs evaluating tonsillectomy in adults.

DEFINITION Tonsillitis is infection of the parenchyma of the palatine tonsils. The definition of severe recurrent tonsillitis is arbitrary, but recent criteria have defined tonsillitis as five or more episodes of true tonsillitis a year, symptoms for at least a year, and episodes that are disabling and prevent normal functioning.[1]

INCIDENCE/ PREVALENCE Recurrent sore throat has an incidence in general practice in the UK of 100/1000 population a year.[2] Acute tonsillitis is more common in childhood.

AETIOLOGY/ RISK FACTORS Common bacterial pathogens include β haemolytic and other streptococci. Bacteria are cultured successfully only from a minority of people with tonsillitis. The role of viruses is uncertain.

PROGNOSIS We found no good data on the natural history of tonsillitis or recurrent sore throat in children or adults. Participants in RCTs who were randomised to medical treatment (courses of antibiotics as required) have shown a tendency towards improvement over time.[3,4] Recurrent severe tonsillits results in significant morbidity, including time lost from school or work.

Please refer to CD-ROM for full text and references.

Wax in ear

Search date August 2002

George Browning

What are the effects of methods to remove symptomatic ear wax?

TRADE OFF BETWEEN BENEFITS AND HARMS

Ear syringing*

There is consensus that ear syringing is effective but we found no RCTs comparing ear syringing versus no treatment or versus alternative treatment. A survey found that 38% of 274 general practitioners reported complications in people receiving ear syringing, including otitis externa, perforation of the tympanic membrane, damage to the skin of the external canal, tinnitus, pain, and vertigo.

UNKNOWN EFFECTIVENESS

Manual removal (other than ear syringing)*

We found no RCTs about mechanical methods of removing ear wax.

Wax softeners

One small RCT, in people with impacted wax, found that active treatment (with wax softeners, sodium bicarbonate, or water) versus no treatment reduced the risk of persisting impaction after 5 days' treatment, but found no significant difference among active treatments. Three RCTs found no consistent evidence that any one type of wax softener was superior to the others. RCTs found insufficient evidence to assess the effects of wax softeners prior to syringing.

*Although many practitioners consider these to be standard treatments, we found no RCTs of these interventions.

DEFINITION Ear wax is normal and becomes a problem only if it produces deafness, pain, or other aural symptoms. Ear wax may also need to be removed if it prevents inspection of the ear drum. The term "impacted"Ⓖ is used in different ways and can merely imply the coexistence of wax obscuring the ear drum with symptoms in that ear.[1,2]

INCIDENCE/ PREVALENCE We found four surveys of the prevalence of impacted waxⓉ.[3–6] The prevalence was higher in men than in women, in the elderly than in the young, and in people with intellectual impairment.[7] One survey found that 289 Scottish general practitioners each saw an average of nine people a month requesting removal of ear wax.[1]

AETIOLOGY/ RISK FACTORS Factors that prevent the normal extrusion of wax from the ear canal (e.g. wearing a hearing aid, using cotton buds) increase the chance of ear wax accumulating.

PROGNOSIS Most ear wax emerges from the external canal spontaneously. Without impaction or adherence to the drum, there is likely to be minimal, if any, hearing loss.

Please refer to CD-ROM for full text and references.

Cardiovascular disease in diabetes

Search date April 2002

Janine Malcolm, Hilary Meggison, and Ronald Sigal

What are the effects of treatments?

BENEFICIAL

Antihypertensive treatment (better than placebo)

One RCT in people with diabetes and high blood pressure (BP 165–220/ < 95 mm Hg) found that hypertensive treatment (nitrendipine or enalapril with or without hydrochlorothiazide) versus placebo significantly reduced all cardiovascular events over a median of 2 years but found no significant reduction in overall mortality. One RCT in people aged 55–80 years with diabetic nephropathy and hypertension found no significant difference with amlodipine versus placebo and with irbesartan versus placebo or amlodipine in cardiovascular composite end points (non-fatal myocardial infarction, heart failure). One RCT in people with diabetes, hypertension, and microalbuminuria found no significant reduction in non-fatal cardiovascular events with irbesartan versus placebo. One systematic review in people aged over 50 years has found that blood pressure lowering in people with diabetes significantly reduces mortality and stroke but has no significant effect on myocardial infarction. One RCT in people with diabetes aged over 55 years with additional cardiac risk factors, previously diagnosed coronary vascular disease, or both, has found that the angiotensin converting enzyme (ACE) inhibitor ramipril versus placebo significantly reduces major cardiovascular events and overall mortality within 4.5 years. One RCT found in people with diabetes and baseline blood pressure less than 140/90 mm Hg found that intensive (target diastolic BP 10 mm Hg below baseline) versus moderate (diastolic BP 80–89 mm Hg) blood pressure lowering significantly reduces cerebral vascular accidents but found no significant difference for cardiovascular death, myocardial infarction, congestive heart failure, or all cause mortality.

Antiplatelet treatment

One RCT in men aged 40–80 years with diabetes has found that aspirin versus placebo significantly reduces the risk of first acute myocardial infarction**G** within 5 years. Another RCT in people with diabetes and prior cardiovascular disease found no significant difference with aspirin versus placebo in the risk of acute myocardial infarction or overall mortality within 5 years. Subgroup analysis in one RCT of people presenting with unstable angina or acute myocardial infarction without ST elevation found that the addition of a glycoprotein IIb/IIIa inhibitor (tirofiban) to heparin significantly reduced the risk of death or myocardial infarction at 180 days. One systematic review has found that aspirin versus placebo significantly reduces the risk of morbidity and death from cardiovascular disease within 2 years in people with diabetes and other risk factors for a cardiovascular event.

Coronary artery bypass graft (CABG) versus percutaneous transluminal coronary angioplasty (PTCA)

One large RCT in people with diabetes and multivessel coronary artery disease has found that CABG versus PTCA significantly reduces mortality or myocardial infarction within 8 years. Another RCT found a non-significant reduction in mortality with CABG versus PTCA at 4 years. A third RCT in people with diabetes and multivessel coronary artery disease found no significant difference between CABG and PTCA with stent in short term outcome (to time of discharge) but at 1 year after the procedure there was significantly greater cumulative incidence of combined death, myocardial infarction, or repeat CABG or PTCA.

Clin Evid Concise 2003;9:114–117.

Lipid regulating agents (statins and fibrates)

One systematic review found that in people with diabetes, lovastatin or gemfibrozil versus placebo did not significantly reduce non-fatal myocardial infarction and death from coronary artery disease. One RCT in people aged 35–65 years with type 2 diabetes and hyperlipidaemia found that bezafibrate versus placebo significantly reduced myocardial infarction or new ischaemic changes on electrocardiogram within 3 years. Another RCT in people with diabetes aged 40–80 years found that simvastatin versus placebo significantly decreased all cause mortalilty, non-fatal myocardial infarction, coronary heart disease death, total stroke, or any revascularisation. It found significant risk reduction in people with diabetes and previous coronary heart disease and in people with diabetes and no prior coronary heart disease. Three RCTs identified by a systematic review found that statins versus placebo significantly decreased cardiovascular event rates (person years needed to treat 120, 95% CI 61 to 4856). One RCT including people with diabetes found a borderline significant difference in relative risk of coronary heart disease death or non-fatal acute myocardial infarction with gemfibrozil versus placebo. One RCT found that in people with type 2 diabetes, dyslipidaemia and at least one coronary lesion, fenofibrate versus placebo did not significantly reduce myocardial infarction or death. One RCT found that in people aged 21–74 years with diabetes who had previously undergone CABG, aggressive versus moderate lipid lowering did not significantly reduce the 4 year life event rate relative risk for myocardial infarction or death.

Lower target blood pressures

Large RCTs including people with diabetes and hypertension have found that tighter control of blood pressure with target diastolic blood pressures of less than or equal to 80 mm Hg reduces the risk of major cardiovascular events.

Stent plus glycoprotein IIb/IIIa inhibitors in people undergoing PTCA

RCTs in people with diabetes undergoing PTCA have found that the combination of stent and a glycoprotein IIb/IIIa inhibitor (abciximab) significantly reduces restenosis rates and serious morbidity.

LIKELY TO BE BENEFICIAL

Angiotensin converting enzyme (ACE) inhibitor versus calcium channel blocker (as initial treatment in hypertension)

One systematic review in people with type 2 diabetes has found that ACE inhibitors versus calcium channel blockers as initial treatment for hypertension significantly reduce cardiovascular events.

Angiotensin II receptor antagonist versus β blocker

Subgroup analysis of one RCT in people with diabetes and left ventricular hypertrophy found that after 4 years, losartan versus atenolol significantly reduced primary cardiovascular composite outcomes (cardiovascular mortality, stroke, myocardial infarction).

Blood glucose control

RCTs found that glucose lowering with insulin, sulphonylureas, or metformin may reduce the risk of first acute myocardial infarction. One large RCT in people with a previous acute myocardial infarction found that intensive versus standard insulin treatment significantly reduced mortality at 3.4 years.

Smoking cessation

We found no RCTs on promotion of smoking cessation. Observational evidence and extrapolation from people without diabetes suggest that promotion of smoking cessation is likely to reduce cardiovascular events.

UNKNOWN EFFECTIVENESS

ACE inhibitor versus β blockers (as initial treatment in hypertension)

One RCT found that an ACE inhibitor captopril versus β blockers or diurectics significantly reduced myocardial infarction, stroke, or death. One large RCT found no significant difference with the ACE inhibitor captopril versus the β blocker atenolol in the number of cardiovascular events over about 8 years.

PTCA versus thrombolysis

One RCT in people with diabetes and prior acute myocardial infarction found that PTCA versus thrombolysis reduced the composite end point of death, reinfarction, and disabling stroke at 30 days, but the difference was not significant.

Screening for high cardiovascular risk

We found no RCTs on screening people with diabetes for cardiovascular risk.

DEFINITION **Diabetes mellitus:** See definition under glycaemic control in diabetes, p 120. **Cardiovascular disease:** Atherosclerotic disease of the heart and/or the coronary, cerebral, or peripheral vessels leading to clinical events such as acute myocardial infarction, congestive heart failure, sudden cardiac death, stroke, gangrene, and/or need for revascularisation procedures.

INCIDENCE/ PREVALENCE Diabetes mellitus is a major risk factor for cardiovascular disease. In the USA, 60–75% of people with diabetes die from cardiovascular causes.[1] The annual incidence of cardiovascular disease is increased in people with diabetes (men: RR 2–3; women: RR 3–4 adjusted for age and other cardiovascular risk factors).[2] About 45% of middle aged and older white people with diabetes have evidence of coronary artery disease, compared with about 25% of people without diabetes in the same populations.[2] In a Finnish population based cohort study (1059 people with diabetes and 1373 people without diabetes, aged 45–64 years), the 7 year risk of acute myocardial infarction was as high in adults with diabetes without previous cardiac disease (20.2/100 person years) as it was in people without diabetes with previous cardiac disease (18.8/100 person years).[3]

AETIOLOGY/ RISK FACTORS Diabetes mellitus increases the risk of cardiovascular disease. Cardiovascular risk factors in people with diabetes include conventional risk factors (age, prior cardiovascular disease, cigarette smoking, hypertension, dyslipidaemia, sedentary lifestyle, family history of premature cardiovascular disease) and more diabetes specific risk factors (elevated urinary protein excretion, poor glycaemic control). Conventional risk factors for cardiovascular disease contribute to increasing the relative risk of cardiovascular disease in people with diabetes to about the same extent as in those without diabetes (see aetiology under primary prevention, p 24). One prospective cohort study (164 women and 235 men with diabetes, mean age 65 years; 437 women and 1099 men without diabetes, mean age 61 years followed for mortality for a mean 3.7 years following acute myocardial infarction) found that more people with diabetes died compared with people without diabetes (116/399 [29%] *v* 204/1536 [13%]; RR 2.2, 95% CI 1.8 to 2.7).[4] It also found that the mortality risk after myocardial infarction associated with diabetes was higher for women than for men (adjusted HR 2.7, 95% CI 1.8 to 4.2 for women *v* 1.3, 95% CI 1 to 1.8 for men). Physical inactivity is a significant risk factor for cardiovascular events in both men and women. One cohort study of women with diabetes found that participation in little (< 1 h/wk) or no physical activity compared with physical activity for at least 7 hours a week was associated with doubling of the risk of a cardiovascular event.[5] Another cohort study (1263 men with diabetes, mean follow up 12 years) found that low baseline cardiorespiratory fitness compared with moderate or high fitness increased overall mortality (RR 2.9, 95% CI 2.1 to 3.6); and overall mortality was higher in those reporting no recreational exercise in the previous 3 months compared with those reporting any recreational physical activity in the same period (RR 1.8, 95% CI 1.3 to 2.5).[6] The absolute risk of cardiovascular disease is almost the same in women as in men with diabetes. Diabetes specific cardiovascular risk factors include the duration of diabetes during adulthood (the years of exposure to diabetes before age 20 years add little to risk of cardiovascular disease); raised blood glucose concentrations (reflected in fasting blood glucose or HbA1c**G**; and any degree of microalbuminuria (albuminuria 30–299 mg/24 h).[7] People with diabetes and microalbuminuria have a higher risk of coronary morbidity and mortality than people with normal levels of urinary albumin and a similar duration of diabetes (RR 2–3).[8,9] Clinical proteinuria increases the risk of major cardiac events in type 2 diabetes (RR 3),[10] and in type 1 diabetes (RR 9),[7,11,12] compared with individuals with the same type of diabetes having normal albumin excretion. An epidemiological analysis of people with diabetes enrolled in the Heart Outcomes Prevention Evaluation (HOPE) clinical trial (3498 people with diabetes and at least 1 other cardiovascular risk factor, age > 55 years, of whom 1140 [32%] had microalbuminuria at baseline, 5 years' follow up) found higher risk for major cardiovascular events in for those with microalbuminuria (albumin : creatinine [ACR] ratio ≥ 2.0 mg/mmol) compared with those without microalbuminuria (adjusted RR 1.97, 95% CI 1.68 to 2.31); and for all cause mortality (RR 2.15, 95% CI 1.78 to 2.60). It also found an association between ACR and the risk of major cardiovascular events (ACR 0.22 to 0.57 mg/mmol: RR 0.85, 95% CI 0.63 to 1.14; ACR 0.58 to 1.62 mg/mmol: RR 1.11, 95% CI 0.86 to 1.43; ACR 1.62 to 1.99 mg/mmol: RR 1.89, 95% CI 1.52 to 2.36).[13]

PROGNOSIS Diabetes mellitus increases the risk of mortality or serious morbidity after a coronary event (RR 1.5–3).[2,3,14,15] This excess risk is partly accounted for by increased prevalence of other cardiovascular risk factors in people with diabetes. A systematic review (search date 1998) found that, in people with diabetes admitted to hospital for acute myocardial infarction, "stress hyperglycaemia" versus lower blood glucose levels was associated with increased mortality in hospital (RR 1.7, 95% CI 1.2 to 2.4).[16] One large prospective cohort study (91 285 men aged 40–84, 5 years' follow up) found higher all-cause and coronary heart disease (CHD) mortality in men with diabetes versus men without coronary artery disease or diabetes (age adjusted RR 3.3, 95% CI 2.6 to 4.1 in men with diabetes and without coronary artery disease *v* RR 2.3%, 95% CI 2.0 to 2.6 in healthy people; RR 5.6, 95% CI 4.9 to 6.3 in men with coronary artery disease but without diabetes *v* RR 2.2%, 95% CI 2.0 to 2.4 in healthy people; RR 12.0, 95% CI 9.9 to 14.6 in men with both risk factors *v* RR 4.7%, 95% CI 4.0 to 5.4 in healthy people). Multivariate analysis did not materially alter these associations.[17] These findings support previous studies. Diabetes mellitus alone is associated with a two fold increase in risk for all cause death, a three fold increase in risk of death from CHD and, in people with pre-existing CHD, a 12-fold increase in risk of death from CHD compared with people with neither risk factor.[17]

Please refer to CD-ROM for full text and references.

Foot ulcers and amputations in diabetes

Search date May 2002

Hertzel Gerstein and Dereck Hunt

What are the effects of preventive interventions?

BENEFICIAL

Screening and referral to foot care clinics (major amputations in those at high risk)

One RCT identified by a systemic review has found that a diabetes screening and protection programme (involving referral to a foot clinic) versus usual care significantly reduces the risk of major amputation after 2 years.

UNKNOWN EFFECTIVENESS

Education (ulcer recurrence and major amputation)

We found no RCTs on the effects of education on prevention of diabetic foot complications. One non-randomised trial found that specific foot care education versus routine diabetes care education significantly decreased ulcer recurrences and major amputations after 2 years.

Therapeutic footwear (ulcer recurrence)

One RCT found no significant difference in foot ulceration rates between therapeutic footwear (fitted with cork or polyurethane inserts) versus usual footwear in people with diabetes and previous foot ulcer but without severe deformity. One non-randomised controlled trial identified by a systematic review found that therapeutic footwear (made according to the Towey guidelines) versus ordinary shoes significantly reduced the recurrence of ulceration after 1 year.

What are the effects of therapeutic interventions?

BENEFICIAL

Pressure off-loading with non-removable cast (non-infected foot ulcer healing)

One RCT identified by a systematic review has found that pressure off-loading**G** with total contact casting versus traditional dressing changes significantly improves non-infected diabetic foot ulcer healing. RCTs have found that pressure off-loading with either total contact casting or non-removable fibreglass casts versus removable casts or shoes significantly improves non-infected diabetic foot ulcer healing at 12 weeks.

LIKELY TO BE BENEFICIAL

Cultured human dermis (non-infected foot ulcer healing)

One systematic review that cultured human dermis**G** (Dermagraft, weekly for 8 wks) versus control increased ulcer healing by 21% at 12 weeks in people with non-infected diabetic foot ulcer, but the result did not reach significance.

Human skin equivalent (chronic neuropathic non-infected foot ulcer healing)

One RCT found that human skin equivalent**G** (Graftskin applied weekly for maximum of 5 wks) versus saline moistened gauze significantly increased ulcer healing rates in people with chronic neuropathic non-infected foot ulceration.

◀ Systemic hyperbaric oxygen (infected ulcers)

One RCT in people with severely infected foot ulcers found that systemic hyperbaric oxygen**G** plus usual care versus usual care alone significantly reduced the risk of foot amputation after 10 weeks. Another small, short term RCT found no significant difference in the risk of major amputation after 2 weeks.

Topical growth factors (non-infected foot ulcer healing)

One systematic review found inconsistent evidence about the effects of four different topical growth factors**G** versus placebo on ulcer healing rates in people with non-infected diabetic foot ulcers.

DEFINITION Diabetic foot ulceration is full thickness penetration of the dermis of the foot in a person with diabetes. Ulcer severity is often classified using the Wagner system. Grade 1 ulceration refers to superficial ulcers that involve the full skin thickness but not any underlying tissues. Grade 2 ulceration refers to deeper ulcers that penetrate down to ligaments and muscle, but do not involve bone or have any abscess formation. Grade 3 ulceration refers to deep ulcers that have evidence of cellulitis or abscess formation, and are often complicated with osteomyelitis. Ulcers with evidence of localised gangrene are classified as Grade 4, and Grade 5 ulcers have extensive gangrene involving the entire foot.

INCIDENCE/ PREVALENCE Studies conducted in Australia, Finland, the UK, and the USA have reported the annual incidence of foot ulcers among people with diabetes as 2.5–10.7%, and the annual incidence of amputation as 0.25–1.8%.[1–10]

AETIOLOGY/ RISK FACTORS Long term risk factors for foot complications, including foot ulcers and amputation, include duration of diabetes, poor glycaemic control, and the presence of microvascular complications (retinopathy, nephropathy, and neuropathy). However, the strongest predictors for development of foot complications are altered foot sensation and previous foot ulcer.[1–8]

PROGNOSIS People with diabetes are at risk of developing complications in the lower extremities. These include foot ulcers, infections, and vascular insufficiency. Amputation of a lower extremity is indicated if complications are severe or do not improve with appropriate treatment. As well as affecting quality of life, these complications form a large proportion of the healthcare costs of diabetes. For people with healed diabetic foot ulcers, the 5 year cumulative rate of ulcer recurrence is 66% and of amputation is 12%.[11]

Please refer to CD-ROM for full text and references.

Glycaemic control in diabetes

Search date December 2002

Clinical Evidence freelance writers

What are the effects of intensive versus conventional glycaemic control?

BENEFICIAL

Intensive control of hyperglycaemia in people aged 13–75 years

Large RCTs have found that diabetic complications increase with HbA1c concentrations above the non-diabetic range.

One systematic review and large subsequent RCTs in people with type 1 or type 2 diabetes have found strong evidence that intensive versus conventional glycaemic control significantly reduces the development and progression of microvascular and neuropathic complications. A second systematic review has found that intensive versus conventional treatment is associated with a small reduction in cardiovascular risk.

RCTs have found that intensive treatment increases the incidence of hypoglycaemia and weight gain, without adverse impact on neuropsychological function or quality of life.

The benefit of intensive treatment is limited by the complications of advanced diabetes (such as blindness, end stage renal disease, or cardiovascular disease), major comorbidity, and reduced life expectancy.

TRADE OFF BETWEEN BENEFITS AND HARMS

Intensive control of hyperglycaemia in people with frequent severe hypoglycaemia

The benefits of intensive treatment of hyperglycaemia are described above.

It is difficult to weigh the benefit of reduced complications against the harm of increased hypoglycaemia. The risk of intensive treatment is increased by a history of severe hypoglycaemia or unawareness of hypoglycaemia, advanced autonomic neuropathy or cardiovascular disease, and impaired ability to detect or treat hypoglycaemia (such as altered mental state, immobility, or lack of social support). For people likely to have limited benefit or increased risk with intensive treatment, it may be more appropriate to negotiate less intensive goals for glycaemic management that reflect the person's self determined goals of care and willingness to make lifestyle modifications.

DEFINITION Diabetes mellitus is a group of disorders characterised by hyperglycaemia (definitions vary slightly, one current US definition is fasting plasma glucose ≥ 7.0 mmol/L or ≥ 11.1 mmol/L 2 h after a 75 g oral glucose load, on 2 or more occasions). Intensive treatment is designed to achieve blood glucose values as close to the non-diabetic range as possible. The components of such treatment are education, counselling, monitoring, self management, and pharmacological treatment with insulin or oral antidiabetic agents to achieve specific glycaemic goals.

INCIDENCE/PREVALENCE Diabetes is diagnosed in about 5% of adults aged 20 years or older in the USA.[1] A further 2.7% have undiagnosed diabetes on the basis of fasting glucose. The prevalence is similar in men and women, but diabetes is more common in some ethnic groups. The prevalence in people aged 40–74 years has increased over the past decade.

AETIOLOGY/ RISK FACTORS Diabetes results from deficient insulin secretion, decreased insulin action, or both. Many processes can be involved, from autoimmune destruction of the β cells of the pancreas to incompletely understood abnormalities that result in resistance to insulin action. Genetic factors are involved in both mechanisms. In type 1 diabetes there is an absolute deficiency of insulin. In type 2 diabetes, insulin resistance and an inability of the pancreas to compensate are involved. Hyperglycaemia without clinical symptoms but sufficient to cause tissue damage can be present for many years before diagnosis.

PROGNOSIS Severe hyperglycaemia causes numerous symptoms, including polyuria, polydipsia, weight loss, and blurred vision. Acute, life threatening consequences of diabetes are hyperglycaemia with ketoacidosis or the non-ketotic hyperosmolar syndrome. There is increased susceptibility to certain infections. Long term complications of diabetes include retinopathy (with potential loss of vision), nephropathy (leading to renal failure), peripheral neuropathy (increased risk of foot ulcers, amputation, and Charcot joints), autonomic neuropathy (cardiovascular, gastrointestinal, and genitourinary dysfunction), and greatly increased risk of atheroma affecting large vessels (macrovascular complications of stroke, myocardial infarction, or peripheral vascular disease). The physical, emotional, and social impact of diabetes and the demands of intensive treatment can also create problems for people with diabetes and their families. One systematic review (search date 1998) of observational studies in people with type 2 diabetes found a positive association between increased blood glucose concentration and mortality.[2] It found no minimum threshold level.

Please refer to CD-ROM for full text and references.

Obesity

Search date May 2002

David Arterburn

What are the effects of drug treatments in adults?

TRADE OFF BETWEEN BENEFITS AND HARMS

Diethlypropion

One systematic review found that diethylpropion versus placebo promotes modest weight loss in healthy obese adults. We found two case reports describing pulmonary hypertension and psychosis with diethylpropion. We found insufficient evidence on weight regain and long term safety. Diethylpropion is no longer marketed in Europe for use in obesity because of a possible link between diethylpropion and heart and lung problems that could not be totally excluded.

Fluoxetine

One systematic review found that fluoxetine versus placebo promotes modest weight loss in healthy obese adults. We found insufficient evidence on weight regain and long term safety of fluoxetine in obesity. One systematic review of antidepressant treatment has found an association between selective serotonin reuptake inhibitors and uncommon but serious adverse events including bradycardia, bleeding, granulocytopenia, seizures, hyponatraemia, hepatotoxicity, serotonin syndrome**G**, and extrapyramidal effects**G**.

Mazindol

One systematic review found that mazindol versus placebo promotes modest weight loss in healthy obese adults. We found one case report of pulmonary hypertension diagnosed 1 year after stopping treatment with mazindol. We found one clinical evaluation of mazindol in people with stable cardiac disease that found an association between mazindol and cardiac events such as atrial fibrillation. We found insufficient evidence on weight regain and long term safety.

Orlistat

Systematic reviews and subsequent RCTs have found that in addition to a low calorie diet, orlistat versus placebo modestly increases weight loss in adults with obesity. Adverse effects such as oily spotting from the rectum, flatulence, and faecal urgency occurred in up to 27% of people taking orlistat. We found insufficient evidence on weight regain and long term safety.

Phentermine

One systematic review found that phentermine versus placebo promotes modest weight loss in healthy obese adults. We found insufficient evidence on weight regain and long term safety. Phentermine is no longer marketed in Europe for use in obesity because a link between phentermine and heart and lung problems could not be totally excluded.

Sibutramine

A systematic review and RCTs have found that sibutramine versus placebo promotes modest weight loss in healthy, obese adults with diabetes, hyperlipidaemia, and hypertension (body mass index**G** 25–40 kg/m^2). One RCT has found that sibutramine is also more effective than placebo for weight maintenance after weight loss in healthy, obese adults but weight regain occurs when sibutramine is discontinued. Sibutramine is no longer marketed in Italy for use in obesity because of concerns about severe adverse reactions including tachycardia, hypertension, arrhythmia, and two deaths due to cardiac arrests. One RCT found that sibutramine achieved greater weight loss than either orlistat or metformin.

Clin Evid Concise 2003;9:122–124.

UNKNOWN EFFECTIVENESS

Sibutramine plus orlistat

One RCT found no significant change in mean body weight over a 16 week period with sibutramine plus orlistat versus sibutramine alone.

LIKELY TO BE INEFFECTIVE OR HARMFUL

Dexfenfluramine

One systematic review found that dexfenfluramine versus placebo promotes weight loss in healthy obese adults. Dexfenfluramine has been associated with valvular heart disease and pulmonary hypertension and is no longer marketed for use in obesity.

Fenfluramine

One systematic review found that fenfluramine versus placebo promotes modest weight loss in healthy obese adults. Fenfluramine has been associated with valvular heart disease and pulmonary hypertension and is no longer marketed for use in obesity.

Fenfluramine plus phentermine

One RCT found that fenfluramine plus phentermine versus placebo promoted weight loss. The combination of fenfluramine plus phentermine has been associated with valvular heart disease and pulmonary hypertension and is no longer marketed for use in obesity.

Phenylpropanolamine

One systematic review found that phenylpropanolamine versus placebo promotes modest weight loss in healthy obese adults. One case control study found that phenylpropanolamine significantly increased the risk of haemorrhagic stroke in the first 3 days of use. Phenylpropanolamine is no longer marketed for use in obesity.

DEFINITION Obesity is a chronic condition characterised by an excess of body fat. It is most often defined by the body mass index (BMI), a mathematical formula that is highly correlated with body fat. BMI is weight in kilograms divided by height in metres squared (kg/m^2). In the USA and the UK, people with BMIs between 25–30 kg/m^2 are categorised as overweight, and those with BMI above 30 kg/m^2 are categorised as obese.[1] Nearly 5 million US adults used prescription weight loss medication in 1996–1998. A quarter of users were not overweight, suggesting that weight loss medication may be inappropriately used. This is thought to be especially the case among women, white people, and Hispanic people.[2]

INCIDENCE/ PREVALENCE Obesity has increased steadily in many countries since 1900. In the UK in 1994, it was estimated that 13% of men and 16% of women were obese.[1,3] In the past decade alone, the prevalence of obesity in the USA has increased from 12% in 1991 to 27% in 1999.[4]

AETIOLOGY/ RISK FACTORS The cause of obesity includes both genetic and environmental factors. Obesity may also be induced by drugs (e.g. high dose glucocorticoids), or be secondary to a variety of neuroendocrine disorders such as Cushing's syndrome and polycystic ovary syndrome.[5]

PROGNOSIS Obesity is a risk factor for several chronic diseases, including hypertension, dyslipidaemia, diabetes, cardiovascular disease, sleep apnoea, osteoarthritis, and some cancers.[1] The relation between increasing body weight and the mortality rate is curvilinear, with mortality rate increasing in people with low body weight. Whether this is caused by increased mortality risk at low body weights or by unintentional weight loss is not clear.[6] Results from five prospective cohort studies and 1991 national statistics suggest that the number of annual deaths attributable to obesity among US adults is about 280 000.[7]

Please refer to CD-ROM for full text and references.

Primary hypothyroidism

Search date August 2002

Lars Kristensen and Birte Nygaard

What are the effects of treatments for clinical (overt) hypothyroidism?

BENEFICIAL

Levothyroxine (L-thyroxine)

We found no RCTs on the effects of levothyroxine (L-thyroxine) versus placebo, although there is consensus that treatment is beneficial. Treating clinical (overt) hypothyroidism with thyroid hormone (levothyroxine; L-thyroxine) can induce hyperthyroidism (reduced thyroid stimulating hormone).

UNKNOWN EFFECTIVENESS

Levothyroxine (L-thyroxine) plus liothyronine

One small RCT found that levothyroxine plus liothyronine versus levothyroxine alone improved some measures of mood and physical symptoms. A second RCT found insufficient evidence about the effects of combination treatment with levothyroxine plus liothyronine.

What are the effects of treatments for subclinical hypothyroidism?

UNKNOWN EFFECTIVENESS

Levothyroxine (L-thyroxine)

One RCT in women with biochemically defined subclinical hypothyroidism found that levothyroxine (L-thyroxine) versus placebo improved dry skin, cold intolerance, and constipation at 1 year, but the RCT was small and the improvement not significant. Another RCT found no significant difference in health related quality of life scores with levothyroxine versus placebo. Two RCTs found inconclusive results about the effect of levothyroxine versus placebo on cognitive function in people with subclinical hypothyroidism. One RCT found that levothyroxine versus placebo significantly improved left ventricular function at 6 months. Treating subclinical hypothyroidism with thyroid hormone (levothyroxine; L-thyroxine) can induce hyperthyroidism (reduced thyroid stimulating hormone).

DEFINITION Hypothyroidism is characterised by low levels of blood thyroid hormone. **Clinical (overt) hypothyroidism** is diagnosed on the basis of characteristic clinical features consisting of mental slowing, depression, dementia, weight gain, constipation, dry skin, hair loss, cold intolerance, hoarse voice, irregular menstruation, infertility, muscle stiffness and pain, bradycardia, hypercholesterolaemia, combined with a raised blood level of thyroid stimulating hormone (TSH) (serum TSH levels > 12 mU/L) and a low serum thyroxine (T_4 **G**) level (serum T_4 < 60 nmol/L). **Subclinical hypothyroidism** is diagnosed when serum TSH is raised (serum TSH > 4 mU/L) but serum thyroxine (T_4) is normal and there are no symptoms or signs, or minor symptoms or signs, of thyroid dysfunction. **Primary hypothyroidism** is seen after destruction of the thyroid gland because of autoimmune causes (most), or iatrogenic causes such as ▶

surgery, radioiodine, and radiation. **Secondary hypothyroidism** is seen after damage of the pituitary gland or hypothalamic function resulting in insufficient production of TSH. Secondary hypothyroidism is not covered in this review. **Euthyroid sick syndrome** is diagnosed when levels of tri-iodothyronine (T_3 Ⓖ) and serum thyroxine (T_4) are low and TSH levels are normal or low. Euthyroid sick syndrome is not covered in this review.

INCIDENCE/ PREVALENCE Hypothyroidism is more common in women than in men (in the UK female : male ratio of 6 : 1). A study (2779 people in UK with a median age of 58 years) found that the incidence of clinical (overt) hypothyroidism was 40/10 000 women per year and 6/10 000 men per year. The prevalence was 9.3% in women and 1.3% in men.[1] In areas with high iodine intake, the incidence of hypothyroidism is higher than in areas with normal to subnormal iodine intake. In Denmark, where there is moderate iodine insufficiency, the overall incidence of hypothyroidism can be 1.4/10 000 a year increasing to 8/10 000 a year in people older than 70 years.[2] The incidence of subclinical hypothyroidism increases with age. Up to 10% of women over the age of 60 years have subclinical hypothyroidism (evaluated from data from the Netherlands and USA).[3,4]

AETIOLOGY/ RISK FACTORS Primary thyroid gland failure can occur as a result of chronic autoimmune thyroiditis, postradioactive iodine treatment, or thyroidectomy. Other causes include drug adverse effects (e.g. amiodarone and lithium), transient hypothyroidism due to silent thyroiditis, subacute thyroiditis, or postpartum thyroiditis.

PROGNOSIS Hypothyroidism results in mental slowing, depression, dementia, weight gain, constipation, dry skin, hair loss, cold intolerance, hoarse voice, irregular menstruation, infertility, muscle stiffness and pain, bradycardia, and hypercholesterolaemia. In people with subclinical hypothyroidism the risk of developing overt hypothyroidism is described in the UK Whickham Survey (25 years' follow up; for women: OR 8, 95% CI 3 to 20; for men: OR 44, 95% CI 19 to 104; if both a raised TSH and positive antithyroid antibodies present; for women: OR 38, 95% CI 22 to 65; for men: OR 173, 95% CI 81 to 370). For women, it found an annual risk of 4.3% a year (if both raised serum TSH and antithyroid antibodies were present), 2.6% a year (if raised serum TSH was present alone); the minimum number of people with raised TSH and antithyroid antibodies who would need to be treated to prevent this progression to clinical (overt) hypothyroidism in one person over 5 years is 5–8.[1] **Cardiovascular disease:** A large cross-sectional study (25 862 people with serum TSH between 5.1–10 mU/L) found significantly higher mean total cholesterol concentrations in hypothyroid people compared with euthyroid people (5.8 *v* 5.6 mmol/L).[3] Another study (124 elderly women with subclinical hypothyroidism, 931 euthyroid women) found a significantly increased risk of myocardial infarction in women with subclinical hypothyroidism (OR 2.3, 95% CI 1.3 to 4.0) and aortic atherosclerosis (OR 1.7, 95% CI 1.1 to 2.6).[4] **Mental health:** Subclinical hypothyroidism is associated with depression.[5] People with subclinical hypothyroidism may have depression that is refractory to both antidepressant drugs and thyroid hormone alone. Memory impairment, hysteria, anxiety, somatic complaint, and depressive features without depression have been described in people with subclinical hypothyroidism.[6]

Please refer to CD-ROM for full text and references.

Acute anterior uveitis

Search date October 2002

André Curi, Kimble Matos, and Carlos Pavesio

What are the effects of topical anti-inflammatory eye drops?

UNKNOWN EFFECTIVENESS

Topical non-steroidal anti-inflammatory drug eye drops

RCTs found no significant difference between non-steroidal anti-inflammatory eye drops versus placebo or steroid eye drops in clinical cure rate.

Topical steroid eye drops

One small RCT found no significant difference in symptom severity after 14 or 21 days with steroid eye drops (betamethasone phosphate/clobetasone butyrate) versus placebo. Two RCTs found no significant difference with prednisolone versus rimexolone in anterior chamber cell count (a marker of disease severity in acute anterior uveitis). One RCT found that prednisolone versus loteprednol significantly increased the proportion of people with fewer than five anterior chamber cells per examination field after 28 days. The results of another RCT comparing prednisolone versus loteprednol were difficult to interpret. RCTs found that rimexolone and loteprednol were less likely than prednisolone to be associated with increased intraocular pressures, although differences were not significant.

DEFINITION Anterior uveitis is inflammation of the uveal tract, and includes iritis and iridocyclitis. It can be classified according to its clinical course into acute or chronic anterior uveitis, or according to its clinical appearance into granulomatous or non-granulomatous anterior uveitis. Acute anterior uveitis is characterised by an extremely painful red eye, often associated with photophobia and occasionally with decreased visual acuity. Chronic anterior uveitis is defined as inflammation lasting more than 6 weeks. It is usually asymptomatic, but many people have mild symptoms during exacerbations.

INCIDENCE/ PREVALENCE Acute anterior uveitis is rare, with an annual incidence of 12/100 000 population.[1] It is particularly common in Finland (annual incidence 22.6/100 000, prevalence 68.7/100 000), probably because of genetic factors such as the high frequency of HLA-B27 in the Finnish population.[2] It has equal sex incidence, and less than 10% of cases occur before the age of 20 years.[2,3]

AETIOLOGY/ RISK FACTORS No cause is identified in 60–80% of people with acute anterior uveitis. Systemic disorders that may be associated with acute anterior uveitis include ankylosing spondylitis; Reiter's syndrome; juvenile chronic arthritis; Kawasaki syndrome; infectious uveitis; Behçet's syndrome; inflammatory bowel disease; interstitial nephritis; sarcoidosis; multiple sclerosis; Wegener's granulomatosis; Vogt-Koyanagi-Harada syndrome; and masquerade syndromes**G**. Acute anterior uveitis also occurs in association with HLA-B27 expression not linked to any systemic disease, and it may also be the manifestation of an isolated eye disorder such as Fuchs' iridocyclitis, Posner-Schlossman syndrome, or Schwartz syndrome. Acute anterior uveitis may also occur following surgery or as an adverse drug or hypersensitivity reaction.[2,3]

Acute anterior uveitis

PROGNOSIS Acute anterior uveitis is often self limiting, but we found no evidence about how often it resolves spontaneously, in which people, or over what time period. Complications include posterior synechiae**G**, cataract, glaucoma, and chronic uveitis. In a study of 154 people (232 eyes) with acute anterior uveitis (119 people HLA-B27 positive), visual acuity was better than 20/60 in 209/232 (90%) eyes, 20/60 or worse in 23/232 (10%) eyes, and worse than 20/200 (classified as legally blind) in 11/232 (5%) eyes.[4]

Please refer to CD-ROM for full text and references.

Age related macular degeneration

Search date March 2002

Jennifer Arnold and Shirley Sarks

What are the effects of preventive interventions?

UNKNOWN EFFECTIVENESS

Laser to drusen

We found insufficient evidence that drusen**G** reduction by laser**G** prevents late AMD — choroidal neovascularisation**G** or geographic atrophy**G**. One RCT and three pilot studies for RCTs found that laser treatment versus no laser treatment to eyes with high risk drusen significantly improved visual acuity after 2 years. A second RCT found that visual acuity with laser treatment versus no laser treatment only improved in a subgroup of eyes with a reduction in the number of drusen of greater than 50%. The second RCT found that, in eyes with unilateral (but not bilateral) drusen, laser versus no treatment significantly increased the short term incidence of choroidal neovascularisation.

What are the effects of treatments for exudative age related macular degeneration?

BENEFICIAL

Photodynamic treatment with verteporfin

Two RCTs in selected people with exudative age related macular degeneration (AMD) found that photodynamic treatment**G** with verteporfin**G** versus placebo significantly reduced the risk of moderate and severe visual loss after 1–2 years. In the first RCT, subgroup analysis suggests the benefit is greatest in people with predominantly classic lesions**G** on fluorescein angiography. In the second RCT, a more modest benefit was seen in the second year of treatment in people with only occult (no classic) lesions on fluorescein angiography. Both RCTs found that photodynamic treatment with verteporfin was associated with an initial loss of vision and photosensitive reactions in a small number of people.

TRADE OFF BETWEEN BENEFITS AND HARMS

Thermal laser photocoagulation

Four large RCTs in people with exudative AMD and well demarcated lesions have found that thermal laser photocoagulation versus no treatment significantly decreases the rate of severe visual loss after 2–3 years and preserves contrast sensitivity. Choroidal neovascularisation recurs within 2 years in about half of those treated. Photocoagulation may reduce visual acuity initially.

UNKNOWN EFFECTIVENESS

Proton beam and scleral plaque radiotherapy

Non-randomised pilot studies found inconclusive evidence about proton beam and scleral plaque (local) radiotherapy used in a variety of dosing and timing schedules.

Submacular surgery

We found insufficient evidence on the effects of submacular surgery**G**. Case series have found that rates of recurrent choroidal neovascularisation are high, and there is a clinically important risk of ocular complications resulting in visual loss and a need for further surgical intervention.

Clin Evid Concise 2003;9:129–130.

Age related macular degeneration

UNLIKELY TO BE BENEFICIAL

External beam radiation

One large RCT in people with exudative AMD comparing low dose external beam radiation versus placebo has found no significant difference in the number of people with moderate visual loss after 1 year. Smaller RCTs comparing both low and high dose external beam radiation versus placebo or no treatment found conflicting evidence. We found insufficient evidence on long term safety, although RCTs found no evidence of toxicity to the optic nerve or retina after 12–24 months.

LIKELY TO BE INEFFECTIVE OR HARMFUL

Subcutaneous interferon alfa-2a

One large RCT found that subcutaneous interferon alfa-2a versus placebo increased visual loss after 1 year, although the difference was not significant, and found evidence of serious ocular and systemic adverse effects.

DEFINITION AMD is the late stage of age related maculopathy**G**. AMD has two forms: atrophic (or dry) AMD, characterised by geographic atrophy; and exudative (or wet) AMD, characterised by choroidal neovascularisation, which eventually causes a disciform scar.

INCIDENCE/PREVALENCE AMD is a common cause of blind registration in industrialised countries. Atrophic AMD is more common than the more sight threatening exudative AMD, affecting about 85% of people with AMD.[1] End stage (blinding) AMD is found in about 2% of all people aged over 50 years, and incidence rises with age (0.7–1.4% of people aged 65–75 years; 11–19% of people aged > 85 years).[2–4]

AETIOLOGY/RISK FACTORS Age is the strongest risk factor. Ocular risk factors for the development of exudative AMD include the presence of soft drusen, macular pigmentary change, and choroidal neovascularisation in the other eye. Systemic risk factors include hypertension, smoking, and a family history of AMD.[5–8] Diet and exposure to ultraviolet light are suspected as aetiological agents, but this remains unproved.

PROGNOSIS AMD impairs central vision, which is required for reading, driving, face recognition, and all fine visual tasks. **Atrophic AMD** progresses slowly over many years, and time to legal blindness**G** is highly variable (usually about 5–10 years).[9,10] **Exudative AMD** is more often threatening to vision; 90% of people with severe visual loss owing to AMD have the exudative type. This condition usually manifests with a sudden worsening and distortion of central vision. A modelling exercise (derived primarily from cohort studies) found the risk of developing exudative AMD in people with bilateral soft drusen was 1–5% at 1 year and 13–18% at 3 years.[11] The observed 5 year rate in a population survey was 7%.[12] Most eyes (estimates vary from 60–90%) with exudative AMD progress to legal blindness and develop a central defect (scotoma) in the visual field.[13–16] Peripheral vision is preserved, allowing the person to be mobile and independent. The ability to read with visual aids depends on the size and density of the central scotoma and the degree to which the person retains sensitivity to contrast. Once exudative AMD has developed in one eye, the other eye is at high risk (cumulative estimated incidence: 10% at 1 year, 28% at 3 years, and 42% at 5 years).[5]

Please refer to CD-ROM for full text and references.

Bacterial conjunctivitis

Search date October 2002

Justine Smith

What are the effects of antibiotic treatment?

BENEFICIAL

Antibiotic treatment in culture positive bacterial conjunctivitis

One systematic review found that antibiotics (polymyxin–bacitracin, ciprofloxacin, or ofloxacin) versus placebo increased rates of both clinical and microbiological cure after 2–5 days. Five RCTs found no significant difference among antibiotics for clinical and microbiological cure. One RCT found that topical netilmicin increased clinical cure rate compared with topical gentamicin.

LIKELY TO BE BENEFICIAL

Empirical antibiotic treatment of suspected bacterial conjunctivitis

One systematic review found limited evidence that topical norfloxacin versus placebo significantly increased rates of clinical and microbiological improvement or cure after 5 days. RCTs comparing different topical antibiotics versus each other found no significant difference in rates of clinical or microbiological cure. One RCT found no significant difference with topical polymyxin–bacitracin ointment versus oral cefixime in the number of people who improved clinically or microbiologically.

DEFINITION Conjunctivitis is any inflammation of the conjunctiva, generally characterised by irritation, itching, foreign body sensation, and tearing or discharge. Bacterial conjunctivitis may usually be distinguished from other types of conjunctivitis by the presence of a yellow–white mucopurulent discharge. There is also usually a papillary reaction (small bumps with fibrovascular cores on the palpebral conjunctiva, appearing grossly as a fine velvety surface). Bacterial conjunctivitis is usually bilateral. This review covers only non-gonococcal bacterial conjunctivitis.

INCIDENCE/ PREVALENCE We found no good evidence on the incidence or prevalence of bacterial conjunctivitis.

AETIOLOGY/ RISK FACTORS Conjunctivitis may be infectious (caused by bacteria or viruses) or allergic. In adults, bacterial conjunctivitis is less common than viral conjunctivitis, although estimates vary widely (viral conjunctivitis has been reported to account for 8–75% of acute conjunctivitis).[1–3] *Staphylococcus* species are the most common pathogens for bacterial conjunctivitis in adults, followed by *Streptococcus pneumoniae* and *Haemophilus influenzae*.[4,5] In children, bacterial conjunctivitis is more common than viral, and is mainly caused by *H influenzae, S pneumoniae*, and *Moraxella catarrhalis*.[6,7]

PROGNOSIS Most bacterial conjunctivitis is self limiting. One systematic review (search date 2002) found clinical cure or significant improvement with placebo within 2–5 days in 64% of people (99% CI 54% to 73%).[8] Some organisms cause corneal or systemic complications, or both; otitis may develop in 25% of children with *H influenzae* conjunctivitis,[9] and systemic meningitis may complicate primary meningococcal conjunctivitis in 18% of people.[10]

Please refer to CD-ROM for full text and references.

Diabetic retinopathy

Search date September 2002

Simon Harding

What are the effects of treatments for diabetic retinopathy?

BENEFICIAL

Control of diabetes (see glycaemic control in diabetes, p 120)

Control of hypertension (see primary prevention, p 21)

Macular photocoagulation in people with clinically significant macular oedema

One large RCT has found that laser photocoagulation to the macula versus no treatment significantly reduces visual loss at 3 years in eyes with macular oedema and mild to moderate diabetic retinopathy, with some evidence of greater benefit in eyes with better vision. Subgroup analysis found that focal laser treatment**G** was significantly more effective in reducing visual loss in eyes with clinically significant macular oedema**G**, particularly in people in whom the centre of the macula was involved or imminently threatened.

Peripheral retinal laser photocoagulation in people with preproliferative (*moderate/severe non-proliferative) retinopathy and maculopathy**

RCTs in eyes with preproliferative retinopathy and maculopathy have found that peripheral retinal photocoagulation versus no treatment significantly reduces the risk of severe visual loss at 5 years.

Peripheral retinal laser photocoagulation in people with proliferative retinopathy

RCTs have found that peripheral retinal photocoagulation versus no treatment significantly reduces the risk of severe visual loss at 2–3 years. One RCT in eyes with high risk proliferative diabetic retinopathy found that low intensity versus standard intensity argon laser significantly reduced vitreous haemorrhage**G** and macular oedema. It found no significant difference between treatments for visual acuity, although it may have lacked power to detect clinically important effects.

Smoking cessation (see primary prevention, p 21)

LIKELY TO BE BENEFICIAL

Grid photocoagulation to zones of retinal thickening in people with diabetic maculopathy

One RCT found a significant improvement in visual acuity in eyes treated with grid photocoagulation versus untreated eyes at 12 months and at 24 months. Photocoagulation versus no photocoagulation reduced the risk of moderate visual loss by 50–70%.

UNKNOWN EFFECTIVENESS

Macular photocoagulation in people with maculopathy but without clinically significant macular oedema

We found no RCTs of macular photocoagulation in this population.

Peripheral retinal laser photocoagulation in people with background or preproliferative (*non-proliferative) retinopathy without maculopathy**

We found no RCTs in people with background or preproliferative**G** retinopathy without maculopathy.

Clin Evid Concise 2003;9:132–133.

What are the effects of treatments for vitreous haemorrhage?

LIKELY TO BE BENEFICIAL

Vitrectomy in people with severe vitreous haemorrhage and proliferative retinopathy (if performed early)

One RCT found that early versus deferred (for 1 year) vitrectomy**G** significantly reduced visual loss at 1, 2, and 3 years in eyes with severe vitreous haemorrhage and proliferative retinopathy. Subgroup analysis showed significant benefit in people with type 1 diabetes but not those with type 2.

UNKNOWN EFFECTIVENESS

Vitrectomy in people with maculopathy

The role of vitrectomy in this population remains unclear.

DEFINITION Diabetic retinopathy is characterised by varying degrees of microaneurysms, haemorrhages, exudates *(hard exudates)*, venous changes, new vessel formation, and retinal thickening. It can involve the peripheral retina or the macula, or both. The range of severity of retinopathy includes background**G** *(mild non-proliferative)*, preproliferative *(moderate/severe non-proliferative)*, proliferative**G**, and advanced retinopathy**G**. Involvement of the macula can be focal**G**, diffuse**G**, ischaemic**G**, or mixed.

INCIDENCE/ PREVALENCE Diabetic eye disease is the most common cause of blindness in the UK, responsible for 12% of registrable blindness in people aged 16–64 years.[1]

AETIOLOGY/ RISK FACTORS Risk factors include age, duration and control of diabetes, raised blood pressure, and raised serum lipids.[2]

PROGNOSIS Natural history studies from the 1960s found that at least half of people with proliferative diabetic retinopathy progressed to Snellen visual acuity**G** of less than 6/60 *(20/200)* within 3-5 years.[3–5] After 4 years' follow up the rate of progression to less than 6/60 *(20/200)* visual acuity in the better eye was 1.5% in people with type 1 diabetes, 2.7% in people with non-insulin requiring type 2 diabetes, and 3.2% in people with insulin requiring type 2 diabetes.[6]

*Terms in italics indicate US definitions.**T**

Please refer to CD-ROM for full text and references.

Glaucoma

Search date August 2002

Rajiv Shah and Richard Wormald

What are the effects of treatments for established primary open angle glaucoma?

LIKELY TO BE BENEFICIAL

Laser trabeculoplasty (*v* medical treatment)

One RCT found that combined treatment with initial laser trabeculoplasty**G** followed by medical treatment versus medical treatment alone significantly reduced intraocular pressure and deterioration in optic disc appearance, and significantly improved visual fields after a mean of 7 years.

Topical medical treatment

One systematic review found limited evidence that topical medical treatments versus placebo significantly reduced intraocular pressure after a minimum of 3 months, but found no significant difference between treatments in visual field loss on long term follow up. The systematic review did not clearly define the medical treatments involved.

TRADE OFF BETWEEN BENEFITS AND HARMS

Surgical trabeculectomy

RCTs found that surgical trabeculectomy**G** versus medical treatment significantly reduced both visual field loss and intraocular pressures, but found no significant difference between treatments in visual acuity after about 5 years. RCTs found that surgical trabeculectomy versus laser trabeculoplasty significantly reduced intraocular pressure, but found conflicting results for changes in visual acuity after 5–7 years. Observational studies have found limited evidence that surgical trabeculectomy may reduce central vision.

UNKNOWN EFFECTIVENESS

Laser trabeculoplasty (*v* surgical treatment)

RCTs found that laser trabeculoplasty reduced intraocular pressures significantly less than surgical trabeculectomy, but found conflicting results for changes in visual acuity after 5–7 years.

What are the effects of lowering intraocular pressure in normal tension glaucoma?

LIKELY TO BE BENEFICIAL

Medical treatments for lowering intraocular pressure in normal pressure glaucoma

One RCT found that surgical or medical treatment significantly reduced progression of visual field loss after 8 years.

TRADE OFF BETWEEN BENEFITS AND HARMS

Surgical treatments for lowering intraocular pressure in normal pressure glaucoma

One RCT found that surgical or medical treatment significantly reduced progression of visual field loss after 8 years. However, it found that surgery significantly increased cataract formation.

Clin Evid Concise 2003;9:134–136.

What are the effects of treatments for acute angle closure glaucoma?

UNKNOWN EFFECTIVENESS

Medical treatments of acute angle closure glaucoma

We found no placebo controlled RCTs, but strong consensus suggests that medical treatments are effective. One RCT found no significant difference in intraocular pressure after 2 hours with low dose pilocarpine versus an intensive pilocarpine regimen versus pilocarpine ocular inserts. We found no RCTs of other medical treatments.

Surgical treatments of acute angle closure glaucoma

We found no placebo controlled RCTs, but strong consensus suggests that surgical treatments are effective. One RCT found no significant difference with surgical iridectomy**G** versus laser iridotomy**G** in visual acuity or intraocular pressure after 3 years.

DEFINITION Glaucoma is a group of diseases that are characterised by progressive optic neuropathy. It is usually bilateral but asymmetric and may occur at any point within a wide range of intraocular pressures. All forms of glaucoma show optic nerve cupping with pallor associated with peripheral visual field loss. **Primary open angle glaucoma** occurs in people with an open drainage angle and no secondary identifiable cause. **Normal tension glaucoma** occurs in people with intraocular pressures that are consistently below 21 mm Hg (a point two standard deviations above the population mean). **Acute angle closure glaucoma** is a rapid and severe rise in intraocular pressure caused by physical obstruction of the anterior chamber drainage angle.

INCIDENCE/ PREVALENCE Glaucoma occurs in 1–2% of white people aged over 40 years, rising to 5% at 70 years. Primary open angle glaucoma accounts for two thirds of those affected, and normal tension glaucoma for about a quarter.[1,2] In black people glaucoma is more prevalent, presents at a younger age with higher intraocular pressures, is more difficult to control, and is the main irreversible cause of blindness.[1,3] Glaucoma related blindness is responsible for 8% of new blind registrations in the UK.[4]

AETIOLOGY/ RISK FACTORS The major risk factor for developing primary open angle glaucoma is raised intraocular pressure. Lesser risk factors include family history and ethnic origin. The relationship between systemic blood pressure and intraocular pressure may be an important determinant of blood flow to the optic nerve head and, as a consequence, may represent a risk factor for glaucoma.[5] Systemic hypotension, vasospasm (including Raynaud's disease and migraine), and a history of major blood loss have been reported as risk factors for normal tension glaucoma in hospital based studies. Risk factors for acute angle closure glaucoma include family history, female sex, being long sighted, and cataract. A recent systematic review failed to find any evidence supporting the theory that routine pupillary dilatation with short acting mydriatics was a risk factor for acute angle closure glaucoma.[6]

PROGNOSIS Advanced visual field loss is found in about 20% of people with primary open angle glaucoma at diagnosis,[7] and is an important risk factor for glaucoma related blindness.[8] Blindness results from gross loss of visual field or loss of central vision. Once early field defects have appeared, and where the intraocular pressure is greater than 30 mm Hg, untreated people may lose the remainder of the visual field in 3 years or less.[9] As the disease progresses, people with glaucoma have difficulty moving from a bright room to a darker room, and judging steps and kerbs. Progression of visual field loss is often slower in normal tension glaucoma. Acute angle glaucoma leads to rapid loss of vision, initially from corneal oedema and subsequently from ischaemic optic neuropathy.

Please refer to CD-ROM for full text and references.

Ocular herpes simplex

Search date December 2002

Nigel H Barker

What are the effects of treatments for epithelial ocular herpes simplex?

BENEFICIAL

Interferons

One systematic review has found that topical interferons (alpha or beta) significantly increase healing after 7 and 14 days compared with placebo. The review found no significant difference between a topical interferon and a topical antiviral agent in healing after 7 days, but found that a topical interferon significantly increased healing after 14 days. "Healing" was not clearly defined.

Topical antiviral agents

One systematic review has found that idoxuridine or vidarabine significantly increases healing after 14 days compared with placebo, and that trifluridine or aciclovir (acyclovir) significantly increases healing compared with idoxuridine after 7 and 14 days. "Healing" was not clearly defined.

UNKNOWN EFFECTIVENESS

Debridement

One systematic review has found no significant difference between debridement and placebo in the proportion of people healed, but has found that debridement plus antiviral treatment versus dibridement alone significantly increases the proportion of people healed after 7 and 14 days. "Healing" was not clearly defined.

What are the effects of treatments for stromal ocular herpes simplex?

BENEFICIAL

Topical corticosteroids

One RCT in people receiving topical antiviral treatment found that topical corticosteroids significantly reduced the progression and shortened the duration of stromal keratitis**G** compared with placebo.

UNLIKELY TO BE BENEFICIAL

Oral aciclovir

One RCT in people receiving topical corticosteroids plus antiviral treatment found no significant difference between oral aciclovir and placebo in rates of treatment failure at 16 weeks.

What are the effects of treatments to prevent recurence of epithelial or stromal ocular herpes simplex?

BENEFICIAL

Long term (1 year) oral aciclovir

One large RCT in people with at least one previous episode of epithelial**G** or stromal keratitis found that long term (1 year) oral aciclovir significantly reduced recurrence after 1 year compared with placebo.

Clin Evid Concise 2003;9:137–139.

UNLIKELY TO BE BENEFICIAL

Short term (3 wks) oral aciclovir

One RCT in people with epithelial keratitis receiving topical trifluridine found no significant difference between short term prophylaxis with oral aciclovir and placebo in the rate of stromal keratitis or iritis at 1 year.

What are the effects of treatments to prevent recurrence of ocular herpes simplex in people with corneal grafts?

LIKELY TO BE BENEFICIAL

Oral aciclovir

One small RCT found limited evidence that prophylactic use of oral aciclovir significantly reduced recurrence and improved graft survival compared with placebo.

DEFINITION Ocular herpes simplex is usually caused by herpes simplex virus type 1 (HSV-1), but also occasionally by type 2 virus (HSV-2). Ocular manifestations of HSV are varied and include blepharitis (inflammation of the eyelids), canalicular obstruction, conjunctivitis, epithelial keratitis, stromal keratitis, iritis, and retinitis. HSV infections are classified as neonatal, primary (HSV in a person with no previous viral exposure), and recurrent (previous viral exposure with humoral and cellular immunity present).

INCIDENCE/ PREVALENCE Infections with HSV are usually acquired in early life. A US study found antibodies against HSV-1 in about 50% of people with high socioeconomic status and 80% of people with low socioeconomic status by the age of 30 years.[1] However, only about 20–25% of people with HSV antibodies had any history of clinical manifestations of ocular or cutaneous herpetic disease.[2] Ocular HSV is the most common cause of corneal blindness in high income countries and the most common cause of unilateral corneal blindness in the world.[3] A 33 year study of the population of Rochester, Minnesota, found the annual incidence of new cases of ocular herpes simplex was 8.4/100 000 (95% CI 6.9 to 9.9) and the annual incidence of all episodes (new and recurrent) was 20.7/100 000 (95% CI 18.3 to 23.1).[4] The prevalence of ocular herpes was 149 cases/100 000 population (95% CI 115 to 183). Twelve per cent of people had bilateral disease.

AETIOLOGY/ RISK FACTORS Epithelial keratitis results from productive, lytic viral infection of the corneal epithelial cells. Stromal keratitis and iritis are thought to result from a combination of viral infection and compromised immune mechanisms. Observational evidence (346 people with ocular HSV in the placebo arm of an RCT) has found that the risk of developing stromal keratitis was 4% in people with no previous history of stromal keratitis (RR 1.0) as compared with 32% (RR 10, 95% CI 4.32 to 23.38) with previous stromal keratitis, but that a history of epithelial keratitis was not a risk factor for recurrent epithelial keratitis.[5] Age, sex, ethnicity, and previous experience of non-ocular HSV disease were not associated with an increased risk of recurrence.[5]

PROGNOSIS HSV epithelial keratitis tends to resolve within 1–2 weeks. In a trial of 271 people treated with topical trifluorothymidine and randomly assigned to receive either oral aciclovir or placebo, the epithelial lesion had resolved completely or was at least less than 1 mm after 1 week of treatment with placebo in 89% of people and after 2 weeks in 99% of people.[6] Stromal keratitis or iritis occurs in about 25% of people following epithelial keratitis.[7] The effects of HSV stromal keratitis include scarring, tissue destruction, neovascularisation, glaucoma, and persistent epithelial defects. Rate of recurrence of ocular herpes for people with one episode is 10% at 1 year, 23% at 2 years, and 50% at 10 years.[8] The risk of recurrent ocular HSV infection (epithelial or stromal) has also been found to increase with the number of previous episodes reported (2 or 3 previous episodes: RR 1.41, 95% CI 0.82 to 2.42; 4 or more previous episodes: RR 2.09, 95% CI 1.24 to 3.50).[5] Of corneal grafts performed in Australia over a 10 year period, 5% were in people with visual disability or with actual or impending corneal perforation following stromal ocular herpes simplex. The recurrence of HSV in a corneal graft has a major effect on graft survival. The Australian Corneal Graft Registry has found that, in corneal grafts performed for HSV keratitis, there was at least one HSV recurrence in 58% of corneal grafts that failed over a follow up period of 9 years.[9]

Please refer to CD-ROM for full text and references.

Trachoma

Search date June 2002

Denise Mabey and Nicole Fraser-Hurt

What are the effects of interventions to prevent scarring trachoma by reducing active trachoma?

LIKELY TO BE BENEFICIAL

Promotion of face washing plus topical tetracycline

One RCT from one systematic review found that promotion of face washing plus topical tetracycline versus topical tetracycline alone significantly reduced the rate of severe trachoma after 1 year, but found no significant difference in the overall rate of trachoma. However, the RCT may lack power to rule out a clinically important effect. One additional large RCT has found that face washing alone versus no intervention did not significantly reduce the proportion of children with trachoma after 3 months, although face washing plus topical tetracycline versus no intervention significantly reduced the proportion of children with trachoma after 3 months.

UNKNOWN EFFECTIVENESS

Antibiotics (*v* placebo or no treatment)

One systematic review found no evidence from moderate to poor quality RCTs that antibiotics versus placebo or no antibiotics significantly reduced active trachoma after 3 and 12 months.

Oral azithromycin (*v* topical tetracycline)

One systematic review found no evidence from six RCTs that oral azithromycin versus topical tetracycline significantly reduced active trachoma after 3 and 12 months.

What are the effects of surgical treatments for scarring trachoma (entropion and trichiasis)?

LIKELY TO BE BENEFICIAL

Bilamellar tarsal rotation (*v* other eyelid surgery) when performed by an experienced operator

We found no RCTs on the effects of surgery to improve visual acuity in people with scarring trachoma. In people with major trichiasis**G**, one RCT found limited evidence that tarsal rotation versus eversion splinting**G**, tarsal advance**G**, or tarsal grooving**G** significantly increased operative success after 2 weeks, but found no significant difference between tarsal rotation versus tarsal advance and rotation**G** in operative success after 2 weeks. A second RCT found that tarsal rotation versus tarsal advance and rotation significantly increased operative success after 25 months. In people with minor trichiasis**G**, one RCT found that tarsal rotation versus cryoablation or electrolysis significantly increased operative success after 25 months.

DEFINITION **Active trachoma** is chronic inflammation of the conjunctiva caused by infection with *Chlamydia trachomatis*. The World Health Organization classification for active trachoma defines mild trachoma (grade TF) as the presence of five or more follicles in the upper tarsal conjunctiva of at least 0.5 mm diameter. Severe trachoma (grade TI) is defined as pronounced inflammatory ▶

thickening of the upper tarsal conjunctiva that obscures more than half of the normal deep vessels. **Scarring trachoma** is caused by repeated active infection by *C trachomatis* in which the upper eyelid is shortened and distorted (entropion) and the lashes abrade the eye (trichiasis). Blindness results from corneal opacification, which is related to the degree of entropion/trichiasis.

INCIDENCE/ PREVALENCE Trachoma is the world's leading cause of preventable blindness and is second only to cataract as an overall cause of blindness.[1] Globally, active trachoma affects an estimated 150 million people, most of them children. About 5.5 million people are blind or at risk of blindness as a consequence. Trachoma is a disease of poverty regardless of geographical region. Scarring trachoma is prevalent in large regions of Africa, the Middle East, south-west Asia, the Indian subcontinent, and Aboriginal communities in Australia, and there are also small foci in Central and South America.[1] In areas where trachoma is constantly present at high prevalence, active disease is found in more than 50% of preschool children and may have a prevalence as high as 60–90%.[2] The prevalence of active trachoma decreases with increasing age, with fewer than 5% of adults showing signs of active disease.[2] Although similar rates of active disease are observed in male and female children, the later sequelae of trichiasis, entropion, and corneal opacification are more common in women than men.[2] As many as 75% of women and 50% of men over the age of 45 years may show signs of scarring disease.[3]

AETIOLOGY/ RISK FACTORS Active trachoma is associated with youth and close contact between people. Discharge from the eyes and nose may be a source of further reinfection.[4] Sharing a bedroom with someone who has active trachoma is a risk factor for infection.[5] Facial contact with flies is held to be associated with active trachoma, but studies reporting this relationship employed weak methods.[6]

PROGNOSIS Corneal damage from trachoma is caused by multiple processes. Scarring may cause an inadequate tear film, and a dry eye may be more susceptible to damage from inturned lashes, leading to corneal opacification. The prevalence of scarring and consequent blindness increases with age, and therefore is most commonly seen in older adults.[7]

Please refer to CD-ROM for full text and references.

Chickenpox

Search date November 2002

George Swingler

What are the effects of preventive interventions?

BENEFICIAL

High dose aciclovir (> 3200 mg/day) in people with HIV infection
One systematic review has found that high dose aciclovir (at least 3200 mg/day) significantly reduces the risk of clinical chickenpox and reduces all cause mortality over 22 months' treatment compared with placebo.

Live attenuated vaccine in healthy children
Two RCTs have found that live attenuated varicella vaccine significantly reduces clinical chickenpox compared with placebo, with no significant increase in adverse effects.

LIKELY TO BE BENEFICIAL

Zoster immune globulin (ZIG) versus human serum globulin in healthy children
One small RCT in children exposed to a sibling with chickenpox found that ZIG🅖 significantly reduced the number of exposed children with clinical chickenpox at 20 days compared with human immune serum globulin (ISG)🅖.

UNKNOWN EFFECTIVENESS

Aciclovir in people with immunocompromise other than HIV
We found no RCTs.

Live attenuated vaccine in immunocompromised people
We found no RCTs in immunocompromised people on the effects of live attenuated varicella vaccine.

ZIG versus varicella zoster immune globulin (VZIG) in immunocompromised children
One RCT in immunocompromised children exposed to a sibling with chickenpox found no significant difference in clinical chickenpox with ZIG compared with VZIG🅖 at 12 weeks.

What are the effects of treatments?

BENEFICIAL

Oral aciclovir in healthy people (given < 24 h of onset of the rash)
Two systematic reviews have found that oral aciclovir compared with placebo reduces the symptoms of chickenpox in healthy people.

LIKELY TO BE BENEFICIAL

Intravenous aciclovir for treatment of chickenpox in children with malignancy
Two RCTs compared intravenous aciclovir versus placebo; one large RCT has found that aciclovir significantly reduces clinical deterioration, and the other small RCT found no significant difference in clinical deterioration.

▶

Clin Evid Concise 2003;9:142–143.

UNKNOWN EFFECTIVENESS

Oral aciclovir in healthy people (given > 24 h after the onset of the rash)
One systematic review and one additional RCT have found that oral aciclovir given beyond 24 hours after onset of rash does not significantly reduce the symptoms of chickenpox compared with placebo.

DEFINITION Chickenpox is due to primary infection with varicella zoster virus (VZV). In healthy people it is usually a mild self limiting illness, characterised by low grade fever, malaise, and a generalised, itchy vesicular rash.

INCIDENCE/ PREVALENCE Chickenpox is extremely contagious. Over 90% of unvaccinated people become infected, but infection occurs at different ages in different parts of the world: over 80% of people have been infected by the age of 10 years in the USA, UK, and Japan, but by 30 years of age in India, Southeast Asia, and the West Indies.[1,2]

AETIOLOGY/ RISK FACTORS Chickenpox is caused by exposure to VZV.

PROGNOSIS **Infants and children:** In healthy children the illness is usually mild and self limiting. In the USA, death rates in infants and children aged 1–14 years with chickenpox are about 7/100 000 and 1.4/100 000, respectively.[3] In Australia, mortality in children aged between 1 and 11 years with chickenpox is about 0.5–0.6/100 000, and in infants with chickenpox it is about 1.2/100 000.[4] Bacterial skin sepsis is the most common complication in children under 5 years of age, and acute cerebellar ataxia is the most common complication in older children; both cause hospital admission in 2–3/10 000 children.[5] **Adults:** Mortality in adults is higher, at about 31/100 000.[3] Varicella pneumonia is the most common complication, causing 20–30 hospital admissions/10 000 adults.[5] Activation of latent VZV infection can cause herpes zoster, also known as shingles (see postherpetic neuralgia, p 170). **Cancer chemotherapy:** One case series (77 children with cancer and chickenpox) found that more children receiving chemotherapy versus those in remission developed progressive chickenpox with multiple organ involvement (19/60 [32%] *v* 0/17 [0%]) and more children died (4/60 [7%] *v* 0/17 [0%]).[6] **HIV infection:** One retrospective case series found that one in four children with HIV who acquired chickenpox in hospital developed pneumonia and 5% died.[7] In a retrospective cohort study (73 children with HIV and chickenpox), infection beyond 2 months occurred in 10 children (14%) and recurrent VZV infections occurred in 38 children (55%).[8] Half of recurrent infections involved generalised rashes and the other half had zoster. **Newborns:** We found no cohort studies of untreated children with perinatal exposure to chickenpox. One cohort study (281 neonates receiving VZIG because their mothers had developed a chickenpox rash during the month before or after delivery) found that 134 (48%) developed a chickenpox rash and 19 (14%) developed severe chickenpox.[9] Severe chickenpox occurred in neonates of mothers whose rash had started during the 7 days before delivery.

Please refer to CD-ROM for full text and references.

Congenital toxoplasmosis

Search date November 2002

Piero Olliaro

What are the effects of treating toxoplasmosis in pregnancy?

UNKNOWN EFFECTIVENESS

Spiramycin and other antiparasitic drugs

Two systematic reviews of cohort studies in women who seroconvert during pregnancy found insufficient evidence on the effects of current antiparasitic treatment compared with no treatment on mother or baby.

DEFINITION Toxoplasmosis is caused by the parasite *Toxoplasma gondii*. Infection is asymptomatic or unremarkable in immunocompetent individuals, but leads to a lifelong antibody response. During pregnancy, toxoplasmosis can be transmitted across the placenta and may cause intrauterine death, neonatal growth retardation, mental retardation, ocular defects, and blindness in later life. Congenital toxoplasmosis (confirmed infection of the fetus or newborn) can present at birth, either as subclinical disease, which may evolve with neurological or ophthalmological disease later in life, or as a disease of varying severity, ranging from mild ocular damage to severe mental retardation.

INCIDENCE/ PREVALENCE Reported rates of toxoplasma seroprevalence vary across and within countries, as well as over time. The risk of primary infection is highest in young people, including young women during pregnancy. We found no cohort studies describing annual seroconversion rates in women of childbearing age nor incidence of primary infection. One systematic review (search date 1996) identified 15 studies that reported rates of seroconversion in non-immune pregnant women ranging from 2.4–16/1000 in Europe and from 2–6/1000 in the USA.[1] France began screening for congenital toxoplasmosis in 1978, and during the period 1980–1995 the seroconversion rate during pregnancy in non-immune women was 4–5/1000.[2]

AETIOLOGY/ RISK FACTORS Toxoplasma infection is usually acquired by ingesting either sporocysts (from unwashed fruit or vegetables contaminated by cat faeces) or tissue cysts (from raw or undercooked meat). The risk of contracting toxoplasma infection varies with eating habits, contact with cats and other pets, and occupational exposure.

PROGNOSIS One systematic review of studies conducted from 1983–1996 found no population based prospective studies of the natural history of toxoplasma infection during pregnancy.[1] One systematic review (search date 1997) reported nine controlled, non-randomised studies, and found that untreated toxoplasmosis acquired during pregnancy was associated with infection rates in children of between 10–100%.[3] We found two European studies that correlated gestation at time of seroconversion with risk of transmission and severity of disease at birth.[4,5] Risk of transmission increased with gestational age at maternal seroconversion, reaching 70–90% for infections acquired after 30 weeks' gestation. In contrast, the risk of the infected infant developing clinical disease was highest when infection occurred early in pregnancy. The highest risk of early signs of disease (including chorioretinitis and hydrocephaly) was about 10%, and occurred with infection between 24 and 30 weeks' gestation.[5] Infants with untreated congenital toxoplasmosis and generalised neurological ▶

abnormalities at birth develop mental retardation, growth retardation, blindness or visual defects, seizures, and spasticity. Children with untreated subclinical infection at birth may have cognitive and motor deficits and visual defects or blindness, which may go undiagnosed for many years. One case control study (845 school children in Brazil) found mental retardation and retinochoroiditis to be significantly associated with positive toxoplasma serology (population attributable risk 6–9%).[6]

Please refer to CD-ROM for full text and references.

Diarrhoea in adults

Search date October 2002

Guy de Bruyn

What are the effects of treatments?

LIKELY TO BE BENEFICIAL

Amino acid oral rehydration solution (ORS) (*v* standard ORS)

One small RCT has found that amino acid ORSⒼ versus standard ORS reduces the total volume and duration of diarrhoea.

Rice based ORS (*v* standard ORS)

One systematic review has found that rice based ORS versus standard ORS significantly reduced the 24 hour stool volume.

UNKNOWN EFFECTIVENESS

Bicarbonate ORS (*v* standard ORS)

Two RCTs found no significant difference in the duration or volume of diarrhoea with bicarbonate ORS versus standard ORS. One RCT found no significant difference in total stool output or duration of diarrhoea with bicarbonate ORS versus an otherwise identical ORS in which the bicarbonate was replaced with chloride.

Reduced osmolarity ORS (*v* standard ORS)

Three RCTs comparing reduced osmolarity ORS versus standard IRS found a small and inconsistent effect on total stool volume and duration of diarrhoea.

TRADE OFF BETWEEN BENEFITS AND HARMS

Antimotility agents

RCTs have found that loperamide hydrochloride and loperamide oxide versus placebo significantly reduce the time to relief of symptoms, but frequently cause constipation. We found insufficient evidence about the effects of other antimotility agents.

Empirical antibiotic treatment in community acquired diarrhoea

RCTs have found that ciprofloxacin versus placebo reduces the duration of community acquired diarrhoea by 1–2 daysⓉ. RCTs found limited evidence that other antibiotics, except for lomefloxacin, reduced duration of diarrhoea compared with placebo. Adverse events varied by agent.

Empirical antibiotic treatment in travellers' diarrhoea

One systematic review and one additional RCT have found that empirical use of antibiotics versus placebo significantly increases cure rate at 3 and 6 days. Antibiotic treatment is associated with prolonged presence of bacterial pathogens in the stool and development of resistant strains.

DEFINITION Diarrhoea is watery or liquid stools, usually with an increase in stool weight above 200 g daily and an increase in daily stool frequency. This chapter covers empirical treatment of suspected infectious diarrhoea in adults.

INCIDENCE/ PREVALENCE An estimated 4000 million cases of diarrhoea occurred worldwide in 1996, resulting in 2.5 million deaths.[1] In the USA, the estimated incidence for infectious intestinal disease is 0.44 episodes per person a year (episode per person every 2.3 years), resulting in about one consultation with a doctor per person every 28 years.[2] A recent community study in the UK reported an incidence of 19 cases per 100 person years, of which 3.3 cases per 100 ▶

person years resulted in consultation with a general practitioner.[3] The epidemiology of travellers' diarrhoea (in people who have crossed a national boundary) is not well understood. Incidence is higher in travellers visiting developing countries, but it varies widely by location and season of travel.[4]

AETIOLOGY/ RISK FACTORS The cause of diarrhoea depends on geographic location, standards of food hygiene, sanitation, water supply, and season. Commonly identified causes of sporadic diarrhoea in adults in developed countries include *Campylobacter*, *Salmonella*, *Shigella*, *Escherichia coli*, *Yersinia*, protozoa, and viruses. No pathogens are identified in more than half of people with diarrhoea. In returning travellers, about 50% of episodes are caused by bacteria such as enterotoxigenic *E coli*, *Salmonella*, *Shigella*, *Campylobacter*, *Vibrio*, enteroadherent *E coli*, *Yersinia*, and *Aeromonas*.[5]

PROGNOSIS In developing countries, diarrhoea is reported to cause more deaths in children under 5 years of age than any other condition.[1] Few studies have examined which factors predict poor outcome in adults. In developed countries, death from infectious diarrhoea is rare, although serious complications, including severe dehydration and renal failure, can occur and may necessitate admission to hospital. Elderly people and those in long term care have an increased risk of death.[6]

Please refer to CD-ROM for full text and references.

HIV infection

Search date March 2002

David Wilkinson and Clinical Evidence freelance writers

What are the effects of preventive interventions?

BENEFICIAL

Early diagnosis and treatment of sexually transmitted diseases (STDs)

One RCT has found that early diagnosis and treatment of STDs significantly reduces the risk of acquiring HIV infection over 2 years.

LIKELY TO BE BENEFICIAL

Postexposure prophylaxis in healthcare workers

One case control study in people exposed to HIV found limited evidence suggesting that postexposure prophylaxis with zidovudine may reduce the risk of HIV infection over 6 months. Evidence from other settings suggests that combining several antiretroviral drugs is likely to be more effective than zidovudine alone.

UNKNOWN EFFECTIVENESS

Presumptive mass treatment of STDs

One RCT found no significant difference with presumptive, mass treatment for STDs versus no treatment in the incidence of HIV over 20 months.

What are the effects of treatments?

BENEFICIAL

Three drug antiretroviral regimens

Two RCTs have found that using a protease inhibitor plus two nucleoside analogue drugs versus two nucleoside analogue drugs alone halves the risk of new AIDS diseases or death over about 1 year. Both RCTs found that the risk of serious adverse effects was similar with three versus two drug regimens. Triple therapy is likely to reduce the risk of drug resistance compared with double therapy.

TRADE OFF BETWEEN BENEFITS AND HARMS

Two drug antiretroviral regimens/single drug antiretroviral regimens

Large RCTs, with follow up of 1–3 years, have found that two drug regimens (zidovudine plus another nucleoside analogue or protease inhibitor drug) versus zidovudine alone significantly reduce the risk of new AIDS defining illnesses and death. Adverse events were common in all treatment groups.

UNKNOWN EFFECTIVENESS

Early versus delayed antiretroviral treatment

We found no RCTs evaluating delayed versus early treatment with two or three drug regimens. RCTs, in people with asymptomatic HIV, conducted when zidovudine was the only drug available found no significant difference between immediate versus delayed treatment in survival at 1 year.

DEFINITION HIV infection refers to infection with the human immunodeficiency virus type 1 or type 2. Clinically, this is characterised by a variable period (average around 8–10 years) of asymptomatic infection, followed by repeated episodes of illness of varying and increasing severity as immune function deteriorates. The type of illness varies greatly by country, availability of specific treatment for HIV, and prophylaxis for opportunistic infections. ▶

Clin Evid Concise 2003;9:148–149.

INCIDENCE/ PREVALENCE Worldwide estimates suggest that, by December 1999, about 50 million people had been infected with HIV, about 16 million people had died as a result, and about 16 000 new HIV infections were occurring each day.[1] About 90% of HIV infections occur in the developing world.[1] Occupationally acquired HIV infection in healthcare workers has been documented in 95 definite and 191 possible cases, although this is likely to be an underestimate.[2]

AETIOLOGY/ RISK FACTORS The major risk factor for transmission of HIV is unprotected heterosexual or homosexual intercourse. Other risk factors include needlestick injury, sharing drug injecting equipment, and blood transfusion. An HIV infected woman may also transmit the virus to her baby. This has been reported in 15–30% of pregnant women with HIV infection. Not everyone who is exposed to HIV will become infected, although risk increases if exposure is repeated, at high dose, or through blood. There is at least a two to five times greater risk of HIV infection among people with sexually transmitted diseases.[3]

PROGNOSIS Without treatment, about half of people infected with HIV will become ill and die from AIDS over about 10 years.

Please refer to CD-ROM for full text and references.

HIV: mother to child transmission

Search date September 2002

Jimmy Volmink

What are the effects of measures to reduce mother to child transmission of HIV?

BENEFICIAL

Antiretroviral drugs

One systematic review has found that zidovudine versus placebo significantly reduces the incidence of HIV in infants. One RCT has found that the longer versus shorter courses of zidovudine (long–long versus short–short courses) given to mother and infant significantly reduces the incidence of HIV in infants. One RCT has found that nevirapine versus zidovudine given to the mother and to her newborn significantly reduces the risk of HIV transmission. One RCT found no additional advantage in giving nevirapine to the mother and baby when transmission rates are already reduced by mothers receiving standard antiretroviral treatment. One RCT has found that zidovudine plus lamivudine versus placebo given in the antenatal and intrapartum period, or in the intrapartum and postpartum period, significantly reduces the risk of transmission of HIV.

LIKELY TO BE BENEFICIAL

Elective caesarean section

One RCT found limited evidence that elective caesarean section versus vaginal delivery in women with HIV reduced the incidence of HIV in infants at 18 months.

TRADE OFF BETWEEN BENEFITS AND HARMS

Avoiding breast feeding

One RCT in women with HIV who had access to clean water and health education has found that versus formula feeding breast feeding significantly reduces the incidence of HIV in infants after 24 months without increasing infant mortality.

UNKNOWN EFFECTIVENESS

Immunotherapy

One RCT found no significant difference in the incidence of HIV in infants of mothers taking hyperimmune globulin versus immunoglobulin without HIV antibody in addition to a standard zidovudine regimen, but it may have been too small to exclude a clinically important difference.

Vaginal microbicides

We found insufficient evidence about the effects of vaginal microbicides on the transmission of HIV to infants.

LIKELY TO BE INEFFECTIVE OR HARMFUL

Vitamin supplements

RCTs found no significant difference in the incidence of HIV at birth, 6 weeks, or 3 months in the infants of pregnant women given vitamin A or multivitamins versus placebo.

DEFINITION Mother to child transmission of HIV-1Ⓖ infection can occur during pregnancy, in the intrapartum period, or postnatally through breast feeding.[1] By contrast, HIV-2Ⓖ is rarely transmitted from mother to child.[2] Infected children usually have no symptoms and signs of HIV at birth, but develop them over subsequent months or years.[3]

Clin Evid Concise 2003;9:150–151.

INCIDENCE/ PREVALENCE A review of 13 cohorts found that the risk of mother to child transmission of HIV without antiviral treatment is on average about 15–20% in Europe, 15–30% in the USA, and 25–35% in Africa.[4] The risk of transmission is estimated to be between 15 and 30% during pregnancy, with an additional risk of about 10–20% postpartum through breast feeding.[5] It has been estimated that 800 000 children below the age of 15 years were newly infected with HIV during 2001, bringing the total number of children with HIV/AIDS to 3 million worldwide.[6] Most of these children were infected from their mother and 90% live in sub-Saharan Africa.

AETIOLOGY/ RISK FACTORS Transmission of HIV to children is more likely if the mother has a high viral load.[1,7,8] Women with detectable viraemia (by p24 antigen or culture) have double the risk of transmitting HIV-1 to their infants than those who do not.[1] Breast feeding has also been shown in prospective studies to be a risk factor.[6,10] Other risk factors include sexually transmitted diseases, chorioamnionitis, prolonged rupture of membranes, and vaginal mode of delivery.[11–15]

PROGNOSIS About 25% of infants infected with HIV progress rapidly to AIDS or death in the first year. Some survive beyond 12 years of age.[3] One European study found a mortality of 15% in the first year of life and a mortality of 28% by the age of 5 years.[16] A recent report estimated the mortality attributable to HIV/AIDS in children under 5 years of age in sub-Saharan Africa after correcting for competing causes of mortality.[17] HIV accounted for 2% of deaths in 1990 rising significantly to almost 8% in 1999. Five countries (Botswana, Namibia, Swaziland, Zambia, and Zimbabwe) had rates of HIV attributable mortality in excess of 30/1000 in children under the age of 5 years.

Please refer to CD-ROM for full text and references.

HIV: opportunistic infections

Search date August 2002

John Ioannidis and David Wilkinson

What are the effects of drug prophylaxis?

BENEFICIAL

Aciclovir (for herpes simplex virus and varicella zoster virus)

One systematic review has found that aciclovir versus placebo significantly reduces herpes simplex virus and varicella zoster virus infection, and reduces overall mortality in people at different clinical stages of HIV infection. It found no reduction in cytomegalovirus.

TMP/SMX (trimethoprim/sulfamethoxazole [sulphamethoxazole]; co-trimoxazole) for *Pneumocystis carinii* pneumonia (PCP)

Systematic reviews have found that TMP/SMX versus placebo or pentamidine significantly reduces the incidence of PCP. Two systematic reviews have found that TMP/SMX versus dapsone (with or without pyrimethamine) reduced incidence of PCP, although only one of these reviews found that the reduction was significant. One systematic review and one subsequent RCT found no significant difference between high and low dose TMP/SMX for PCP prophylaxis, although adverse effects were more common with the higher dose.

Tuberculosis prophylaxis versus placebo

Systematic reviews have found that in people who are HIV and tuberculin skin test positive, antituberculosis prophylaxis versus placebo significantly reduces the frequency of tuberculosis over 2–3 years. The reviews have found no evidence of benefit in people who are HIV positive but tuberculin skin test negative. One RCT found that the benefit of prophylaxis diminished with time after treatment was stopped.

LIKELY TO BE BENEFICIAL

Atovaquone (no difference from dapsone or aerosolised pentamidine for PCP in people intolerant of TMP/SMX)

We found no RCTs of atovaquone versus placebo. RCTs found no significant difference in the incidence of PCP with atovaquone versus dapsone or versus aerosolised pentamidine, both of which are regarded as effective in people intolerant of TMP/SMX.

Azithromycin (for *Mycobacterium avium* complex [MAC])

One RCT has found that azithromycin versus placebo significantly reduces the incidence of MAC.

Azithromycin (for PCP)

One RCT has found that azithromycin, either alone or in combination with rifabutin versus rifabutin alone, reduces the risk of PCP in people receiving standard PCP prophylaxis.

Clarithromycin (for MAC)

One RCT has found that clarithromycin versus placebo significantly reduces the incidence of MAC.

Clarithromycin, rifabutin, and ethambutol (*v* clarithromycin plus clofazimine) for MAC in people with previous MAC

One RCT found that clarithromycin, rifabutin and ethambutol reduced MAC relapse compared with clarithromycin plus clofazimine.

Clin Evid Concise 2003;9:152–155.

Discontinuing prophylaxis for MAC in people with CD4 > 100/mm^3 on highly active antiretroviral treatment (HAART)

Two RCTs in people taking HAART found that discontinuation of prophylaxis for MAC disease did not increase the incidence of MAC disease.

Discontinuing prophylaxis for PCP and toxoplasmosis in people with CD4 > 200/mm^3 on HAART

One systematic review of two unblinded RCTs in people taking HAART found that discontinuation of prophylaxis did not increase the incidence of PCP. Two unblinded RCTs found that discontinuation of prophylaxis did not increase the incidence of toxoplasmosis.

Ethambutol added to clarithromycin plus clofazimine (for MAC in people with previous MAC)

One RCT found that adding ethambutol to clarithromycin and clofazimine reduced MAC relapse compared with clarithromycin plus clofazimine.

Itraconazole (for *Penicillium marneffei*)

Two RCTs have found that itraconazole versus placebo significantly reduces the incidence of relapse of *P marneffei* infection**Ⓖ** and candidiasis.

TRADE OFF BETWEEN BENEFITS AND HARMS

Combination treatment (rifabutin plus either clarithromycin or azithromycin) for MAC

One RCT has found that rifabutin plus clarithromycin versus rifabutin alone significantly reduces the incidence of MAC. Another RCT has found that rifabutin plus azithromycin versus azithromycin alone or rifabutin alone significantly reduces the incidence of MAC at 1 year. One systematic review and two subsequent RCTs found that toxicity, including uveitis, was more common with combination treatment compared with clarithromycin or rifabutin alone.

Fluconazole or itraconazole (for invasive fungal disease)

RCTs in people with advanced HIV disease have found that both fluconazole and itraconazole versus placebo significantly reduce the incidence of invasive fungal infections. One RCT found that fluconazole versus clotrimazole reduced the incidence of invasive fungal disease and mucocutaneous candidiasis. One RCT found no significant difference between high and low dose fluconazole.

Isoniazid tuberculosis prophylaxis for 6–12 months (*v* combination treatment for 2 months — similar benefits, fewer harms)

RCTs found no evidence of a difference in effectiveness between regimens using combinations of tuberculosis drugs for 2–3 months and those using isoniazid alone for 6–12 months. One RCT found that multidrug regimens increased the number of people with adverse reactions resulting in cessation of treatment.

Oral ganciclovir (in people with severe CD4 depletion)

One RCT has found that oral ganciclovir versus placebo significantly reduces the incidence of cytomegalovirus in people with severe CD4 depletion. It found that 25% of taking ganciclovir developed severe neutropenia. A second RCT found no significant differences between treatments.

UNKNOWN EFFECTIVENESS

Addition of rifabutin to clarithromycin plus ethambutol (for MAC in people with previous MAC)

One RCT found no significant difference in survival between clarithromycin plus ethambutol with versus without rifabutin in people with previous MAC.

Famciclovir (for recurrent herpes simplex virus)

One small RCT found that famciclovir versus placebo reduced the rate of viral shedding, but provided insufficient evidence on the effect of famciclovir on herpes simplex virus recurrence.

Itraconazole (for histoplasmosis)

We found no RCTs.

Stopping prophylaxis for cytomegalovirus in people with CD4 > 100/mm^3 on HAART

We found insufficient evidence on the effects of discontinuation of maintenance treatment for cytomegalovirus retinitis or other end organ disease in people taking HAART.

TMP/SMX for toxoplasmosis

One RCT found no significant difference between TMP/SMX versus placebo for preventing toxoplasmosis. One systematic review has found no significant difference between TMP/SMX versus dapsone (with or without pyrimethamine) for incidence of toxoplasmosis.

LIKELY TO BE INEFFECTIVE OR HARMFUL

Clofazimine added to ethambutol plus clarithromycin (*v* clofazimine plus ethambutol for MAC in people with previous MAC)

One RCT found that adding clarithromycin to clofazimine and ethambutol significantly increased mortality compared with clofazimine plus ethambutol.

Itraconazole (*v* fluconazole for maintenance treatment of cryptococcal meningitis)

One RCT has found that itraconazole versus fluconazole significantly increases the relapse of cryptococcal meningitis.

Valaciclovir (*v* aciclovir for cytomegalovirus)

One RCT has found that valaciclovir versus aciclovir reduces the incidence of cytomegalovirus, but may be associated with increased mortality.

DEFINITION Opportunistic infections are intercurrent infections that occur in people infected with HIV. Prophylaxis aims to avoid either the first occurrence of these infections (primary prophylaxis) or their recurrence (secondary prophylaxis, maintenance treatment). This review includes PCP, *Toxoplasma gondii* encephalitis, *Mycobacterium tuberculosis*, MAC disease, CMV disease (most often retinitis), infections from other herpes viruses (herpes simplex virus and varicella zoster virus), and invasive fungal disease (*Cryptococcus neoformans*, *Histoplasma capsulatum*, and *P marneffei*).

INCIDENCE/ PREVALENCE The incidence of opportunistic infections is high in people with immune impairment. Data available before the introduction of HAART suggest that, with a CD4 < 250/mm^3, the 2 year probability of developing an opportunistic infection is 40% for PCP, 22% for CMV, 18% for MAC, 6% for toxoplasmosis, and 5% for cryptococcal meningitis.[1] The introduction of HAART has reduced the rate of opportunistic infections. A recent cohort study found that the introduction of HAART decreased the incidence of PCP by 94%, CMV by 82%, and MAC by 64%, as presenting AIDS events. HAART decreased the incidence of events subsequent to the diagnosis of AIDS by 84% for PCP, 82% for CMV, and 97% for MAC.[2]

AETIOLOGY/ RISK FACTORS Opportunistic infections are caused by a wide array of pathogens and result from immune defects induced by HIV. The risk of developing opportunistic infections increases dramatically with progressive impairment of the immune system. Each opportunistic infection has a different threshold of immune impairment, beyond which the risk increases substantially.[1] Opportunistic pathogens may infect the immunocompromised host *de novo*, but usually they are simply reactivations of latent pathogens in such hosts.

PROGNOSIS Prognosis depends on the type of opportunistic infection. Even with treatment they may cause serious morbidity and mortality. Most deaths owing to HIV infection are caused by opportunistic infections.

Please refer to CD-ROM for full text and references.

Influenza

Search date March 2002

Clinical Evidence freelance writers

What are the effects of antiviral treatment of influenza in adults?

LIKELY TO BE BENEFICIAL

Oral amantadine for early treatment of influenza A in adults (duration of symptoms reduced)

One systematic review and three additional RCTs have found that oral amantadine versus placebo reduces the duration of influenza A symptoms by about 1 day. We found insufficient evidence about adverse effects in this setting. We found no good evidence of benefit if amantadine is started more than 2 days after symptom onset.

Oral rimantadine for early treatment of influenza A in adults (duration of symptoms reduced)

One systematic review has found that oral rimantadine versus placebo reduces the duration of influenza A symptoms by about 1 day. We found insufficient evidence about adverse effects in this setting. We found no good evidence of benefit if rimantadine is started more than 2 days after symptom onset.

Orally inhaled zanamivir for early treatment of influenza A and B in adults (duration of symptoms reduced)

One systematic review has found that orally inhaled zanamivir versus placebo reduces the duration of influenza symptoms by about 1 day. Adverse effects were similar in people taking zanamivir and in people taking placebo. We found no good evidence of benefit if zanamivir is started more than 2 days after symptom onset.

Oral oseltamivir for early treatment of influenza A and B in adults (duration of symptoms reduced)

Two RCTs have found that oral oseltamivir versus placebo reduces the duration of influenza symptoms by about 1 day. Oral oseltamivir versus placebo increases the incidence of nausea and vomiting. We found no good evidence of benefit if oseltamivir is started more than 1.5 days after symptom onset.

UNKNOWN EFFECTIVENESS

All antivirals (reduction of serious influenza complications)

We found insufficient evidence about the effects of antiviral agents on reducing serious complications of influenza, but we found strong evidence that influenza immunisation reduces the risk of complications and death in people at high risk for complications from influenza, including elderly people (see influenza vaccine under community acquired pneumonia, p 313).

DEFINITION Influenza is caused by infection with influenza viruses. Uncomplicated influenza is characterised by the abrupt onset of fever, chills, non-productive cough, myalgias, headache, nasal congestion, sore throat, and fatigue.[1] Influenza is usually diagnosed clinically. Not all people infected with influenza viruses become symptomatic. People infected with other pathogens may have symptoms identical to those of influenza.[2] The percentage of infections resulting in clinical illness can vary from about 40–85%, depending on age ▶

and pre-existing immunity to the virus.[3] Influenza can be confirmed by viral culture, immunofluorescence staining, enzyme immunoassay, or rapid diagnostic testing of nasopharyngeal, nasal or throat swab specimens, or by serologic testing of paired sera. Some rapid tests detect influenza A only, some detect and distinguish between influenza A and B, whereas others detect but do not distinguish between influenza A and B.

INCIDENCE/ PREVALENCE In temperate areas of the Northern Hemisphere, influenza activity typically peaks between late December and early March whereas, in temperate areas of the Southern Hemisphere, influenza activity typically peaks between May and September. In tropical areas, influenza can occur throughout the year.[2] The annual incidence of influenza varies yearly, and depends partly on the underlying level of population immunity to circulating influenza viruses.[1] One localised study in the USA found that serological conversion with or without symptoms occurred in 10–20% a year, with the highest infection rates in people aged under 20 years.[4] Attack rates are higher in institutions and in areas of overcrowding.[5]

AETIOLOGY/ RISK FACTORS Influenza viruses are transmitted primarily from person to person through respiratory droplets disseminated during sneezing, coughing, and talking.[1,6]

PROGNOSIS The incubation period of influenza is 1–4 days and infected adults are usually contagious from the day before symptom onset until 5 days after symptom onset. The signs and symptoms of uncomplicated influenza usually resolve within a week, although cough and fatigue may persist.[1] Complications include otitis media, bacterial sinusitis, secondary bacterial pneumonia, and, less commonly, viral pneumonia and respiratory failure. Complications are also caused by exacerbation of underlying disease.[1,2] In the USA each year, over 110 000 admissions to hospital and about 20 000 deaths are related to influenza.[2] The risk of hospitalisation is highest in people 65 years or older, in very young children, and in those with chronic medical conditions.[1,7,8] Over 90% of influenza related deaths during recent seasonal epidemics in the USA have been in people 65 years or older.[1] During influenza pandemics, morbidity and mortality may be high in younger age groups.[1] Severe illness is more common with influenza A infections than influenza B infections.[1]

Please refer to CD-ROM for full text and references.

Leprosy

Search date November 2001

Diana Lockwood

What are the effects of preventive interventions?

BENEFICIAL

Bacillus Calmette Guerin (BCG) vaccine

One RCT and three population based controlled clinical trials found that BCG vaccination versus no intervention or placebo significantly reduced the incidence of leprosy for up to 16 years. The degree of protection varied between countries, with higher protection in Uganda than Burma (now Myanmar).

BCG plus killed *Mycobacterium*

One RCT found that in people with a BCG scar, BCG plus killed *Mycobacterium leprae* versus placebo significantly reduced the incidence of leprosy over 5–9 years. In people without a BCG scar, the RCT found that the addition of *M leprae* to BCG did not reduce the incidence of leprosy. Another RCT found that BCG plus killed *M leprae* versus saline significantly reduced the incidence of leprosy over about 7 years.

LIKELY TO BE BENEFICIAL

ICRC vaccine

One RCT found that ICRC vaccine**G** versus placebo significantly reduced the incidence of leprosy over about 7 years. The effect was higher than that observed with BCG alone, and similar to that observed with BCG plus killed *M leprae*.

UNKNOWN EFFECTIVENESS

***Mycobacterium w* vaccine**

One RCT found that *Mycobacterium w* vaccine versus placebo marginally reduced the incidence of leprosy over about 7 years.

What are the effects of treatments?

BENEFICIAL

Dapsone plus rifampicin for paucibacillary leprosy*

We found no systematic review or RCT on multidrug treatment for paucibacillary leprosy. We found no RCT comparing dapsone plus rifampicin versus dapsone alone. Observational studies found that in people taking dapsone plus rifampicin for 6 months, up to 38% of lesions had resolved at 1 year and relapse rates were low for up to 8 years.

Rifampicin plus dapsone plus clofazimine for multibacillary leprosy*

We found no systematic review or RCT. We found no RCT comparing rifampicin plus clofazimine plus dapsone versus dapsone alone, or versus dapsone plus rifampicin. Observational studies found that multidrug treatment for 24 months improved skin lesions and was associated with a low relapse rate.

UNLIKELY TO BE BENEFICIAL

Single dose versus multiple dose treatment for single lesion leprosy (both increase cure rates but multiple more than single dose)

One RCT found that 6 months treatment with rifampicin monthly plus dapsone daily significantly increased the cure rate at 18 months compared with a single dose of rifampicin plus minocycline plus ofloxacin. Adverse effects were similar with both regimens.

*Observational evidence only, RCTs unlikely to be conducted.

DEFINITION Leprosy is a chronic granulomatous disease caused by *Mycobacterium leprae*, and primarily affects the peripheral nerves and skin. The clinical outcome of infection is determined by the individual's immune response to *M leprae*. A spectrum of disease types are seen. At the tuberculoid end of the Ridley–Jopling scale, cell mediated immunity is good and there are few skin lesions. At the lepromatous end of the scale there is diminished reactivity for *M leprae* resulting in uncontrolled bacterial multiplication, and skin and mucosal infiltration. Peripheral nerve damage occurs across the spectrum. Between the poles are the unstable borderline tuberculoid and borderline lepromatous forms. Classification is based on the clinical appearance and bacterial index of lesions Ⓖ. The World Health Organization field classification is based on the number of skin lesions: single lesion leprosy (1 lesion), paucibacillary leprosy (2–5 skin lesions), and multibacillary leprosy (> 5 skin lesions).[1]

INCIDENCE/ PREVALENCE Worldwide, about 720 000 new cases of leprosy are reported each year,[2] and about 2 million people have leprosy related disabilities. Six major endemic countries (India, Brazil, Myanmar, Madagascar, Nepal, and Mozambique) account for 88% of all new cases. Cohort studies show a peak of disease presentation between 10–20 years of age.[3] After puberty there are twice as many male as female cases.

AETIOLOGY/ RISK FACTORS *M leprae* is discharged from the nasal mucosa of people with untreated lepromatous leprosy, and transmitted through the nasal mucosa with subsequent spread of mycobacteria to skin and nerves. It is a hardy organism and has been shown to survive in the Indian environment for many months.[4] Risk factors include household contact with a person with leprosy. We found no good evidence of a relationship between HIV infection, nutrition, and socio-economic status.[5]

PROGNOSIS Complications of leprosy include nerve damage, immunological reactions, and bacillary infiltration. In the absence of treatment, tuberculoid and borderline tuberculoid infections will resolve spontaneously. Other people with borderline tuberculoid and borderline lepromatous leprosy slowly develop lepromatous infection. Many people have peripheral nerve damage at the time of diagnosis, ranging from 15% in Bangladesh to 55% in Ethiopia. Immunological reactions can occur with or without antibiotic treatment. Further nerve damage occurs through immune mediated reactions and neuritis. Erythema nodosum leprosum is an immune complex mediated reaction causing fever, malaise, and neuritis, which is reported to occur in 20% of people with lepromatous leprosy and 15% with borderline lepromatous leprosy.[8] Secondary impairments (wounds, contractures, and digit resorption) occur in 33–56% of people with established nerve damage.[9] We found no recent information on mortality.

Please refer to CD-ROM for full text and references.

Lyme disease

Search date May 2002

Edward Hayes

What are the effects of preventive interventions and treatments?

BENEFICIAL

Prophylactic treatment of tick bite

Combined results from RCTs have found that prophylactic antibiotics versus placebo for the treatment of tick bite reduce the incidence of Lyme disease.

Three doses of recombinant Osp–A Lyme disease vaccine with adjuvant in immunocompetent people aged 15–70 years exposed to North American strains of Borrelia burgdorferi

One RCT has found that a vaccine (consisting of recombinant outer surface protein A [Osp–A] of *Borrelia burgdorferi* combined with adjuvantⒼ) versus placebo significantly reduces the incidence of Lyme disease in people at high risk of developing Lyme disease within North America.

LIKELY TO BE BENEFICIAL

Penicillin (better than placebo for Lyme arthritis)

One RCT in people with Lyme arthritis has found that penicillin versus placebo significantly increases resolution of Lyme arthritis at 3 weeks.

Cefotaxime (more effective than penicillin for late neurological Lyme disease)

One RCT found weak evidence from subgroup analysis of people with late Lyme disease that cefotaxime versus penicillin significantly increased the number of people with full recovery at 2 years.

Cefotaxime (more effective than penicillin for Lyme arthritis)

One RCT found weak evidence from subgroup analysis of people with Lyme arthritis that cefotaxime versus penicillin significantly increased the number of people with full recovery at 2 years.

Ceftriaxone (more effective than penicillin for Lyme arthritis)

One RCT found weak evidence from subgroup analysis of people with Lyme arthritis that ceftriaxone versus penicillin significantly improved symptoms at 3 months.

Doxycycline (as effective as amoxicillin and probenecid for Lyme arthritis)

One RCT in people with Lyme arthritis has found no significant difference between doxycycline versus amoxicillin plus probenicid in resolution of Lyme arthritis.

UNKNOWN EFFECTIVENESS

Ceftriaxone (in late neurological Lyme disease)

One RCT found weak evidence from subgroup analysis in people with late neurological Lyme disease and found that there was no significant difference between ceftriaxone versus cefotaxime in the proportion of people who were asymptomatic at 8 months after treatment.

Clin Evid Concise 2003;9:160–162.

Ceftriaxone plus doxycycline (in people with late neurological Lyme disease who had been previously treated)

One RCT comparing ceftriaxone plus doxycycline versus placebo in people with previously treated Lyme disease and persistent neurological symptoms found no significant difference in health related quality of life at interim analysis at 180 days; therefore the RCT was terminated.

Lyme disease vaccine in Europe or Asia

We found no evidence about the effectiveness of recombinant outer surface protein A (Osp–A) vaccine in European or Asian populations. There is heterogeneity of the species that cause Lyme disease in Europe and Asia. The vaccine may not be as effective in European or Asian populations as it is in North American.

LIKELY TO BE INEFFECTIVE OR HARMFUL

Oral antibiotic treatment of people with Lyme arthritis plus neuroborreliosis

Some people have developed symptoms of neuroborreliosis after oral antibiotic treatment of Lyme arthritis.

DEFINITION Lyme disease is an inflammatory illness resulting from infection with spirochetes of the *Borrelia burgdorferi* genospecies transmitted to humans by ticks. Some infected people have no symptoms. The characteristic manifestation of early Lyme disease is erythema migrans: a circular rash at the site of the infectious tick attachment that expands over a period of days to weeks in 80–90% of people with Lyme disease. Early disseminated infection may cause secondary erythema migrans, disease of the nervous system (facial palsy or other cranial neuropathies, meningitis, and radiculoneuritis), musculoskeletal disease (arthralgia), and, rarely, cardiac disease (myocarditis or transient atrioventricular block). Untreated or inadequately treated Lyme disease can cause late disseminated manifestations weeks to months after infection. These late manifestations include arthritis, polyneuropathy, and encephalopathy. Diagnosis of Lyme disease is based primarily on clinical findings and a high likelihood of exposure to infected ticks. Serological testing may be helpful in people with endemic exposure who have clinical findings consistent with later stage disseminated Lyme disease.

INCIDENCE/ PREVALENCE Lyme disease occurs in temperate regions of North America, Europe, and Asia. It is the most commonly reported vector borne disease in the USA, with over 16 000 cases reported a year.[1] Most cases occur in the northeastern and northcentral states, with a reported annual incidence in endemic states as high as 67.9/100 000 people.[1] In highly endemic communities, the incidence of Lyme disease may exceed 1000/100 000 people a year.[2] In some countries of Europe, the incidence of Lyme disease has been estimated to be over 100/100 000 people a year.[3] Foci of Lyme disease have been described in northern forested regions of Russia, in China, and in Japan.[4] Transmission cycles of *B burgdorferi* have not been described in tropical areas or in the Southern hemisphere.[4]

AETIOLOGY/ RISK FACTORS Lyme disease is caused by infection with any of the *B burgdorferi* sensu lato genospecies. Virtually all cases of Lyme disease in North America are the result of infection with *B burgdorferi*. In Europe, Lyme disease may be caused by *B burgdorferi*, *B garinii,* and *B afzelii*. The infectious spirochetes are transmitted to humans through the bite of certain *Ixodes* ticks.[4] Humans who have frequent or prolonged exposure to the habitats of infected *Ixodes* ticks are at highest risk of acquiring Lyme disease. Individual risk depends on the likelihood of being bitten by infected tick vectors, which varies with the density of vector ticks in the environment, the prevalence of infection in ticks, and the extent of a person's contact with infected ticks. The risk of Lyme disease is often concentrated in focal areas. In the USA, risk is highest in certain counties within northeastern and northcentral states during the months of April to July.[2] People become infected when they engage in activities in wooded or bushy areas that are favourable habitats for ticks, and deer and rodent hosts.

PROGNOSIS Lyme disease is rarely fatal. Untreated Lyme arthritis resolves at a rate of 10–20% a year; over 90% of facial palsies due to Lyme disease resolve spontaneously, and most cases of Lyme carditis resolve without sequelae.[5] However, untreated Lyme disease can result in arthritis (50% of untreated people), meningitis or neuropathies (15% of untreated people), carditis (5–10% of untreated people with erythema migrans), and, rarely, encephalopathy.

Please refer to CD-ROM for full text and references.

Malaria in endemic areas

Search date October 2002

Aika Omari and Paul Garner

What are the effects of medical treatment for complicated falciparum malaria in non-pregnant people?

LIKELY TO BE BENEFICIAL

Artemether (v quinine)

Two systematic reviews and one subsequent RCT found no significant difference between artemether versus quinine for preventing death in people with severe malaria.

High first dose quinine

One systematic review and one additional RCT found no significant difference in mortality between quinine regimens with high initial quinine dose versus no loading dose. The systematic review found that high first dose of quinine reduced parasite and fever clearance timesⒼ compared with no loading dose.

Quinine

We found no RCTs comparing quinine versus placebo or no treatment, but there is consensus that treatment is likely to be beneficial.

Rectal artemisinin (as effective as quinine)

One systematic review found no significant difference in mortality with rectal artemisinin versus quinine.

UNKNOWN EFFECTIVENESS

Chloroquine versus quinine

Two RCTs in children found no significant difference in mortality with chloroquine versus quinine. However, these RCTs were conducted in the Gambia between 1988 and 1994, when chloroquine resistance was uncommon.

Desferrioxamine mesylate

One systematic review found weak evidence that desferrioxamine mesylate versus placebo reduced the risk of persistent seizures in children with cerebral malaria. However, we were unable to draw reliable conclusions.

Exchange blood transfusion

One systematic review has found no suitable RCTs.

Initial blood transfusion

One systematic review found no significant difference in deaths in clinically stable children who received an initial blood transfusion for malaria anaemia and found more adverse events.

Intramuscular versus intravenous quinine

One RCT in children found no significant difference with intramuscular versus intravenous quinine in recovery times or deaths in Kenya in 1990.

Sulfadoxine–pyrimethamine versus quinine

One RCT found that sulfadoxine–pyrimethamine versus quinine cleared parasites faster in children with complicated non-cerebral malaria in 1992–1994 in the Gambia, but found no significant difference in mortality.

LIKELY TO BE INEFFECTIVE OR HARMFUL

Dexamethasone

One systematic review has found no significant difference in mortality with dexamethasone versus placebo, but gastrointestinal bleeding and seizures were more common with dexamethasone.

DEFINITION Severe malaria is caused by the protozoan infection of red blood cells with *Plasmodium falciparum*Ⓖ. Clinically complicated malaria presents with life threatening conditions, which include coma, severe anaemia, renal failure, respiratory distress syndrome, hypoglycaemia, shock, spontaneous haemorrhage, and convulsions. The diagnosis of cerebral malaria should be considered where there is encephalopathy in the presence of malaria parasites. A strict definition of cerebral malaria requires the presence of unrousable coma, and no other cause of encephalopathy (e.g. hypoglycaemia, sedative drugs) in the presence of *P falciparum* infection.[1] This review does not currently include the treatment of malaria in pregnancy.

INCIDENCE/ PREVALENCE Malaria is a major health problem in the tropics with 300–500 million clinical cases occurring annually, and an estimated 1.1–2.7 million deaths occur each year as a result of severe malaria.[2] Over 90% of deaths occur in children below 5 years of age, mainly from cerebral malaria and anaemia.[2] In areas where malaria transmission is stable (endemic), those most at risk of acquiring severe malaria are children under 5 years old, because adults and older children have partial immunity that offers some protection. In areas where malaria transmission is unstable (non-endemic), severe malaria affects both adults and children. Non-immune travellers and migrants are also at risk from developing severe malaria.

AETIOLOGY/ RISK FACTORS Malaria is transmitted by the bite of infected female anopheline mosquitoes. Certain genes are associated with resistance to severe malaria. Human leukocyte antigens (HLA), namely HLA-Bw53 and HLA-DRB1*1302, protect against severe malaria. However, the associations of HLA antigens with severe malaria are limited to specific populations.[3,4] Haemoglobin S[3] and haemoglobin C[5] are also protective against severe malaria. Genes, such as the tumour necrosis factor gene have also been associated with an increased susceptibility to severe malaria (see aetiology under malaria: prevention in travellers, p 165).[6]

PROGNOSIS In children under 5 years of age with cerebral malaria, the estimated case fatality of treated malaria is 19%, although reported hospital case fatality may be as high as 10–40%.[1,7] Neurological sequelae persisting for more than 6 months occur in more than 2% of the survivors, and include ataxia, hemiplegia, speech disorders, behavioural disorders, epilepsy, and blindness. Severe malarial anaemia has a case fatality rate higher than 13%.[7] In adults, the mortality of cerebral malaria is 20%; this rises to 50% in pregnancy,[8] and neurological sequelae occur in about 3% of survivors.[9]

Please refer to CD-ROM for full text and references.

Malaria: prevention in travellers

Search date March 2002

Ashley Croft

What are the effects of treatments?

BENEFICIAL

Insecticide treated nets

We found no RCTs in travellers. One systematic review in residents of a malaria endemic area has found that nets treated with insecticide significantly reduce the number of mild episodes of malaria and reduced child mortality.

LIKELY TO BE BENEFICIAL

Doxycycline in adults

Two RCTs in soldiers have found that doxycycline versus placebo significantly reduces the risk of malaria.

Insecticide treated clothing

Two RCTs in soldiers and refugee householders have found that permethrin treated fabric (clothing or sheets) significantly reduces the incidence of malaria.

Mefloquine in adults

One RCT in soldiers comparing mefloquine versus placebo found that mefloquine had a 100% protective efficacy. One RCT of mefloquine versus atovaquone plus proguanil found no cases of clinical malaria throughout the trial, but found a significantly higher rate of neuropsychiatric harm with mefloquine.

UNKNOWN EFFECTIVENESS

Aerosol insecticides

One large observational study in travellers found insufficient evidence on the effects of aerosol insecticides in preventing malaria. Two RCTs in malaria endemic areas found that indoor spraying of aerosol insecticides reduced clinical malaria.

Air conditioning and electric fans

One large observational study found that air conditioning significantly reduced the incidence of malaria. One small observational study found that electric fans reduced the number of culicine mosquitos in indoor spaces.

Atovaquone plus proguanil

One RCT found no significant difference between atovaquone plus proguanil versus chloroquine plus proguanil in preventing malaria. One RCT found no significant difference between atovaquone plus proguanil versus mefloquine in preventing malaria.

Chloroquine

We found no RCTs about the effects of chloroquine in travellers. One RCT in Austrian workers residing in Nigeria found no significant difference between chloroquine versus sulfadoxine plus pyrimethamine in the incidence of malaria at 6–22 months.

Chloroquine plus proguanil

One RCT found no significant difference between chloroquine plus proguanil versus proguanil alone or versus chloroquine plus other antimalaria drugs in the incidence of *Plasmodium falciparum* malaria. One RCT found no significant difference between chloroquine plus proguanil versus atovaquone plus proguanil in preventing malaria.

Clin Evid Concise 2003;9:165–167.

Full length clothing

One observational study found that wearing trousers and long sleeved shirts significantly reduced the incidence of malaria.

Insecticide treated nets in pregnant travellers

We found no RCTs of the effects of insecticide treated nets on pregnant travellers. One RCT of pregnant residents found inconclusive evidence on the effects of permethrin treated nets in preventing malaria.

Mosquito coils and vaporising mats

We found no systematic review and no RCTs of the effects of coils and vaporising mats in preventing malaria in travellers. One RCT of coils and one observational study of pyrethroid vaporising mats found that these devices reduced numbers of mosquitoes in indoor spaces.

Pyrimethamine plus dapsone

We found no RCTs in travellers. One RCT in Thai soldiers comparing pyrimethamine plus dapsone versus proguanil plus dapsone found no significant difference in *P falciparum* infection rates over 40 days.

Smoke

We found no RCTs of the effects of smoke in preventing malaria. One controlled clinical trial found that smoke repelled mosquitoes during the evening.

Topical insect repellents

We found no systematic review and no RCTs on the effects of topical insect repellents in preventing malaria. One very small crossover RCT found that DEET preparations protected against mosquito bites.

Vaccines

We found no RCTs in travellers. One systematic review of antimalaria vaccines in residents of malaria endemic areas has found that the SPf66 vaccine versus placebo significantly reduces first attacks of malaria.

Antimalaria drugs in airline pilots or pregnant travellers; biological control measures; insect buzzers and electrocuters; insecticides in airline pilots; insecticide treated clothing in pregnant travellers; mefloquine in children; topical insect repellents in pregnant travellers

We found no RCTs on the effects of these interventions.

LIKELY TO BE INEFFECTIVE OR HARMFUL

Amodiaquine

We found insufficient evidence on the effect of amodiaquine on malaria in travellers. However, we found limited observational evidence that amodiaquine may cause liver damage and hepatitis.

Doxycycline in children

We found no RCTs in child travellers on the use of doxycycline. Case reports in young children found adverse effects with doxycycline.

Insect repellents containing DEET in children

We found no RCTs on the effects of DEET in preventing malaria in child travellers. Case reports in young children found serious adverse effects with DEET.

Sulfadoxine plus pyrimethamine

We found insufficient evidence on the effect of these drugs on malaria in travellers. One retrospective cohort study suggested that sulfadoxine plus pyrimethamine was associated with severe cutaneous reactions and a risk of mortality.

Malaria: prevention in travellers

DEFINITION Malaria is caused by a protozoan infection of red blood cells with one of four species of the genus *Plasmodium*: *P falciparum*, *P vivax*, *P ovale,* and *P malariae*.[1] Clinically, malaria may present in different ways, but is usually characterised by fever (which may be swinging), tachycardia, rigors, and sweating. Anaemia, hepatosplenomegaly, cerebral involvement, renal failure, and shock may occur.[2,3]

INCIDENCE/ PREVALENCE Each year there are 300–500 million clinical cases of malaria. About 40% of the world's population is at risk of acquiring the disease.[2,3] Each year 25–30 million people from non-tropical countries visit malaria endemic areas, of whom 10 000–30 000 contract malaria.[4,5] Most RCTs of malaria prevention have been carried out on soldiers and travellers. The results of these trials may not be applicable to people such as refugees and migrants, who are likely to differ in their health status and their susceptibility to disease and adverse drug effects.

AETIOLOGY/ RISK FACTORS Malaria is mainly a rural disease, requiring nearby standing water. It is transmitted by bites of infected female anopheline mosquitoes, mainly at dusk and during the night.[1,6–8] In cities, mosquito bites are usually from female culicine mosquitoes, which are not vectors of malaria.[9] Malaria is resurgent in most tropical countries and risk to travellers is increasing.[10] The sickle cell trait has been shown to convey some protection against malaria in non-immune carriers of that trait. Non-immune adults with the sickle cell trait who develop severe malaria have lower parasite densities, fewer complications (e.g. cerebral malaria), and a reduced mortality compared with adults without the trait.[11] There is little good evidence on the degree of protection afforded by the sickle cell trait.[12]

PROGNOSIS Ninety per cent of tourists and business travellers who contract malaria do not become ill until after they return home.[5] "Imported malaria" is easily treated if diagnosed promptly, and follows a serious course in only about 12% of people.[13,14] The most severe form is cerebral malaria, with a case fatality rate in adult travellers of 2–6% mainly because of delays in diagnosis.[3,15]

Please refer to CD-ROM for full text and references.

Meningococcal disease

Search date June 2002

J Correia and C A Hart

What are the effects of treatments?

LIKELY TO BE BENEFICIAL

Prophylactic antibiotics in contacts

We found no RCTs about the effects of prophylactic antibiotics on the incidence of meningococcal disease among contacts. RCTs are unlikely to be performed because the intervention has few associated risks whereas meningitis has high associated risks. Observational evidence suggests that antibiotics reduce the risk of meningococcal disease. We found no evidence to address the question of which contacts should be treated.

UNKNOWN EFFECTIVENESS

Antibiotics for throat carriage (reduce carriage but unknown effect on risk of disease)

RCTs have found that antibiotics versus placebo significantly increase the number of people with eradication of meningococcus in the throat. We found no evidence that eradicating throat carriage reduces the risk of meningococcal disease.

Pre-admission parenteral antibiotics in suspected cases

We found no RCTs on the effect of pre-admission antibiotics. It is unlikely that RCTs will be performed because of the unpredictably rapid course of meningococcal disease in some people, the intuitive risks involved in delaying treatment, and the relatively low risk of causing harm. Most of the observational studies we found show a trend toward benefit with antibiotics, but at least one found contradictory results.

DEFINITION Meningococcal disease is any clinical condition caused by *Neisseria meningitidis* (the meningococcus) groups A, B, C, or other serogroups. These conditions include purulent conjunctivitis, septic arthritis, meningitis, and septicaemia with or without meningitis.

INCIDENCE/ PREVALENCE Meningococcal disease is sporadic in temperate countries, and is most commonly caused by group B or C meningococci. The incidence in the UK varies from 2–8 cases/100 000 people a year,[1] and in the USA from 0.6–1.5/100 000 people.[2] Occasional outbreaks occur among close family contacts, secondary school pupils, and students living in halls of residence. Sub-Saharan Africa has regular epidemics because of serogroup A, particularly in countries lying between The Gambia in the west and Ethiopia in the east (the "meningitis belt"), where incidence during epidemics reaches 500/100 000 people.[3]

AETIOLOGY/ RISK FACTORS The meningococcus infects healthy people and is transmitted by close contact: probably by exchange of upper respiratory tract secretions Ⓣ.[4–12] Risk of transmission is greatest during the first week of contact.[7] Risk factors include crowding and exposure to cigarette smoke.[13] Children younger than 2 years have the highest incidence, with a second peak between ages 15–24 years. There is currently an increased incidence of meningococcal disease among university students, especially among those in their first term and living in catered accommodation,[14] although we found no accurate numerical estimate of risk from close contact in, for example, halls of residence. Close contacts of ▶

an index case have a much higher risk of infection than people in the general population.[7,10,11] The risk of epidemic spread is higher with groups A and C meningococci than with group B meningococci.[4–6,8] It is not known what makes a meningococcus virulent, but certain clones tend to predominate at different times and in different groups. Carriage of meningococcus in the throat has been reported in 10–15% of people; recent acquisition of a virulent meningococcus is more likely to be associated with invasive disease.

PROGNOSIS Mortality is highest in infants and adolescents, and is related to disease presentation: case fatality rates are 19–25% in septicaemia, 10–12% in meningitis plus septicaemia, and less than 1% in meningitis alone.[15–17]

Please refer to CD-ROM for full text and references.

Postherpetic neuralgia

Search date September 2002

Tim Lancaster, David Wareham, and John Yaphe

What are the effects of interventions to prevent postherpetic neuralgia?

LIKELY TO BE BENEFICIAL

Oral antiviral agents (aciclovir, famciclovir, valaciclovir, netivudine)

One systematic review of RCTs has found limited evidence that aciclovir given for 7–10 days reduces pain at 1–3 months. One RCT found that famciclovir versus placebo significantly reduced pain duration after acute herpes zoster. One RCT has found that valaciclovir versus aciclovir significantly reduced the prevalence of postherpetic neuralgia at 6 months. One RCT found no significant difference in outcomes between netivudine and aciclovir. One RCT found no significant difference in the resolution of postherpetic neuralgia between valaciclovir and famciclovir.

UNKNOWN EFFECTIVENESS

Amitriptyline

One small RCT found that amitriptyline versus placebo started within 48 hours of rash onset and continued for 90 days reduced the prevalence of postherpetic neuralgia at 6 months, but the difference did not reach significance.

Adenosine monophosphate; amantadine; cimetidine; inosine pranobex; levodopa

RCTs found insufficient evidence on the effects of these interventions.

UNLIKELY TO BE BENEFICIAL

Topical antiviral agents (idoxuridine)

One systematic review has found that idoxuridine versus placebo or versus oral aciclovir increases short term pain relief in acute herpes zoster, but found no significant difference in pain at 6 months.

LIKELY TO BE INEFFECTIVE OR HARMFUL

Corticosteroids

Systematic reviews have found conflicting evidence about the effects of corticosteroids alone on postherpetic neuralgia. One RCT found limited evidence that high dose steroids added to antiviral agents may be of short term benefit in acute herpes zoster, but found no significant effect on pain at 6 months. There is concern that corticosteroids may cause dissemination of herpes zoster.

What are the effects of treatments in established postherpetic neuralgia?

BENEFICIAL

Gabapentin

One systematic review identified one RCT, which found that gabapentin versus placebo significantly relieves pain after 8 weeks' treatment. One subsequent RCT found similar results.

Clin Evid Concise 2003;9:170–172.

Tricyclic antidepressants

Two systematic reviews have found that tricyclic antidepressants versus placebo significantly increase pain relief in postherpetic neuralgia after 6 weeks.

UNKNOWN EFFECTIVENESS

Oxycodone (oral opioid)

One systematic review found limited evidence that oral oxycodone versus placebo may reduce pain after 4–8 weeks, but may be associated with more adverse effects.

Topical anaesthesia

We found insufficient evidence from three RCTs about the effects of lidocaine (lignocaine).

Topical counterirritants

Two systematic reviews and one small RCT found limited evidence that capsaicin versus placebo may improve pain relief, but also causes painful skin reactions in some people.

Tramadol

One systematic review found limited evidence from one small RCT that tramadol reduced pain more than clomipramine after 6 weeks.

LIKELY TO BE INEFFECTIVE OR HARMFUL

Dextromethorphan

One systematic review and one subsequent RCT found no evidence that dextromethorphan was more effective than placebo or lorazepam after 3–6 weeks.

Epidural morphine

One small RCT found that epidural morphine versus placebo reduced pain by more than 50% but the reduction was not maintained beyond 36 hours. Epidural morphine caused intolerable opioid effects in 75% of people.

DEFINITION Postherpetic neuralgia is pain that sometimes follows resolution of acute herpes zoster and healing of the zoster rash. It can be severe, accompanied by itching, and follows the distribution of the original infection. Herpes zoster is an acute infection caused by activation of latent varicella zoster virus (human herpes virus 3) in people who have been rendered partially immune by a previous attack of chickenpox. Herpes zoster infects the sensory ganglia and their areas of innervation. It is characterised by pain along the distribution of the affected nerve and crops of clustered vesicles over the area.

INCIDENCE/ PREVALENCE In a UK general practice survey of 3600-3800 people, the annual incidence of herpes zoster was 3.4/1000.[1] Incidence varied with age. Herpes zoster was relatively uncommon in people under the age of 50 years (< 2/1000 a year), but rose to 5–7/1000 a year in people aged 50–79 years, and 11/1000 in people aged 80 years or older. In a population based study of 590 cases in Rochester, Minnesota, USA, the overall incidence was lower (1.5/1000) but there were similar increases in incidence with age.[2] Prevalence of postherpetic neuralgia depends on when it is measured after acute infection, and there is no agreed time point for diagnosis.

AETIOLOGY/ RISK FACTORS The main risk factor for postherpetic neuralgia is increasing age. In a UK general practice study (involving 3600–3800 people, 321 cases of acute herpes zoster) there was little risk in those under the age of 50 years, but postherpetic neuralgia developed in over 20% of people who had had acute herpes zoster aged 60–65 years and in 34% aged over 80 years.[1] No other risk factor has been found to predict consistently which people with herpes zoster will experience continued pain. In a general practice study in Iceland (421 people followed for up to 7 years after an initial episode of herpes zoster), the risk of postherpetic neuralgia was 1.8% (95% CI 0.6% to 4.2%) for people under 60 years of age and the pain was mild in all cases.[2] The risk of severe pain after 3 months in people aged over 60 years was 1.7% (95% CI 0% to 6.2%).

PROGNOSIS About 2% of people with acute herpes zoster in the UK general practice survey had pain for more than 5 years.[1] Prevalence of pain falls as time elapses after the initial episode. Among 183 people aged over 60 years in the placebo arm of a UK trial, the prevalence of pain was 61% at 1 month, 24% at 3 months, and 13% at 6 months after acute infection.[3] In a more recent RCT, the prevalence of postherpetic pain in the placebo arm at 6 months was 35% in 72 people over 60 years of age.[4]

Please refer to CD-ROM for full text and references.

Tuberculosis

Search date April 2002

Paul Garner and Alison Holmes

What are the effects of interventions in newly diagnosed pulmonary tuberculosis and multidrug resistant tuberculosis?

BENEFICIAL

Short course chemotherapy (as good as longer courses)
RCTs in people with newly diagnosed tuberculosis found no evidence of a difference in relapse rates with standard short course (6 months) versus longer term (8–9 months) chemotherapy.

LIKELY TO BE BENEFICIAL

Intermittent short course chemotherapy (as good as daily treatment)
Limited evidence from two RCTs in people with newly diagnosed tuberculosis found no significant difference in cure rates with daily versus twice or three times weekly short course chemotherapy regimens.

Pyrazinamide
RCTs found that, in people with newly diagnosed tuberculosis, regimens containing pyrazinamide versus other regimens speed up sputum clearance in the first 2 months, but have found conflicting evidence about effects on relapse rates.

UNKNOWN EFFECTIVENESS

Comparative benefits of different regimens in multidrug resistant tuberculosis
We found no RCTs in people with newly diagnosed tuberculosis comparing different drug regimens for multidrug resistant tuberculosis.

Regimens containing quinolones
We found insufficient evidence in people with newly diagnosed tuberculosis comparing regimens containing quinolones versus existing regimens.

LIKELY TO BE INEFFECTIVE OR HARMFUL

Chemotherapy for less than 6 months
One systematic review in people with newly diagnosed tuberculosis found limited evidence that reducing the duration of chemotherapy to less than 6 months significantly increased relapse rates.

What are the effects of interventions to improve adherence and screening attendance?

LIKELY TO BE BENEFICIAL

Cash incentives
One systematic review has found that cash incentives versus usual care significantly improve attendance among people living in deprived circumstances. Two subsequent RCTs found conflicting results on the effect of cash incentives on treatment completion.

Community health advisors
One RCT found that health advisors recruited from the community versus usual care significantly increased attendance for treatment.

Clin Evid Concise 2003;9:173–174.

Defaulter actionsⒼ

RCTs have found that intensive action (repeated home visits and reminder letters) versus routine action (single reminder letter and home visit) for defaulters significantly improves completion of treatment.

Health education by a nurse

One RCT found that health education by a nurse versus an educational leaflet significantly improved treatment completion.

UNKNOWN EFFECTIVENESS

Prompts and contracts to improve reattendance for Mantoux test reading

One RCT in healthy people found that telephone prompts to return for Mantoux test reading versus no prompts slightly increased the number of people who reattended, but the difference was not significant. Another RCT in healthy people found that a verbal commitment versus no commitment significantly increased reattendance for Mantoux reading.

Health education by a doctor; prompts to adhere to treatment; sanctions for non-adherence; staff training

We found insufficient evidence on the effects of these interventions.

UNLIKELY TO BE BENEFICIAL

Directly observed treatment

One systematic review and one additional RCT found no significant difference between directly observed treatment versus self treatment in cure or treatment completion; therefore a policy of directly observed treatment for all people with tuberculosis is unlikely to be beneficial.

DEFINITION Tuberculosis is caused by *Mycobacterium tuberculosis* and can affect many organs. Specific symptoms relate to site of infection and are generally accompanied by fever, sweats, and weight loss.

INCIDENCE/ PREVALENCE About a third of the world's population is infected with *M tuberculosis*. The organism kills more people than any other infectious agent. The World Health Organization estimates that 95% of cases are in developing countries, and that 25% of avoidable deaths in developing countries are caused by tuberculosis.[1]

AETIOLOGY/ RISK FACTORS Social factors include poverty, overcrowding, homelessness, and inadequate health services. Medical factors include HIV and immunosuppression.

PROGNOSIS Prognosis varies widely and depends on treatment.[2]

Please refer to CD-ROM for full text and references.

Acute renal failure

Search date April 2002

John A Kellum, Martine Leblanc, and Ramesh Venkataraman

What are the effects of interventions to prevent acute renal failure in people at high risk?

BENEFICIAL

Low osmolality contrast media (better than standard)

One systematic review comparing low osmolality contrast media**G** versus standard contrast media has found that the development of acute renal failure or need for dialysis are rare events. However, nephrotoxicity (evaluated by serum creatinine) was less likely with low osmolality contrast media, especially in people with underlying renal impairments.

LIKELY TO BE BENEFICIAL

Fluids

We found no RCTs of fluids versus no intervention to prevent acute renal failure. However, dehydration is an important risk factor for acute renal failure and recommended volumes of fluid have little potential for harm. One RCT found that hydration with 0.9% sodium chloride intravenous infusion versus hydration with 0.45% sodium chloride intravenous infusion significantly reduced the incidence of contrast media associated nephropathy.

Single (better than multiple doses of aminoglycosides)

One RCT found that single daily dosing versus standard preparations and dosing of aminoglycosides significantly reduced nephrotoxicity**G**.

UNKNOWN EFFECTIVENESS

Acetylcysteine

One small RCT found limited evidence that acetylcysteine versus placebo significantly reduced the incidence of acute renal failure induced by contrast media.

Lipid formulations of amphotericin (better than standard formulations)

One RCT found limited evidence that lipid versus standard formulations of amphotericin may cause less nephrotoxicity. We found no evidence about the long term safety of lipid formulations of amphotericin**G**.

UNLIKELY TO BE BENEFICIAL

Mannitol

Small RCTs in people with traumatic rhabdomyolysis, or undergoing coronary artery bypass, vascular, or biliary tract surgery, found that mannitol versus hydration alone did not reduce acute renal failure. One RCT found that mannitol versus 0.9% sodium chloride infusion increased the risk of acute renal failure, but the difference was not significant.

Theophylline in acute renal failure induced by contrast media

RCTs found that theophylline versus placebo does not prevent acute renal failure induced by contrast media when people are adequately hydrated. ▶

Clin Evid Concise 2003;9:175–178.

LIKELY TO BE INEFFECTIVE OR HARMFUL

Calcium channel blockers for early allograft dysfunction

One large RCT found no significant difference with calcium channel blockers versus placebo in reducing graft dysfunction in renal transplantation. We found no RCTs of the effects of calcium channel blockers in other forms of acute renal failure.

Dopamine

One systematic review and one subsequent RCT have found that dopamine versus placebo does not prevent the onset of acute renal failure, the need for dialysis, or mortality.

Loop diuretics

One systematic review has found that loop diuretics versus fluids alone do not prevent acute renal failure. One RCT in people with acute tubular necrosis induced by contrast media found that diuretics versus 0.9% sodium chloride infusion significantly increased acute renal failure. Another RCT found that diuretics versus 0.9% sodium chloride infusion significantly increased acute renal failure after cardiac surgery.

Natriuretic peptides

One large RCT found no significant difference with natriuretic peptides versus placebo in the prevention of acute renal failure induced by contrast media. Subgroup analysis in another RCT found that atrial natriuretic peptide versus placebo reduced dialysis free survival in non-oliguric people.

What are the effects of treatments in critically ill people with acute renal failure?

LIKELY TO BE BENEFICIAL

Biocompatible dialysis membranes (better than non-biocompatible membranes)

Limited evidence from RCTs suggests that biocompatible**G** membranes versus non-biocompatible membranes reduce mortality.

High dose continuous replacement renal therapy (better than low dose)

One RCT found good evidence that high dose versus low dose continuous renal replacement therapy**G** (haemofiltration) significantly reduces mortality. One RCT found evidence that high dose haemofiltration reduced mortality compared to low dose haemofiltration in continuous renal replacement therapy. A small prospective study found that intensive (daily) intermittent haemodialysis reduced mortality in people with acute renal failure when compared to conventional alternate-day haemodialysis.

UNKNOWN EFFECTIVENESS

Continuous versus single intermittent renal replacement therapy

One systematic review of all prior randomised and observational studies comparing intermittent to continuous renal replacement therapies found no difference between therapies overall, but found a survival benefit with continuous renal replacement therapy when the analysis was restricted to the subgroup of studies that compared people with similar baseline severity of illness. Weaknesses of the included studies preclude a definitive conclusion.

Combined diuretics and albumin; continuous versus bolus diuretics

We found insufficient evidence on the effects of these interventions.

UNLIKELY TO BE BENEFICIAL

Fenoldopam

We found no systematic review or RCTs evaluating the effects of fenoldopam, but its use has been associated with hypotension.

Loop diuretics

RCTs in people with oliguric acute renal failure found no significant difference in renal recovery, number of days spent on dialysis, or mortality with loop diuretics versus placebo. Loop diuretics have been associated with ototoxicity and low renal perfusion.

LIKELY TO BE INEFFECTIVE OR HARMFUL

Dopamine

One systematic review has found no significant difference in mortality, onset of acute renal failure, or need for dialysis with dopamine versus control. One additional RCT found that low dose dopamine versus placebo did not reduce renal dysfunction. Dopamine has been associated with important adverse effects, including extravasation necrosis, gangrene, tachycardia, and conduction abnormalities.

Natriuretic peptides

RCTs have found no significant difference with atrial natriuretic peptide or ularitide (urodilantin) versus placebo in dialysis free survival in oliguric and non-oliguric people. One of the RCTs found that atrial natriuretic peptide may reduce survival in non-oliguric people.

DEFINITION Acute renal failure is characterised by abrupt and sustained decline in glomerular filtration rate Ⓖ,[1] which leads to accumulation of urea and other chemicals in the blood. There is no clear consensus on a biochemical definition,[2] but most studies define it as a serum creatinine of 2–3 mg/dL (200–250 μmol/L), an elevation of more than 0.5 mg/dL (45 μmol/L) over a baseline creatinine below 2 mg/dL (170 μmol/L) or a twofold increase of baseline creatinine. "Severe" acute renal failure has been defined as a serum concentration of creatinine above 5.5 mg/dL (500 μmol/L) or as requiring renal replacement therapy. Acute renal failure is usually classified according to the location of the predominant primary pathology (prerenal, intrarenal, and postrenal failure). People who are critically ill are those who are unstable and at imminent risk of death, which usually implies that they are people who need to be in, or have been admitted to, the intensive care unit.

INCIDENCE/PREVALENCE Two prospective observational studies (2576 people) have found that established acute renal failure affects nearly 5% of people in hospital and as many as 15% of critically ill people depending on the definitions used.[3,4]

AETIOLOGY/RISK FACTORS **For acute renal failure prevention:** Risk factors for acute renal failure that are consistent across multiple aetiologies include hypovolaemia, hypotension, sepsis, pre-existing renal, hepatic, or cardiac dysfunction, diabetes mellitus, and exposure to nephrotoxins (e.g. aminoglycosides, amphotericin, immunosuppressive agents, non-steroidal anti-inflammatory drugs, angiotensin converting enzyme inhibitors, intravenous contrast media) Ⓣ. Isolated episodes of acute renal failure are rarely seen in critically ill people, but are usually part of multiple organ dysfunction syndromes Ⓖ. Acute renal failure requiring dialysis is rarely seen in isolation (< 5% of people). The kidneys are often the first organs to fail.[5] In the perioperative setting, acute renal failure risk factors include prolonged aortic clamping, emergency rather than elective surgery, and use of higher volumes (> 100 mL) of intravenous contrast media. One study (3695 people) using multiple logistic regression identified these independent risk factors: baseline creatinine clearance below 47 mL/minute (OR 1.20, 95% CI

1.12 to 1.30), diabetes (OR 5.5, 95% CI 1.4 to 21.0), and identified a marginal effect for doses of contrast media above 100 mL (OR 1.01, 95% CI 1.00 to 1.01). The mortality rate of people with acute renal failure requiring dialysis was 36% during hospitalisation.[6] **For acute renal failure in critically ill people:** Prerenal acute renal failure Ⓖ is caused by reduced blood flow to the kidney from renal artery disease, systematic hypotension, or maldistribution of blood flow. Intrarenal acute renal failure Ⓖ is caused by parenchymal injury (acute tubular necrosis, interstitial nephritis, embolic disease, glomerulonephritis, vasculitis, or small vessel disease). Postrenal acute renal failure Ⓖ is caused by urinary tract obstruction. Observational studies (in several hundred people from Europe, North America, and West Africa with acute renal failure) found a prerenal cause in 40–80%, an intrarenal cause in 10–50%, and a postrenal cause in the remaining 10%.[7–11] Prerenal acute renal failure is the commonest type of acute renal failure in people who are critically ill,[7,12] but acute renal failure in this context is usually part of multisystem failure, and most frequently due to acute tubular necrosis resulting from ischaemic or nephrotoxic injury, or both.[13,14]

PROGNOSIS One retrospective study (1347 people with acute renal failure) found that mortality was less than 15% in people with isolated acute renal failure.[15] One recent prospective study (> 700 people) found that, in people with acute renal failure, overall mortality and the need for dialysis was higher in an intensive care unit than in a non-intensive care unit setting, despite no significant difference between the groups in mean maximal serum creatinine (need for dialysis 71% in intensive care unit *v* 18%; $P < 0.001$; mortality 72% in intensive care unit *v* 32%; $P = 0.001$).[16]

Please refer to CD-ROM for full text and references.

Benign prostatic hyperplasia

Search date March 2002

Clinical Evidence writers on benign prostatic hyperplasia

What are the effects of treatments?

BENEFICIAL

α Blockers

Systematic reviews and two subsequent RCTs have found that α blockers are more effective than placebo for improving lower urinary tract symptoms. Systematic reviews and subsequent RCTs found no significant differences among different α blockers. Two RCTs found limited evidence that α blockers were more effective in improving symptoms than 5α reductase inhibitors. We found no direct comparison of α blockers with surgical treatment.

5α Reductase inhibitors

One systematic review and one subsequent RCT have found that 5α reductase inhibitors are more effective than placebo for improving lower urinary tract symptoms and reducing complications in men with benign prostatic hyperplasia, especially in men with larger prostates. Two RCTs found limited evidence that 5α reductase inhibitors were less effective at improving symptoms than α blockers. We found no direct comparison of 5α reductase inhibitors with surgical treatment.

Saw palmetto plant extracts

One systematic review has found that self rated improvement is better in men taking saw palmetto compared with placebo. It found no significant difference in symptom scores between saw palmetto and finasteride.

Transurethral microwave thermotherapy

RCTs have found that transurethral microwave thermotherapy versus sham treatment significantly reduces symptoms. One systematic review and one RCT found limited evidence that transurethral resection relieved short term symptoms more than transurethral microwave thermotherapy. One RCT found limited evidence that transurethral microwave thermotherapy improved symptoms more than α blockers over 18 months.

Transurethral resection

We found limited evidence from two RCTs that transurethral resection was more effective than watchful waiting for improving symptoms and reducing complications, and did not increase the risk of erectile dysfunction or incontinence. One systematic review found greater symptom improvement with transurethral resection versus visual laser ablation, but transurethral resection was associated with a higher risk of blood transfusion.

LIKELY TO BE BENEFICIAL

β–sitosterol plant extract

One systematic review found that β–sitosterol plant extract versus placebo significantly improved lower urinary tract symptoms in the short term.

UNKNOWN EFFECTIVENESS

Rye grass pollen extract

One systematic review found limited evidence that rye grass pollen extract versus placebo increased self rated improvement and reduced nocturia in the short term. ▶

Clin Evid Concise 2003;9:179–180.

Transurethral resection versus less invasive surgical techniques

We found limited evidence from two RCTs that transurethral resection is more effective than watchful waiting for improving symptoms and reducing complications, and did not increase the risk of erectile dysfunction or incontinence. Two systematic reviews and subsequent RCTs found no significant differences between transurethral resection and transurethral incision or between transurethral resection and electrical vaporisation for symptoms. One systematic review found greater symptom improvement with transurethral resection versus visual laser ablation, but transurethral resection was associated with a higher risk of blood transfusion.

Transurethral resection versus transurethral needle ablation

We found limited evidence from one RCT that transurethral resection versus transurethral needle ablation reduced symptoms of benign prostatic hyperplasia, although transurethral needle ablation caused fewer adverse effects.

DEFINITION Benign prostatic hyperplasia is defined histologically. Clinically, it is characterised by lower urinary tract symptoms (urinary frequency, urgency, a weak and intermittent stream, needing to strain, a sense of incomplete emptying, and nocturia), and can lead to complications, including acute urinary retention.

INCIDENCE/ PREVALENCE Estimates of the prevalence of symptomatic benign prostatic hyperplasia range from 10–30% for men in their early 70s, depending on how benign prostatic hyperplasia is defined.[1]

AETIOLOGY/ RISK FACTORS The mechanisms by which benign prostatic hyperplasia causes symptoms and complications are unclear, although bladder outlet obstruction is an important factor.[2] The best documented risk factors are increasing age and functioning testes.[3]

PROGNOSIS Community and practice based studies suggest that men with lower urinary tract symptoms can expect slow progression of the symptoms.[4,5] However, symptoms can wax and wane without treatment. In men with symptoms of benign prostatic hyperplasia, rates of acute urinary retention range from 1–2% a year.[5–7]

Please refer to CD-ROM for full text and references.

Chronic prostatitis

Search date June 2002

Jeffrey Stern and Anthony Schaeffer

What are the effects of treatments for chronic bacterial prostatitis?

LIKELY TO BE BENEFICIAL

α Blockers (when added to antimicrobials)

We found limited evidence from one RCT suggesting that adding α blockers to antimicrobials versus antimicrobials alone may significantly improve symptoms and reduce recurrence.

UNKNOWN EFFECTIVENESS

Oral antimicrobial drugs

We found no RCTs of the effects of oral antimicrobial drugs. Retrospective cohort studies report cure rates of 0–88% depending on the drug used and the duration of treatment.

Local injection of antimicrobials; radical prostatectomy; transurethral resection

We found no RCTs on the effects of these interventions.

What are the effects of treatments for chronic abacterial prostatitis?

UNKNOWN EFFECTIVENESS

Allopurinol

One systematic review found limited evidence from one small RCT that allopurinol versus placebo significantly improved symptoms over about 8 months.

Anti-inflammatory medications (pentosan polysulfate sodium)

One RCT found no significant difference with pentosan polysulfate sodium versus placebo in symptoms, but the RCT may have been too small to rule out a clinically important difference.

α Blockers

One systematic review found limited evidence suggesting that α blockers versus placebo may significantly improve maximal flow time and pain.

5α-Reductase inhibitors

One systematic review of one small RCT found insufficient evidence on the effects of 5α reductase inhibitors.

Transurethral microwave thermotherapy

One systematic review found limited evidence from one RCT suggesting that transurethral microwave thermotherapy versus sham treatment may significantly improve quality of life at 3 months and symptoms over 21 months (NNT 2 for symptom improvement, 95% CI 2 to 6).

Biofeedback; prostatic massage; Sitz bath

We found no good evidence on these interventions.

Chronic prostatitis

DEFINITION **Chronic bacterial prostatitis** is characterised by a positive culture of expressed prostatic secretions. It can be symptomatic (recurrent urinary tract infection, or suprapubic, lower back, or perineal pain), asymptomatic, or associated with minimal urgency, frequency, and dysuria. **Chronic abacterial prostatitis** is characterised by pelvic or perineal pain, often associated with urinary urgency, nocturia, weak urinary stream, frequency, dysuria, hesitancy, dribbling after micturition, interrupted flow, and inflammation (white cells) in prostatic secretions. Symptoms can also include suprapubic, scrotal, testicular, penile, or lower back pain or discomfort, known as prostodynia in the absence of inflammation in prostatic secretions.

INCIDENCE/ PREVALENCE One US community based study (58 955 visits by men ≥ 18 years of age to office based physicians) estimated that 9% of men have a diagnosis of chronic prostatitis at any one time.[1] Another study found that, of men with genitourinary symptoms, 8% presenting to urologists and 1% presenting to primary care physicians are diagnosed with chronic prostatitis.[2] Most cases of chronic prostatitis are abacterial. Acute bacterial prostatitis, although easy to diagnose and treat, is rare.

AETIOLOGY/ RISK FACTORS Organisms commonly implicated in bacterial prostatitis include *Escherichia coli*, other Gram negative *Enterobacteriaceae*, occasionally *Pseudomonas* species, and rarely Gram positive enterococci. The cause of abacterial prostatitis is unclear, but autoimmunity could be involved.[3]

PROGNOSIS One recent study found that chronic abacterial prostatitis had an impact on quality of life similar to that from angina, Crohn's disease, or a previous myocardial infarction.[4]

Please refer to CD-ROM for full text and references.

Erectile dysfunction

Search date April 2002

Clinical Evidence freelance writers

What are the effects of treatments?

BENEFICIAL

Intracavernosal alprostadil

One large RCT found that intracavernosal alprostadil versus placebo significantly increased the chance of a satisfactory erection.

Intraurethral alprostadil (in men who had responded to a single test dose)

One large RCT (in men who had previously responded to alprostadil) found limited evidence that intraurethral alprostadil (prostaglandin E1) significantly increased the chances of successful sexual intercourse and at least one orgasm over 3 months. About a third of men suffered penile ache. We found no direct comparisons of intraurethral alprostadil with either intracavernosal alprostadil or oral drug treatments.

Sildenafil

One systematic review has found that sildenafil versus placebo significantly increases the number of men reporting improved erection and successful intercourse. Additional RCTs have found similar results. We found no RCTs directly comparing sildenafil versus other treatments. Adverse effects, including headaches, flushing, and dyspepsia are reported in up to a quarter of men. Deaths have been reported in men on concomitant treatment with oral nitrates.

Yohimbine

One systematic review has found that yohimbine versus placebo significantly improves self reported sexual function and penile rigidity at 2–10 weeks. We found no RCTs directly comparing yohimbine versus other treatments. Transient adverse effects are reported in up to a third of men.

UNKNOWN EFFECTIVENESS

L-arginine

One small RCT found no significant difference in sexual function with L-arginine versus placebo, but it may have been too small to exclude a clinically important difference.

Penile prostheses; vacuum devices

We found insufficient evidence on the effects of penile prostheses and vacuum devices.

Topical alprostadil

Two quasi randomised trials found limited evidence that topical alprostadil versus placebo increased the number of men with erections sufficient for intercourse.

Trazodone

One small RCT found no significant difference in erections or libido with trazodone versus placebo, but it may have been too small to exclude a clinically important difference.

Clin Evid Concise 2003;9:183–184.

Erectile dysfunction

DEFINITION Erectile dysfunction has largely replaced the term "impotence". It is defined as the persistent inability to obtain or maintain sufficient rigidity of the penis to allow satisfactory sexual performance.

INCIDENCE/ PREVALENCE We found little good epidemiological information, but current normative data suggest that age is the variable most strongly associated with erectile dysfunction, and that up to 30 million men in the USA may be affected.[1] Even among men in their 40s, nearly 40% report at least occasional difficulty obtaining or maintaining erection, whereas this approaches 70% in 70 year olds.

AETIOLOGY/ RISK FACTORS It is now believed that about 80% of cases of erectile dysfunction have an organic cause, the rest being psychogenic in origin. Risk factors include increasing age, smoking, and obesity. Erectile problems fall into three categories: failure to initiate; failure to fill, caused by insufficient arterial inflow into the penis to allow engorgement and tumescence because of vascular insufficiency; and failure to store because of veno-occlusive dysfunction.

PROGNOSIS We found no good evidence on prognosis in untreated organic erectile dysfunction.

Please refer to CD-ROM for full text and references.

Prostate cancer (metastatic)

Search date January 2002

M Dror Michaelson, James A Talcott, and Matthew R Smith

What are the effects of treatments in men with metastatic prostate cancer?

LIKELY TO BE BENEFICIAL

Androgen deprivation

We found limited evidence from RCTs suggesting that androgen deprivation versus no initial treatment reduced mortality. One systematic review and one subsequent RCT found no evidence of a difference between different types of androgen deprivation (orchidectomy**G**, diethylstilbestrol, and luteinising hormone releasing hormone agonists).

Combined androgen blockade (androgen deprivation and non-steroidal antiandrogen) compared with androgen deprivation alone

Inconclusive evidence from four systematic reviews suggests that there could be a 2–5% improvement in 5 year survival associated with combined androgen blockade (androgen deprivation plus a non-steroidal antiandrogen) versus androgen deprivation alone.

UNKNOWN EFFECTIVENESS

Intermittent androgen deprivation

We found no RCTs assessing the long term effects of intermittent versus continuous androgen deprivation on mortality, morbidity, or quality of life.

LIKELY TO BE INEFFECTIVE OR HARMFUL

Deferred androgen deprivation

One small RCT found that immediate androgen deprivation versus deferring androgen deprivation until disease progression becomes apparent in men with stage D1 prostate cancer after radical prostectomy significantly increased overall survival after a median of 7 years. Subgroup analysis from a larger RCT, without formal surveillance criteria, found no significant difference in survival after about 10 years. This RCT also found that deferred androgen deprivation resulted in higher rates of complications.

What are the effects of treatments in men with symptomatic androgen independent metastatic disease?

LIKELY TO BE BENEFICIAL

Chemotherapy (palliation but no evidence of an effect on survival)

RCTs have found that chemotherapy plus corticosteroids versus corticosteroids alone reduces pain, lengthens palliation, and improves quality of life, but found no improvement in overall survival.

External beam radiation (palliation but no evidence of an effect on survival)

We found no RCTs comparing external beam radiation versus palliative treatments other than radionuclides. Observational evidence suggests complete pain relief in about a quarter of people, and placebo controlled RCTs would probably be considered unethical. A systematic review of one RCT in men with symptomatic ▶

bone metastases found no significant difference in survival between external beam radiation versus strontium-89; however, strontium-89 was associated with significantly fewer new sites of pain, and reduced need for additional radiotherapy.

Radionuclides (palliation but no clear evidence of an effect on survival)

One systematic review found one small RCT in men with symptomatic bone metastases, which found no significant difference in survival between external beam radiation plus placebo versus external beam radiation plus strontium-89. However, strontium-89 significantly reduced the number of new sites of pain. A second RCT in men with symptomatic bone metastases found no significant difference in survival between external beam radiation versus strontium-89; however, strontium-89 was associated with significantly fewer new sites of pain, and reduced need for additional radiotherapy. One small subsequent RCT in men with painful bone metastases found that samarium-153 versus placebo significantly reduced pain scores. A second small subsequent RCT in a selected population found an improvement in survival with strontium-89 versus placebo, but the results are difficult to generalise.

UNKNOWN EFFECTIVENESS

Bisphosphonates

One systematic review of two poor quality RCTs found insufficient evidence about the effects of bisphosphonates.

DEFINITION See prostate cancer (non-metastatic), p 188. Androgen independent metastatic disease is defined as disease that progresses despite androgen deprivation.

INCIDENCE/ PREVALENCE See prostate cancer (non-metastatic), p 188.

AETIOLOGY/ RISK FACTORS See prostate cancer (non-metastatic), p 188.

PROGNOSIS Prostate cancer metastasises predominantly to bone. Metastatic prostate cancer can result in pain, weakness, paralysis, and death.

Please refer to CD-ROM for full text and references.

Prostate cancer (non-metastatic)

Search date June 2002

Timothy Wilt

What are the effects of treatments for clinically localised prostate cancer?

UNKNOWN EFFECTIVENESS

Androgen suppression

We found no RCTs assessing the effects of primary treatment with early androgen suppression**G** in the absence of symptoms on length or quality of life in men with clinically localised prostate cancer. One RCT found limited evidence that androgen suppression with bicalutamide reduced disease progression after a median of 2.6 years compared with placebo, but interpreting the results was difficult because men with prostate cancer of different stages were included in the trial.

External beam radiation

We found no RCTs comparing external beam radiation versus watchful waiting. One small RCT found limited evidence that external beam radiation increased the risk of metastases compared with radical prostatectomy**G**.

Radical prostatectomy

One small RCT found no significant difference in survival between radical prostatectomy and watchful waiting. One RCT found limited evidence that radical prostatectomy reduced the risk of metastases compared with external beam radiation. Radical prostatectomy carries the risks of major surgery and of sexual and urinary dysfunction.

Watchful waiting

One small RCT found no significant difference in survival between radical prostatectomy and watchful waiting. We found no information from RCTs on quality of life.

Androgen suppression in asymptomatic men with raised prostate specific antigen concentrations after early treatment; brachytherapyG; cryosurgery

We found no RCTs on the effects of these interventions.

What are the effects of treatments for locally advanced prostate cancer?

BENEFICIAL

Early androgen suppression in addition to external beam radiation (improves survival compared with radiation and deferred androgen suppression)

One systematic review in men with locally advanced disease treated with radiotherapy has found that immediate androgen suppression increases survival at 5 years compared with deferred androgen suppression. One RCT found no significant difference in overall survival or local disease control after orchidectomy, whether or not it was combined with radiotherapy, but the results are difficult to interpret.

Clin Evid Concise 2003;9:187–189.

Prostate cancer (non-metastatic)

LIKELY TO BE BENEFICIAL

Androgen suppression initiated at diagnosis

RCTs found limited evidence that androgen suppression initiated at diagnosis compared with no initial treatment or deferred androgen suppression may improve long term survival (generally about 10 years). One RCT found limited evidence that immediate androgen suppression reduced complications compared with deferred androgen suppression.

Immediate androgen suppression after radical prostatectomy and pelvic lymphadenectomy in men with node-positive prostate cancer (compared with radical prostatectomy and deferred androgen suppression)

One RCT in men with node positive prostate cancer has found that immediate androgen suppression compared with deferred androgen suppression after radical prostatectomy and pelvic lymphadenectomy reduces mortality over a median of 7.1 years, and reduces the risk of a detectable prostate specific antigen.

DEFINITION Prostatic cancer is staged according to two systems: the tumour, node, metastasis (TMN) classification system and the American urologic staging system**T**. Non-metastatic prostate cancer can be divided into clinically localised disease and locally advanced disease. Clinically localised disease is prostate cancer thought, after clinical examination, to be confined to the prostate gland. Locally advanced disease is prostate cancer that has spread outside the capsule of the prostate gland but has not yet spread to other organs. Metastatic disease is prostate cancer that has spread outside the prostate gland to either local, regional, or systemic lymph nodes, seminal vesicles, or to other body organs (e.g. bone, liver, brain) and is not connected to the prostate gland. We consider clinically localised and locally advanced disease here. Metastatic disease is covered in a separate chapter (see metastatic prostate cancer, p 185).

INCIDENCE/ PREVALENCE Prostate cancer is the most common non-dermatological malignancy worldwide and is the second most common cause of cancer death in men in the USA.[1] There were an estimated 180 400 new cases and 31 900 deaths in the USA in 2000.[2] Autopsy data from the 1980s found microscopic prostate cancer in about 42% of men aged 75 years.[3] These data suggest that the risk of clinically evident prostate cancer is about 10%, and that of fatal prostate cancer is 3%.[3]

AETIOLOGY/ RISK FACTORS Risk factors for prostate cancer include age, family history of prostate cancer, black race, and possibly higher dietary consumption of fat and meat, low intake of lycopene (from tomato products), low intake of fruit, and high dietary calcium. In the USA, black men have about a 60% higher incidence than white men.[4] The prostate cancer incidence for black men living in the USA is about 90/100 000 in men aged less than 65 years and about 1300/100 000 in men aged 65–74 years. For white men, incidence is about 44/100 000 in men aged less than 65 years and 900/100 000 in men aged 65–74 years.[4]

PROGNOSIS The chance that men with well to moderately differentiated, palpable, clinically localised prostate cancer will remain free of symptomatic progression is 70% at 5 years and 40% at 10 years.[5] The risk of symptomatic disease progression is higher in men with poorly differentiated prostate cancer.[6] One retrospective analysis of a large surgical series in men with clinically localised prostate cancer found that the median time from the increase in prostate specific antigen (PSA) concentration to the development of metastatic disease was 8 years.[7] Time to PSA progression, PSA doubling time, and Gleason score**G** were predictive of the probability and time to development of metastatic disease. Once men developed metastatic disease, the median actuarial time to death was

5 years.[7] Morbidity from local or regional disease progression includes haematuria, bladder obstruction, and lower extremity oedema. In the USA, population based studies found that death rates from prostate cancer have declined by only about 1/100 000 men since 1992, despite widespread testing for PSA and increased rates of radical prostatectomy and radiotherapy.[8,9] Regions of the USA with the greatest decreases in mortality are those with the lowest rates of testing for PSA and treatment with radical prostatectomy or radiation.[9] Countries with low rates of testing and treatment do not have consistently higher age adjusted rates of death from prostate cancer than countries with high rates of testing and treatment such as the USA.

Please refer to CD-ROM for full text and references.

Anorexia nervosa

Search date August 2002

Janet Treasure and Ulrike Schmidt

What are the effects of treatments?

UNKNOWN EFFECTIVENESS

Inpatient versus outpatient treatment setting (in people not so severely ill as to warrant emergency intervention)

Limited evidence from one small RCT found that outpatient treatment was as effective as inpatient treatment**G** in increasing weight and improving Morgan Russell scale**G** global scores at 1, 2, and 5 years in people who did not need emergency intervention.

Oestrogen treatment (for prevention of fractures)

We found no good evidence about the effects of hormonal treatment on fracture rates in people with anorexia. One small RCT found no significant effect of oestrogen versus no treatment on bone mineral density in people with anorexia.

Psychotherapies

We found insufficient evidence from small RCTs to compare psychotherapies**G** versus dietary counselling**G** or versus each other. One small RCT found limited evidence that focal analytical therapy or family therapy**G** versus usual treatment significantly increased the number of people recovered or improved as assessed by the Morgan Russell scale at 1 year.

Selective serotonin reuptake inhibitors (fluoxetine)

We found insufficient evidence from two small RCTs to compare fluoxetine versus placebo in people with anorexia.

Zinc

One small RCT found limited evidence that zinc may improve daily body mass index**G** gain compared with placebo in people managed in an inpatient setting. However, we were unable to draw firm conclusions.

LIKELY TO BE INEFFECTIVE OR HARMFUL

Cisapride

One small RCT found no significant difference with cisapride versus placebo in weight gain at 8 weeks. Cisapride has now been restricted in many countries because of concerns about cardiac irregularities, including ventricular tachycardia, torsades de pointes, and sudden death.

Cyproheptadine

Three small RCTs found no significant difference with cyproheptadine versus placebo in weight gain.

Neuroleptic drugs that increase the QT interval

We found no RCTs. The QT interval may be prolonged in people with anorexia nervosa, and many neuroleptic drugs (haloperidol, pimozide, sertindole, thioridazine, chlorpromazine, and others) also increase the QT interval. Prolongation of the QT interval may be associated with increased risk of ventricular tachycardia, torsades de pointes, and sudden death.

Tricyclic antidepressants

Two small RCTs found no evidence of benefit with amitriptyline compared with placebo. They found that amitriptyline was associated with more adverse effects, such as palpitations, dry mouth, and blurred vision.

Clin Evid Concise 2003;9:190–192.

DEFINITION Anorexia nervosa is characterised by a refusal to maintain weight at or above a minimally normal weight (< 85% of expected weight for age and height, or body mass index**G** < 17.5 kg/m^2), or a failure to show the expected weight gain during growth. In association with this, there is often an intense fear of gaining weight, preoccupation with weight, denial of the current low weight and its adverse impact on health, and amenorrhoea. Two subtypes of anorexia nervosa, binge–purge and restricting, have been defined.[1]

INCIDENCE/ PREVALENCE A mean incidence in the general population of 19/100 000 a year in females and 2/100 000 a year in males has been estimated from 12 cumulative studies.[2] The highest rate was in female teenagers (age 13–19 years), where there were 50.8 cases/100 000 a year. A large cohort study of Swedish school children (4291 people, aged 16 years) were screened by weighing and subsequent interview, and the prevalence of anorexia nervosa cases (defined using DSM-III and DSM-III-R criteria) was found to be 7/1000 for girls and 1/1000 for boys.[3] Little is known of the incidence or prevalence in Asia, South America, or Africa.

AETIOLOGY/ RISK FACTORS Anorexia nervosa has been related to family, biological, social, and cultural factors.[4] Studies have found that anorexia nervosa is associated with a family history of anorexia nervosa (HR 11.4, 95% CI 1.1 to 89.0), of bulimia nervosa (adjusted HR 3.5, 95% CI 1.1 to 14.0),[5] depression, generalised anxiety disorder, obsessive compulsive disorder, or obsessive compulsive personality disorder (adjusted RR 3.6, 95% CI 1.6 to 8.0).[6] A twin study suggested that anorexia nervosa may be related to genetic factors but it was unable to estimate reliably the contribution of non-shared environmental factors. Specific aspects of childhood temperament thought to be related include perfectionism, negative self evaluation, and extreme compliance.[7] Perinatal factors include prematurity (OR 3.2, 95% CI 1.6 to 6.2), particularly if the baby was small for gestational age (OR 5.7, 95% CI 1.4 to 4.1).

PROGNOSIS One prospective study followed up 51 people with teenage-onset anorexia nervosa, about half of whom received no or minimal treatment (< 8 sessions). After 10 years, 14/51 people (27%) had a persistent eating disorder, three (6%) had ongoing anorexia nervosa, and six (12%) had experienced a period of bulimia nervosa. People with anorexia nervosa were significantly more likely to have an affective disorder than controls matched for sex, age, and school (lifetime risk of affective disorder 96% in people with anorexia *v* 23% with controls, ARI 73%, 95% CI 60% to 85%). Obsessive compulsive disorder was, similarly, significantly more likely in people with anorexia nervosa compared with controls (ARI 10%, 95% CI 10% to 41%). However, in 35% of people with obsessive compulsive disorder and anorexia nervosa, obsessive compulsive disorder preceded the anorexia. About half of all participants continued to have poor psychosocial functioning at 10 years (assessed using the Morgan Russell scale and Global Assessment of Functioning Scale).[8] A summary of treatment studies (68 studies published between 1953 and 1989, 3104 people, length of follow up 1–33 years) found that 43% of people recover completely (range 7–86%), 36% improve (range 1–69%), 20% develop a chronic eating disorder (range 0–43%), and 5% die from anorexia nervosa (range 0–21%).[9] Favourable prognostic factors include an early age at onset and a short interval between onset of symptoms and the beginning of treatment. Unfavourable prognostic factors include vomiting, bulimia, profound weight loss, chronicity, and a history of premorbid developmental or clinical abnormalities. The all cause standardised mortality ratio of eating disorders (anorexia nervosa and bulimia nervosa) has been estimated at 538, about three times higher than other psychiatric illnesses.[10] The average annual risk of mortality was 0.59% a year in females in

10 eating disorder populations (1322 people) with a minimum follow up of 6 years.[11] The mortality risk was higher for people with lower weight and with older age at presentation. Young women with anorexia nervosa are at an increased risk of fractures later in life.[12]

Please refer to CD-ROM for full text and references.

Bulimia nervosa

Search date April 2002

Phillipa Hay and Josue Bacaltchuk

What are the effects of treatments?

LIKELY TO BE BENEFICIAL

Antidepressant medication (tricyclic antidepressants, monoamine oxidase inhibitors, and fluoxetine)

Systematic reviews and one subsequent RCT have found short term reduction in bulimic symptoms (significant for vomiting only in the subsequent RCT) and a small reduction in depressive symptoms with tricyclic and monoamine oxidase inhibitor antidepressants. One systematic review and one subsequent RCT found that fluoxetine versus placebo significantly reduces bulimic symptoms in the short term.

Cognitive behavioural therapy

Systematic reviews have found that cognitive behavioural therapy**G** versus remaining on a waiting list significantly reduces specific symptoms of bulimia nervosa**G** (binge eating**G**, purging, disturbed eating patterns), and improves non-specific symptoms such as depression. One review and subsequent RCTs found no clear benefit from cognitive behavioural therapy versus other psychotherapies.

Combination treatment with an antidepressant and psychotherapy

One systematic review has found that combination treatment (antidepressants plus psychotherapy) versus antidepressants alone reduces binge frequency and depressive symptoms but found no significant effect on remission rates. It has also found that combination treatment versus psychotherapy alone improves short term remission from binge eating and depressive symptoms but has no significant effect on binge eating frequency.

Other psychotherapies

One systematic review and one subsequent RCT have found that non-cognitive behavioural psychotherapy versus being on a waiting list significantly improves the symptoms of bulimia nervosa.

UNKNOWN EFFECTIVENESS

Antidepressants as maintenance

We found insufficient evidence to assess the effects of antidepresssants for maintenance.

Other antidepressants (venlafaxine, mirtazapine, and reboxetine)

We found no RCTs on the effects of venlafaxine, mirtazapine, and reboxetine.

Selective serotonin reuptake inhibitors (other than fluoxetine)

We found no good evidence on selective serotonin reuptake inhibitors other than fluoxetine.

Bulimia nervosa

DEFINITION Bulimia nervosa is an intense preoccupation with body weight and shape, with regular episodes of uncontrolled overeating of large amounts of food (binge eating) associated with use of extreme methods to counteract the feared effects of overeating. If a person also meets the diagnostic criteria for anorexia nervosa, then the diagnosis of anorexia nervosa takes precedence.[1] Bulimia nervosa can be difficult to identify because of extreme secrecy about binge eating and purgative behaviour. Weight may be normal but there is often a history of anorexia nervosa or restrictive dieting. Some people alternate between anorexia nervosa and bulimia nervosa.

INCIDENCE/ PREVALENCE In community based studies, the prevalence of bulimia nervosa is between 0.5% and 1.0% in young women, with an even social class distribution.[2–4] About 90% of people diagnosed with bulimia nervosa are women. The numbers presenting with bulimia nervosa in industrialised countries increased during the decade that followed its recognition in the late 1970s and "a cohort effect" is reported in community surveys,[2,5,6] implying an increase in incidence. The prevalence of eating disorders such as bulimia nervosa is lower in non-industrialised populations[7] and varies across ethnic groups. African-American women have a lower rate of restrictive dieting than white American women, but have a similar rate of recurrent binge eating.[8]

AETIOLOGY/ RISK FACTORS Young women from the developed world who restrict their dietary intake are at greatest risk of developing bulimia nervosa and other eating disorders. One community based case control study compared 102 people with bulimia nervosa with 204 healthy controls and found higher rates of the following in people with the eating disorder: obesity, mood disorder, sexual and physical abuse, parental obesity, substance misuse, low self esteem, perfectionism, disturbed family dynamics, parental weight/shape concern, and early menarche.[9] Compared with a control group of 102 women who had other psychiatric disorders, women with bulimia nervosa had higher rates of parental problems and obesity.

PROGNOSIS A 10 year follow up study (50 people with bulimia nervosa from a former trial of mianserin treatment) found that 52% had fully recovered, and only 9% continued to experience full symptoms of bulimia nervosa.[10] A larger study (222 people from a trial of antidepressants and structured, intensive group psychotherapy, 101 of whom were from a controlled trial of imipramine and a structure intensive cognitive behavioural group psychotherapy) found that, after a mean follow up of 11.5 years, 11% still met criteria for bulimia nervosa, whereas 70% were in full or partial remission.[11] For the people from the controlled trial, being in either the imipramine, psychotherapy plus imipramine, or psychotherapy plus placebo groups, versus the placebo only group, was associated with significantly better psychosocial adjustment, but not bulimic symptoms, at follow up. Short term studies found similar results: about 50% of people made a full recovery, 30% made a partial recovery, and 20% continued to be symptomatic.[12] There are few consistent predictors of longer term outcome. Good prognosis has been associated with shorter illness duration, a younger age of onset, higher social class, and a family history of alcohol abuse.[10] Poor prognosis has been associated with a history of substance misuse,[13] premorbid and paternal obesity,[14] and, in some studies, personality disorder.[15–18] One study (102 people) of the natural course of bulimia nervosa found that 31% still had the disorder at 15 months and 15% at 5 years.[19] Only 28% received treatment during the follow up period. In an evaluation of response to cognitive behavioural therapy, early progress (by session 6) best predicted outcome.[20] A subsequent systematic review of the outcome literature found no consistent evidence to support early intervention and a better prognosis.[21]

Please refer to CD-ROM for full text and references.

Dementia

Search date October 2002

James Warner, Rob Butler, and Pramod Prabhakaran

What are the effects of treatments on cognitive symptoms of dementia?

People in dementia RCTs are often not representative of people in routine settings. Few RCTs are conducted in primary care and few are conducted in people with types of dementia other than Alzheimer's disease.

BENEFICIAL

Donepezil

One systematic review and two subsequent RCTs have found that, compared with placebo, donepezil improves cognitive function and global clinical state at up to 52 weeks in people with mild to moderate Alzheimer's disease. The review found no significant difference in patient rated quality of life at 12 or 24 weeks between donepezil and placebo. One RCT in people with mild to moderate Alzheimer's disease found no significant difference in cognitive function at 12 weeks between donepezil and rivastigmine, although significantly fewer people taking donepezil withdrew from the trial for any cause.

Galantamine

RCTs identified by a systematic review, and one additional RCT, have found that galantamine improves cognitive function compared with placebo in people with Alzheimer's disease or vascular dementia.

LIKELY TO BE BENEFICIAL

Ginkgo biloba

RCTs found limited evidence that ginkgo biloba improved cognitive function compared with placebo in people with Alzheimer's disease.

Oestrogen (in women)

One systematic review has found that, in women with mild to moderate Alzheimer's disease, oestrogen improves cognition over 7–12 months treatment compared with no oestrogen.

Reality orientation

One systematic review of small RCTs found that reality orientation**G** improved cognitive function compared with no treatment in people with various types of dementia.

Selegiline

One systematic review has found that, in people with mild to moderate Alzheimer's disease, selegiline improves cognitive function, behavioural disturbance, and mood compared with placebo, but has found no significant difference in global clinical state.

TRADE OFF BETWEEN BENEFITS AND HARMS

Physostigmine

One systematic review in people with Alzheimer's disease found limited evidence that slow release physostigmine improved cognitive function compared with placebo, but adverse effects, including nausea, vomiting, diarrhoea, dizziness, and stomach pain, were common.

Rivastigmine

One systematic review and one additional RCT have found that rivastigmine improves cognitive function compared with placebo in people with Alzheimers disease or Lewy body dementia, but adverse effects such as nausea, vomiting, and anorexia are common. Subgroup analysis from one RCT in people with Alzheimer's disease suggests that people with vascular risk factors may respond better to rivastigmine than those without. One RCT in people with mild to moderate Alzheimer's disease found no significant difference in cognitive function at 12 weeks between donepezil and rivastigmine, although rivastigmine significantly increased the proportion of people who withdrew from the trial for any cause.

UNKNOWN EFFECTIVENESS

Lecithin

Small, poor RCTs identified by a systematic review provided insufficient evidence to assess lecithin in people with Alzheimer's disease.

Music therapy

Poor studies identified by a systematic review provided insufficient evidence to assess music therapy.

Nicotine

One systematic review found no RCTs of adequate quality on the effects of nicotine.

Non-steroidal anti-inflammatory drugs

One RCT in people with Alzheimer's disease found no significant difference in cognitive function after 25 weeks' treatment with diclofenac plus misoprostol compared with placebo. Another RCT in people with Alzheimer's disease found that indometacin (indomethacin) improved cognitive function after 6 months' treatment compared with placebo.

Reminiscence therapy

One systematic review provided insufficient evidence to assess reminiscence therapy**G**.

Tacrine

Systematic reviews found limited evidence that tacrine improved cognitive function and global state in Alzheimer's disease compared with placebo, but adverse effects, including nausea and vomiting, diarrhoea, anorexia, and abdominal pain, were common.

Vitamin E

One RCT in people with moderate to severe Alzheimer's disease found no significant difference in cognitive function after 2 years' treatment with vitamin E compared with placebo. However, it found that vitamin E reduced mortality, institutionalisation, loss of ability to perform activities of daily living, and the proportion of people who developed severe dementia.

What are the effects of treatments on behavioural and psychological symptoms of dementia?

LIKELY TO BE BENEFICIAL

Carbamazepine

One RCT found that carbamazepine reduced agitation and aggression compared with placebo in people with various types of dementia.

Olanzapine

One RCT in people with Alzheimer's disease found that olanzapine (5–10 mg daily) reduced agitation, hallucinations, and delusions compared with placebo.

Reality orientation

One systematic review of small RCTs found that reality orientation significantly improved behaviour compared with no treatment in people with various types of dementia.

Risperidone

One RCT in people with moderate to severe dementia, including Alzheimer's disease and vascular dementia, found that risperidone significantly improved behavioural and psychological symptoms over 12 weeks compared with placebo, but another RCT in people with severe dementia and agitation found no significant difference in symptoms over 13 weeks.

UNKNOWN EFFECTIVENESS

Cholinesterase inhibitors

One RCT in people with mild to moderate Alzheimer's disease found no significant difference in psychiatric symptoms at 3 months between galantamine and placebo, but another RCT found that galantamine significantly improved psychiatric symptoms at 6 months compared with placebo. One RCT in people with moderate to severe Alzheimer's disease found that donepezil significantly improved functional and behavioural symptoms at 24 weeks compared with placebo, but another RCT in people with mild to moderate Alzheimer's disease found no significant difference in psychiatric symptoms at 24 weeks between donepezil and placebo.

Haloperidol

One systematic review in people with various types of dementia found no significant difference in agitation between haloperidol and placebo, but found limited evidence that haloperidol may reduce aggression.

Sodium valproate

One RCT found that sodium valproate reduced agitation over 6 weeks in people with dementia, but another RCT found no significant difference in aggressive behaviour over 8 weeks between sodium valproate and placebo.

Trazodone

One RCT in people with Alzheimer's disease found no significant difference between trazodone and haloperidol in reducing agitation. Another RCT in people with dementia and agitated behaviour found no significant difference in agitation among trazodone, haloperidol, behavioural management techniques, and placebo. The RCTs may have been too small to exclude a clinically important difference.

DEFINITION **Dementia** is characterised by chronic, global, non-reversible impairment of cerebral function. It usually results in loss of memory (initially of recent events), loss of executive function (such as the ability to make decisions or sequence complex tasks), and changes in personality. **Alzheimer's disease** is a type of dementia characterised by an insidious onset and slow deterioration, and involves speech, motor, personality, and executive function impairment. It should be diagnosed after other systemic, psychiatric, and neurological causes of dementia have been excluded clinically and by laboratory investigation. **Vascular dementia** is multi-infarct dementia involving a stepwise deterioration of executive function with or without language and motor dysfunction occurring as a result of cerebral arterial occlusion. It usually occurs in the presence of vascular risk factors (diabetes, hypertension, and smoking). Characteristically, it has a more sudden onset and stepwise progression than Alzheimer's disease. **Lewy body dementia** is a type of dementia involving insidious impairment of executive functions with (1) Parkinsonism, (2) visual hallucinations, and (3) fluctuating cognitive abilities and increased risk of falls or autonomic failure.[1,2] Careful clinical examination of people with mild to moderate dementia, and the use of established diagnostic criteria, has an antemortem positive predictive value of 70–90% compared with the gold standard of postmortem diagnosis.[3,4]

INCIDENCE/ PREVALENCE About 6% of people aged over 65 years and 30% of people aged over 90 years have some form of dementia.[5] Dementia is rare before the age of 60 years. The most common types of dementia are Alzheimer's disease, vascular dementia, mixed vascular and Alzheimer's disease, and Lewy body dementia. Alzheimer's disease and vascular dementia (including mixed dementia) are each estimated to account for 35–50% of dementia, and Lewy body dementia is estimated to account for up to 20% of dementia in the elderly, varying with geographical, cultural, and racial factors.[1,5–10]

AETIOLOGY/ RISK FACTORS **Alzheimer's disease:** The cause of Alzheimer's disease is unclear. A key pathological process is deposition of abnormal amyloid in the central nervous system.[11] Most people with the relatively rare condition of early onset Alzheimer's disease (before age 60 years) show an autosomal dominant inheritance due to mutations on presenelin or amyloid precursor protein genes. Several genes (*APP*, *PS-1*, and *PS-2*) have been identified. Later onset dementia is sometimes clustered in families, but specific gene mutations have not been identified. Head injury, Down's syndrome, and lower premorbid intellect may be risk factors for Alzheimer's disease. **Vascular dementia** is related to cardiovascular risk factors, such as smoking, hypertension, and diabetes. **Lewy body dementia:** The aetiology of Lewy body dementia is unknown. Brain acetylcholine activity is reduced in many forms of dementia, and the level of reduction correlates with cognitive impairment. Many treatments for Alzheimer's disease enhance cholinergic activity.[1,6]

PROGNOSIS **Alzheimer's disease:** Alzheimer's disease usually has an insidious onset with progressive reduction in cerebral function. Diagnosis is difficult in the early stages. Average life expectancy after diagnosis is 7–10 years.[10] **Lewy body dementia:** People with Lewy body dementia have an average life expectancy of around 6 years after diagnosis.[5] Behavioural problems, depression, and psychotic symptoms are common in all types of dementia.[12,13] Eventually, most people with dementia find it difficult to perform simple tasks without help.

Please refer to CD-ROM for full text and references.

Depressive disorders

Search date July 2002

John Geddes, Rob Butler, and Simon Hatcher

What are the effects of treatments?

We found no reliable direct evidence that one type of treatment (drug or non-drug) is superior to another in improving symptoms of depression. However, we found strong evidence that some treatments are effective, whereas the effectiveness of others remains uncertain. Of the interventions examined, prescription antidepressant drugs and electroconvulsive therapy are the only treatments for which there is good evidence of effectiveness in severe and psychotic depressive disorders. We found no RCTs comparing drug and non-drug treatments in severe depressive disorders.

BENEFICIAL

Cognitive therapy (in mild to moderate depression)

One systematic review in younger and older adults has found that cognitive therapy**G** significantly improves the symptoms of depression compared with no treatment.

Continuation drug treatment in mild to moderate depression (reduces risk of relapse in mild to moderate depression)

One systematic review and subsequent RCTs in younger and older adults have found that continuation treatment**G** with antidepressant drugs compared with placebo for 4–6 months after recovery significantly reduces the risk of relapse. One RCT in people aged over 60 years has found that continuation treatment with dosulepin (dothiepin) significantly reduces the risk of relapse over 2 years compared with placebo.

Electroconvulsive therapy (in severe depression)

Two systematic reviews and additional RCTs in people aged over 16 years have found that electroconvulsive therapy significantly improves symptoms in severe depression compared with simulated electroconvulsive therapy.

Interpersonal psychotherapy (in mild to moderate depression)

One large RCT has found that interpersonal psychotherapy**G** significantly improves rates of recovery from depression after 16 weeks compared with antidepressants or standard care.

Prescription antidepressant drugs (in mild to moderate and severe depression)

Systematic reviews in people aged 16 years or over have found that antidepressant drugs are effective in acute treatment of all grades of depressive disorders compared with placebo. Systematic reviews have found no significant difference in outcomes with different kinds of antidepressant drug. One systematic review in people aged 55 years or over with all grades of depressive disorder has found that tricyclic antidepressants, selective serotonin reuptake inhibitors, or monoamine oxidase inhibitors significantly reduce the proportion of people who fail to recover over 26–49 days compared with placebo. We found no specific evidence on adverse effects in older adults. However, the drugs differ in their adverse event profiles.

One systematic review found that monoamine oxidase inhibitors were less effective than tricyclic antidepressants in people with severe depressive disorders, but may be more effective in atypical depressive disorders with biological features such as increased sleep, increased appetite, mood reactivity, and rejection sensitivity. ▶

One systematic review found that selective serotonin reuptake inhibitors were associated with a lower rate of adverse effects compared with tricyclic antidepressants, but the difference was small. Another systematic review and one retrospective cohort study found no strong evidence that fluoxetine was associated with increased risk of suicide compared with tricyclic antidepressants or placebo. One RCT and observational data suggest that abrupt withdrawal of selective serotonin reuptake inhibitors is associated with symptoms including dizziness, nausea, paraesthesia, headache, and vertigo, and that these symptoms are more likely with drugs with a short half life, such as paroxetine.

Tricyclic antidepressants

One systematic review found that tricyclic antidepressants were associated with higher rates of adverse effects compared with selective serotonin reuptake inhibitors, but the difference was small.

LIKELY TO BE BENEFICIAL

Care pathways (in mild to moderate depression)

Five RCTs in people aged over 18 years found limited evidence that the effectiveness of antidepressant treatment may be improved by several approaches, including collaborative working between primary care clinicians and psychiatrists plus intensive patient education, case management, telephone support, and relapse prevention programmes. One RCT found that a clinical practice guideline and practice based education did not improve either detection or outcome of depression compared with usual care.

Combining prescription antidepressant drug and psychological treatment (in mild to moderate and severe depression)

One non-systematic review of RCTs in people aged 18–80 years has found that, in people with severe depression, adding drug treatment to interpersonal psychotherapy or to cognitive therapy compared with either psychological treatment alone improves symptoms, but found no significant difference in symptoms in people with mild to moderate depression. Subsequent RCTs in younger and older adults with mild to moderate depression have found that combining antidepressants plus psychotherapy improves symptoms significantly more than either antidepressants or psychotherapy alone. One RCT in older adults with mild to moderate depression found that cognitive behavioural therapy**G** plus desipramine improved symptoms significantly more than desipramine alone.

Non-directive counselling (in mild to moderate depression)

One systematic review in people aged over 18 years with recent onset psychological problems, including depression, found that brief, non-directive counselling**G** significantly reduced symptom scores in the short term (< 6 months) compared with usual care, but found no significant difference in scores in the long term (> 6 months).

Problem solving treatment (in mild to moderate depression)

RCTs have found that problem solving treatment**G** significantly improves symptoms over 3–6 months compared with placebo or control, and have found no significant difference in symptoms between problem solving treatment and drug treatment.

St John's Wort (in mild to moderate depression)

Systematic reviews in people with mild to moderate depressive disorders have found that St John's Wort (*Hypericum perforatum*) significantly improves depressive symptoms over 4–12 weeks compared with placebo, and have found no significant difference in symptoms with St John's Wort compared with prescription antidepressant drugs. The results of the reviews should be interpreted with caution because the RCTs did not use standardised preparations of St John's Wort, and doses of antidepressants varied. One large subsequent RCT in people aged over 18 with major depressive disorder found no significant difference in depressive symptoms at 8 weeks between a standardised preparation of St John's Wort and placebo or sertraline, but it is likely to have been underpowered to detect a clinically important difference.

UNKNOWN EFFECTIVENESS

Befriending (in mild to moderate depression)
One small RCT provided insufficient evidence to assess befriending**G**.

Bibliotherapy (in mild to moderate depression)
One systematic review of RCTs in younger and older adults recruited by advertisement found limited evidence that bibliotherapy**G** may reduce mild depressive symptoms compared with waiting list control or standard care. Another systematic review in people with combined anxiety and depression, anxiety, or chronic fatigue found that bibliotherapy may improve symptoms over 2–6 months compared with standard care. It is unclear whether people in the RCTs identified by the reviews are clinically representative of people with depressive disorders.

Care pathways versus usual care for long term outcomes (in mild to moderate depression)
One RCT found that a multifaceted "quality improvement programme" significantly improved symptoms and increased the proportion of people who returned to work over 1 year compared with usual care, but found no significant difference in outcomes at 2 years.

Cognitive therapy versus antidepressants for long term outcomes (in mild to moderate depression)
One systematic review and one additional RCT in younger and older adults found limited evidence by combining relapse rates across different RCTs that cognitive therapy may reduce the risk of relapse over 2 years compared with antidepressants.

Exercise (in mild to moderate depression)
One systematic review found limited evidence from poor RCTs that exercise may improve symptoms compared with placebo, and may be as effective as cognitive therapy or anitdepressants.

Psychological treatments (cognitive therapy, interpersonal psychotherapy, and problem solving treatment) in severe depression
RCTs provided insufficient evidence to assess psychological treatments in severe depression.

DEFINITION **Depressive disorders** are characterised by persistent low mood, loss of interest and enjoyment, and reduced energy. They often impair day to day functioning. Most of the RCTs assessed in this review classify depression using the *Diagnostic and statistical manual of mental disorders* (DSM IV)[1] or the *International classification of mental and behavioural disorders* (ICD-10).[2] DSM IV divides depression into major depressive disorder or dysthymic disorder. **Major depressive disorder** is characterised by one or more major depressive episodes (i.e. at least 2 wks of depressed mood or loss of interest accompanied by at least 4 additional symptoms of depression). **Dysthymic disorder** is characterised by at least 2 years of depressed mood for more days than not, accompanied by additional symptoms that do not reach the criteria for major depressive disorder.[1] ICD-10 divides depression into mild to moderate or severe depressive episodes.[2] **Mild to moderate depression** is characterised by depressive symptoms and some functional impairment. **Severe depression** is characterised by additional agitation or psychomotor retardation with marked somatic symptoms.[2] In this review, we use both DSM IV and ICD-10 classifications, but treatments are considered to have been assessed in severe depression if the RCT included inpatients. **Older adults:** Older adults are generally defined as people aged 65 years or older. However, some of the RCTs of older people in this review included people aged 55 years or over. The presentation of depression in older adults may be atypical: low mood may be masked and anxiety or memory impairment may be the principal presenting symptoms. Dementia should be considered in the differential diagnosis of depression in older adults.[3]

INCIDENCE/ PREVALENCE Depressive disorders are common, with a prevalence of major depression between 5% and 10% of people seen in primary care settings.[4] Two to three times as many people may have depressive symptoms but do not meet DSM IV criteria for major depression. Women are affected twice as often as men. Depressive disorders are the fourth most important cause of disability worldwide and they are expected to become the second most important cause by the year 2020.[5,6] **Older adults:** Between 10% and 15% of older people have depressive symptoms, although major depression is relatively rare in older adults.[7]

AETIOLOGY/ RISK FACTORS The causes are uncertain but include both childhood events and current psychosocial adversity.

PROGNOSIS About half of people suffering a first episode of major depressive disorder experience further symptoms in the next 10 years.[8] **Older adults:** One systematic review (search date 1996, 12 prospective cohort studies, 1268 people, mean age 60 years) found that the prognosis may be especially poor in elderly people with a chronic or relapsing course of depression.[9] Another systematic review (search date 1999, 23 prospective cohort studies in people aged > 65 years, including 5 identified by the first review) found that depression in older people was associated with increased mortality (15 studies; pooled OR 1.73, 95% CI 1.53 to 1.95).[10]

Please refer to CD-ROM for full text and references.

Generalised anxiety disorder

Search date October 2002

Christopher Gale and Mark Oakley-Browne

What are the effects of treatments?

LIKELY TO BE BENEFICIAL

Buspirone

RCTs have found that buspirone versus placebo significantly improves symptoms compared with placebo over 4–9 weeks. RCTs found no significant difference in symptoms over 6–8 weeks with buspirone versus antidepressants, diazepam, or hydroxyzine, but the studies may have lacked power to detect clinically important differences among treatment.

Certain antidepressants (imipramine, opipramol, paroxetine, trazodone, venlafaxine)

One systematic review and four additional RCTs have found that antidepressants (imipramine, opipramol, paroxetine, trazodone, and venlafaxine) versus placebo significantly improve symptoms over 4–8 weeks. RCTs found no significant difference among these antidepressants or between antidepressants and benzodiazepines or buspirone. RCTs and observational studies have found that antidepressants are associated with sedation, dizziness, nausea, falls, and sexual dysfunction.

Cognitive therapy

Two systematic reviews have found limited evidence that cognitive behavioural therapy**G**, using a combination of interventions, such as exposure, relaxation, and cognitive restructuring, improves anxiety and depression over 4–12 weeks compared with waiting list control, anxiety management training alone, relaxation training alone, or non-directive psychotherapy. Two subsequent RCTs found no significant difference in symptoms for cognitive therapy**G** versus applied relaxation at 13 weeks and 24 months.

TRADE OFF BETWEEN BENEFITS AND HARMS

Benzodiazepines

One systematic review and one subsequent RCT found limited evidence that benzodiazepines versus placebo reduced symptoms over 2–9 weeks. However, RCTs and observational studies found that benzodiazepines increased the risk of dependence, sedation, industrial accidents, and road traffic accidents. One non-systematic review found that, if used in late pregnancy or while breast feeding, benzodiazepines may cause adverse effects in neonates. One RCT found no significant difference in symptoms of anxiety with sustained release alprazolam versus bromazepam, and another RCT found no significant difference in overall symptoms with mexazolam versus alprazolam. Limited evidence from RCTs found no significant difference in symptoms over 6–8 weeks with benzodiazepines versus buspirone, abecarnil, or antidepressants. One systematic review of poor quality RCTs found insufficient evidence about the effects of long term treatment with benzodiazepines.

Kava

One systematic review in people with anxiety, including generalised anxiety disorder (GAD), found that kava versus placebo significantly reduced symptoms of anxiety over 4 weeks. Observational evidence suggests that kava may be associated with hepatotoxicity.

▶

Clin Evid Concise 2003;9:203–205.

UNKNOWN EFFECTIVENESS

Abecarnil

RCTs found conflicting evidence of the effects of abecarnil versus placebo in improving symptoms.

Antipsychotic drugs

We found limited evidence from one RCT that trifluoperazine significantly reduced anxiety compared with placebo after 4 weeks, but caused more drowsiness, extrapyramidal reactions, and other movement disorders.

Applied relaxation

We found no RCTs of applied relaxation**G** versus placebo or no treatment. One RCT found no significant difference in symptoms at 13 weeks for applied relaxation versus cognitive behaviour therapy.

β Blockers

We found no RCTs on the effects of β blockers.

Hydroxyzine

Two RCTs compared hydroxyzine versus placebo and found different results. After about 1 month, one RCT found that hydroxyzine versus placebo significantly improved symptoms of anxiety, but the other found no significant difference between treatments. One further RCT found no significant difference for hydroxyzine versus buspirone after 28 days. We found no RCTs of longer term treatment.

DEFINITION GAD is defined as excessive worry and tension about every day events and problems, on most days, for at least 6 months, to the point where the person experiences distress or has marked difficulty in performing day-to-day tasks.[1] It may be characterised by the following symptoms and signs: increased motor tension (fatigability, trembling, restlessness, and muscle tension); autonomic hyperactivity (shortness of breath, rapid heart rate, dry mouth, cold hands, and dizziness); and increased vigilance and scanning (feeling keyed up, increased startling, and impaired concentration), but not panic attacks.[1] One non-systematic review of epidemiological and clinical studies found marked reduction of quality of life and psychosocial functioning in people with anxiety disorders (including GAD).[2] It also found that people with GAD have low overall life satisfaction and some impairment in ability to fulfil roles, social tasks, or both.[2]

INCIDENCE/ PREVALENCE One overview found that the prevalence of GAD among adults in the community is 1.5–3.0%.[3] It found that 3–5% of adults have had GAD in the past year and 4–7% have had GAD during their life. One non-systematic review identified the US National Comorbidity Survey, which found that over 90% of people diagnosed with GAD had a co-morbid diagnosis, including dysthymia (22%), depression (39–69%), somatisation, other anxiety disorders, bipolar disorder, or substance abuse.[4] The reliability of the measures used to diagnose GAD in epidemiological studies is unsatisfactory.[5,6] One US study, with explicit diagnostic criteria (DSM-III-R), estimated that 5% of people will develop GAD at some time during their lives.[6] A recent cohort study of people with depressive and anxiety disorders found that 49% of people initially diagnosed with GAD retained this diagnosis over 2 years.[7] One non-systematic review found that the incidence of GAD in men is only half the incidence in women.[8] One non-systematic review of seven epidemiological studies found reduced prevalence of anxiety disorders in older people.[9] Another non-systematic review of 20 observational studies in younger and older adults suggested that autonomic arousal to stressful tasks is decreased in older people, and that older people become accustomed to stressful tasks more quickly than younger people.[10]

AETIOLOGY/ RISK FACTORS One community study and a clinical study have found that GAD is associated with an increase in the number of minor stressors, independent of demographic factors,[11,12] but this finding was common in people with other diagnoses in the clinical population.[7] One non-systematic review (5 case control studies) of psychological sequelae to civilian trauma found that rates of GAD reported in four of the five studies were increased significantly compared with a control population (rate ratio 3.3, 95% CI 2.0 to 5.5).[13] One systematic review of cross-sectional studies found that bullying (or peer victimisation) was associated with a significant increase in the incidence of GAD (effect size 0.21).[14] One systematic review (search date not stated) of the genetic epidemiology of anxiety disorders (including GAD) identified two family studies and three twin studies.[15] The family studies (45 index cases, 225 first degree relatives) found a significant association between GAD in the index cases and in their first degree relatives (OR 6.1, 95% CI 2.5 to 14.9). The twin studies (13 305 people) estimated that 32% (95% CI 24% to 39%) of the variance to liability to GAD was explained by genetic factors.[15]

PROGNOSIS One systematic review found that 25% of adults with GAD will be in full remission after 2 years, and 38% will have a remission after 5 years.[3]

Please refer to CD-ROM for full text and references.

Obsessive compulsive disorder

Search date May 2002

G Mustafa Soomro

What are the effects of initial treatments in adults?

BENEFICIAL

Behavioural therapy

One systematic review and one subsequent RCT have found that behavioural therapy**G** improves symptoms compared with relaxation. Two observational studies found that improvement was maintained for up to 2 years. Another systematic review found no significant difference in symptoms with behavioural therapy versus cognitive therapy**G**. One additional RCT found limited evidence that group behavioural therapy versus group cognitive therapy improved symptoms after 3 months.

Cognitive therapy

One systematic review has found no significant difference in symptoms with cognitive therapy versus behavioural therapy. One subsequent RCT found limited evidence that group cognitive therapy improved symptoms less than group behavioural therapy after 12 weeks.

Drug treatment (fluvoxamine) plus behavioural therapy

Systematic reviews have found that monotherapy with drug therapy (serotonin reuptake inhibitors) or behavioural therapy improve symptoms. But RCTs have found only limited evidence that behavioural therapy plus fluvoxamine reduces symptoms more than behavioural therapy alone.

Selective and non-selective serotonin reuptake inhibitors

Systematic reviews and subsequent RCTs have found that serotonin reuptake inhibitors**G** versus placebo significantly improve symptoms after 12 weeks. One observational study found that most people relapsed within 7 weeks of stopping treatment with clomipramine (a non-selective serotonin reuptake inhibitor**G**). RCTs have found no consistent evidence of different efficacy among serotonin reuptake inhibitors. One systematic review and two subsequent RCTs have found that serotonin reuptake inhibitors reduce symptoms significantly more than other types of antidepressants. RCTs have found that clomipramine is associated with more adverse effects than selective serotonin reuptake inhibitors.

What are the effects of treatments in adults who have not responded to initial serotonin reuptake inhibitors?

LIKELY TO BE BENEFICIAL

Addition of antipsychotics in people who have not responded to serotonin reuptake inhibitors

Two small RCTs in people unresponsive to serotonin reuptake inhibitors have found that the addition of antipsychotics versus placebo significantly improves symptoms.

DEFINITION Obsessive compulsive disorder (OCD) involves obsessions or compulsions (or both) that are not caused by drugs or a physical disorder, and which cause significant personal distress or social dysfunction. **Obsessions** are recurrent and persistent ideas, images, or impulses that cause pronounced anxiety and that the person perceives to be self produced. **Compulsions** are intentional repetitive behaviours or mental acts performed in response to obsessions or ▶

according to certain rules, and are aimed at reducing distress or preventing certain imagined dreaded events. Obsessions and compulsions are usually recognised as pointless and are resisted by the person. (There are minor differences in the criteria for OCD between the third, revised third, and fourth editions of the *Diagnostic and Statistical Manual*: DSM–III, DSM–III–R, and DSM–IV.)[1]

INCIDENCE/ PREVALENCE One national, community based survey of OCD in the UK (1993, 10 000 people) found a prevalence of 1% in men and 1.5% in women.[2] A survey in the USA (18 500 people) found a lifetime prevalence of OCD of between 1.9 and 3.3% in 1984.[3] An international study found a lifetime prevalence of 3% in Canada, 3.1% in Puerto Rico, 0.3–0.9% in Taiwan, and 2.2% in New Zealand.[2]

AETIOLOGY/ RISK FACTORS Behavioural, cognitive, genetic, and neurobiological factors are implicated in OCD.[4–10]

PROGNOSIS One study (144 people followed for a mean of 47 years) found that an episodic**G** course was more common during the initial years (about 1–9 years), but a chronic**G** course was more common afterwards.[11] Over time, the study found that 39–48% of people had symptomatic improvement. A 1 year prospective cohort study found 46% of people had an episodic course and 54% had a chronic course.[12]

Please refer to CD-ROM for full text and references.

Panic disorder

Search date May 2002

Shailesh Kumar and Mark Oakley Browne

What are the effects of drug treatments?

BENEFICIAL

Selective serotonin reuptake inhibitors

Systematic reviews and one additional RCT have found that selective serotonin reuptake inhibitors versus placebo improve symptoms in panic disorder. One RCT found that discontinuation of sertraline in people with a good response significantly increased exacerbation of symptoms.

Tricyclic antidepressants (imipramine)

One systematic review and subsequent RCTs have found that imipramine versus placebo significantly improves symptoms. One RCT found that imipramine significantly reduced relapse rates over 12 months.

TRADE OFF BETWEEN BENEFITS AND HARMS

Benzodiazepines

One systematic review and one additional RCT have found that alprazolam versus placebo significantly reduces the number of panic attacks and improves symptoms. However, benzodiazepines are associated with a wide range of adverse effects both during their use and after treatment has been withdrawn.

UNKNOWN EFFECTIVENESS

Buspirone

RCTs found insufficient evidence on the effects of buspirone versus placebo.

Monoamine oxidase inhibitors

We found no RCTs on the effects of monoamine oxidase inhibitors.

DEFINITION A panic attack is a period in which there is sudden onset of intense apprehension, fearfulness, or terror often associated with feelings of impending doom. Panic disorder occurs when there are recurrent, unpredictable attacks followed by at least 1 month of persistent concern about having another panic attack, worry about the possible implications or consequences of the panic attacks, or a significant behavioural change related to the attacks.[1] The term panic disorder excludes panic attacks attributable to the direct physiological effects of a general medical condition, substance, or another mental disorder. Panic disorder is sometimes categorised as with or without agoraphobia.[1] Alternative categorisations focus on phobic anxiety disorders and specify agoraphobia with or without panic disorder.[2]

INCIDENCE/ PREVALENCE Panic disorder often starts around 20 years of age (between late adolescence and the mid 30s).[3] Lifetime prevalence is between 1–3%, and panic disorder is more common in women than in men.[4] An Australian community study found 1 month prevalence rates for panic disorder (with or without agoraphobia) of 0.4% using International Classification of Diseases (ICD-10) diagnostic criteria and of 0.5% using Diagnostic and Statistical Manual (DSM-IV) diagnostic criteria.[5]

AETIOLOGY/ RISK FACTORS Stressful life events tend to precede the onset of panic disorder,[6,7] although a negative interpretation of these events in addition to their occurrence has been suggested as an important aetiological factor.[8] Panic disorder is associated with major depression,[9] social phobia, generalised anxiety disorder, obsessive ▶

compulsive disorder,[10] and a substantial risk of drug and alcohol abuse.[11] It is also associated with avoidant, histrionic, and dependent personality disorders.[10]

PROGNOSIS The severity of symptoms in people with panic disorder fluctuates considerably, with periods of no attacks, or only mild attacks with few symptoms, being common. There is often a long delay between the initial onset of symptoms and presentation for treatment. Recurrent attacks may continue for a number of years, especially if associated with agoraphobia. Reduced social or occupational functioning varies among people with panic disorder and is worse in people with associated agoraphobia. Panic disorder is also associated with an increased rate of attempted but unsuccessful suicide.[12]

Please refer to CD-ROM for full text and references.

Post-traumatic stress disorder

Search date September 2002

Jonathan Bisson

What are the effects of preventive psychological interventions?

LIKELY TO BE BENEFICIAL

Multiple episode cognitive behavioural therapy in people with acute stress disorder

Two small RCTs in people with acute stress disorder after a traumatic event (accident or non-sexual assault) found that five sessions of cognitive behavioural therapy**G** significantly reduces the proportion of people with post-traumatic stress disorder after 6 months compared with supportive counselling**G**.

UNKNOWN EFFECTIVENESS

Multiple episode cognitive behavioural therapy in all people exposed to a traumatic event

One RCT in bus drivers who had been attacked in the past 5 months found that cognitive behavioural therapy significantly improved measures of anxiety and intrusive symptoms at 6 months compared with usual care, but found no significant difference in measures of depression or avoidance symptoms. Another RCT comparing cognitive behavioural therapy versus standard care in people who had been exposed to a traumatic event in the past 5–12 months found no significant difference in overall symptoms of post-traumatic stress disorder at 6 months.

Multiple episode memory restructuring

One RCT provided insufficient evidence to assess memory restructuring compared with supportive care in people exposed to a traumatic event in the past 24 hours.

Multiple episode trauma support

Two RCTs provided insufficient evidence to assess collaborative care**G** interventions involving emotional, social, and practical support in people exposed to a traumatic event in the past 1 day to 1 week.

UNLIKELY TO BE BENEFICIAL

Single episode psychological interventions ("debriefing") in all people exposed to a traumatic event

RCTs in people who had been exposed to a traumatic event in the previous month found no significant difference between a single session of psychological debriefing**G** and no debriefing in the incidence of post-traumatic stress disorder at 3 months or 1 year.

What are the effects of treatments?

BENEFICIAL

Cognitive behavioural therapy

RCTs have found that cognitive behavioural therapy significantly improves post-traumatic stress disorder symptoms, anxiety, and depression compared with no treatment or supportive counselling.

Eye movement desensitisation and reprocessing

RCTs have found that eye movement desensitisation and reprocessing Ⓖ improves symptoms compared with waiting list control or relaxation treatment debriefingⒼ. Two RCTs found no significant difference in symptoms between eye movement desensitisation and reprocessing compared with exposure therapy.

Paroxetine

One systematic review and subsequent RCTs found that paroxetine reduced symptoms at 3 months compared with placebo.

Sertraline

One systematic review and subsequent RCTs found that sertraline significantly reduced symptoms at 3–7months compared with placebo.

LIKELY TO BE BENEFICIAL

Fluoxetine

Two RCTs found that fluoxetine may reduce symptoms at 3 months compared with placebo.

UNKNOWN EFFECTIVENESS

Affect managementⒼ; drama therapyⒼ; hypnotherapyⒼ; inpatient programmes; other drug treatments (brofaromine, amitriptyline, lamotrigine, imipramine, phenelzine, nefazodone, carbamazepine, antipsychotics, benzodiazepines); psychodynamic psychotherapyⒼ; supportive counselling

We found insufficient evidence about the effects of these interventions in improving symptoms.

DEFINITION Post-traumatic stress disorder can occur after a major traumatic event. Symptoms include upsetting thoughts and nightmares about the traumatic event, avoidance behaviour, numbing of general responsiveness, increased irritability, and hypervigilance for at least 1 month.[1] Acute stress disorder occurs within the first month after a major traumatic event and requires the presence of symptoms for at least 2 days. It is similar to post-traumatic stress disorder but more dissociative symptoms are required to make the diagnosis.

INCIDENCE/ PREVALENCE One large cross-sectional study in the USA found that 1/10 women and 1/20 men experience post-traumatic stress disorder at some stage in their lives.[2]

AETIOLOGY/ RISK FACTORS Risk factors include major trauma, such as rape, a history of psychiatric disorders, acute distress and depression after the trauma, lack of social support, and personality factors (such as neuroticism).[3]

PROGNOSIS One large cross-sectional study in the USA found that over a third of sufferers continued to satisfy the criteria for a diagnosis of post-traumatic stress disorder 6 years after diagnosis.[2] However, cross-sectional studies provide weak evidence about prognosis.

Please refer to CD-ROM for full text and references.

Schizophrenia

Search date April 2002

Zia Nadeem, Andrew McIntosh, and Stephen Lawrie

What are the effects of treatments?

BENEFICIAL

Continuation of medication for 6–9 months after an acute episode

Systematic reviews have found that continuing antipsychotic medication for at least 6 months after an acute episode significantly reduces relapse rates, and that some benefit of continuing medication is apparent for up to 2 years.

Family interventions to reduce relapse rates

One systematic review has found that family intervention versus usual care significantly reduces relapse rates at 12 and 24 months. Seven families would have to be treated to avoid one additional relapse (and likely hospitalisation) in the family member with schizophrenia. One RCT found that fewer people receiving a multiple family versus single family intervention relapsed over 2 years, but the difference did not quite reach significance.

Psychoeducational interventions to reduce relapse rates

One systematic review has found that psychoeducation versus control intervention significantly reduces relapse rates at 9–18 months.

LIKELY TO BE BENEFICIAL

Behavioural therapy for improving adherence

One RCT found that behavioural interventions versus usual treatment improved adherence to antipsychotic medication over 3 months. Two RCTs found that behavioural interventions versus psychoeducational therapy improved adherence.

"Compliance" therapy

One RCT found limited evidence that compliance therapy❻ versus non-specific counselling may increase adherence to antipsychotic medication at 6 and 18 months.

Psychoeducational interventions to improve adherence

One systematic review found limited evidence that psychoeducation versus usual care improved adherence with antipsychotic medication. Two RCTs found that psychoeducational therapy improved adherence less than behavioural therapy.

TRADE OFF BETWEEN BENEFITS AND HARMS

Chlorpromazine

One systematic review has found that chlorpromazine versus placebo significantly reduces the proportion of people who have no improvement or have marked/worse severity of illness at 6 months on a psychiatrist rated scale. The review found that clopramazine versus placebo caused significantly more adverse effects, such as sedation, acute dystonia, and parkinsonism.

Clozapine

Two systematic reviews found that clozapine versus standard antipsychotic drugs improved symptoms over 4–10 weeks, and may improve symptoms in the longer term. However, RCTs found that clozapine may be associated with blood dyscrasias. Three systematic reviews found no strong evidence about the effectiveness or safety of clozapine versus new antipsychotic drugs. One systematic review in people resistant to standard treatment has found that clozapine versus standard treatment improves symptoms after 12 weeks and after 2 years.

Clin Evid Concise 2003;9:212–214.

◀ **Depot bromperidol decanoate**

One systematic review found no significant difference in the proportion of people who needed additional medication or left the study early over 6–12 months with bromperidol versus haloperidol or fluphenazine decanoate. One RCT found no significant difference in anticholinergic adverse effects at 12 months with depot bromperidol decanoate versus fluphenazine, and two RCTs found no significant difference in movement disorders over 6–12 months with bromperidol versus haloperidol or fluphenazine.

Depot haloperidol decanoate

One RCT found that depot haloperidol decanoate versus placebo reduced the need for additional medication at 4 months. One systematic review has found that haloperidol versus placebo is associated with with acute dystonia, akathisia, and parkinsonism.

Depot pipotiazine palmitate

One RCT found no significant difference with depot pipotiazine (pipothiazine) palmitate versus standard antipsychotic drugs in symptoms or in the proportion of people requiring anticholenergic drugs at 18 months. RCTs found no significant difference with depot pipotiazone versus antipsychotic drugs in the proportion of people who left the trial early.

Haloperidol

One systematic review has found that haloperidol versus placebo significantly increases physician rated global improvement for up to 2 years, but is associated with acute dystonia, akathisia, and parkinsonism.

Amisulpride; loxapine; molindone; olanzapine; pimozide; quetiapine; risperidone; sulpiride; thioridazine; ziprasidone; zotepine

Systematic reviews have found that these antipsychotic drugs are as effective as standard antipsychotic drugs, and have different profiles of adverse effects.

UNKNOWN EFFECTIVENESS

Cognitive behavioural therapy to reduce relapse rates

Limited evidence from RCTs found no significant difference in relapse rates with the addition of cognitive behavioural therapy to standard care alone.

Polyunsaturated fatty acids

One small RCT found limited evidence that polyunsaturated fatty acids versus placebo reduced the subsequent use of antipsychotic medication after 12 weeks.

Social skills training to reduce relapse rates

Limited evidence from a systematic reviews of RCTs and observational studies suggests that social skills training versus usual care may reduce relapse rates.

Benperidol; perazine

Systematic reviews of poor quality RCTs found insufficient evidence about the effects of these interventions.

UNLIKELY TO BE BENEFICIAL

Family interventions to improve adherence

One systematic review has found that family therapy versus usual care is unlikely to improve adherence to antipsychotic medication. ▶

Schizophrenia

DEFINITION Schizophrenia is characterised by the "positive symptoms"Ⓖ of auditory hallucinations, delusions, and thought disorder, and the "negative symptoms"Ⓖ of demotivation, self neglect, and reduced emotion.[1]

INCIDENCE/ PREVALENCE Onset of symptoms typically occurs in early adult life (average age 25 years) and is earlier in men than women. Prevalence worldwide is 2–4/1000. One in 100 people will develop schizophrenia in their lifetime.[2,3]

AETIOLOGY/ RISK FACTORS Risk factors include a family history (although no major genes have been identified); obstetric complications; developmental difficulties; central nervous system infections in childhood; cannabis use; and acute life events.[2] The precise contributions of these factors and ways in which they may interact are unclear.

PROGNOSIS About three quarters of people suffer recurrent relapse and continued disability, although outcomes were worse in the pretreatment era.[4] Outcome may be worse in people with insidious onset and delayed initial treatment, social isolation, or a strong family history; in people living in industrialised countries; in men; and in people who misuse drugs.[3] Drug treatment is generally successful in treating positive symptoms, but up to a third of people derive little benefit and negative symptoms are notoriously difficult to treat. About half of people with schizophrenia do not adhere to treatment in the short term. The figure is even higher in the longer term.[5]

Please refer to CD-ROM for full text and references.

Ankle sprain

Search date March 2002

Peter Struijs and Gino Kerkhoffs

What are the effects of treatments for acute ankle ligament ruptures?

BENEFICIAL

Functional treatment

One systematic review and one subsequent RCT found limited evidence that functional treatment**G** versus minimal treatment significantly reduced the risk of the ankle giving way. One systematic review and two RCTs comparing functional treatment versus surgery found conflicting evidence. One systematic review found that functional treatment versus immobilisation**G** significantly improved six outcome measures at either short (up to 6 weeks), intermediate (6 weeks to 1 year), or long term (over 1 year) follow up. Effects were less marked at long term follow up. Another systematic review found that functional treatment versus immobilisation resulted in significantly less persistent subjective instability but no significant difference in pain. We found insufficient evidence comparing different functional treatments.

LIKELY TO BE BENEFICIAL

Immobilisation

One systematic review found that functional treatment versus immobilisation significantly improved six outcome measures at either short (up to 6 weeks), intermediate (6 weeks to 1 year), or long term (over 1 year) follow up. Effects were less marked at long term follow up. One other systematic review found functional treatment versus immobilisation resulted in significantly less persistent subjective instability but no significant difference in pain. One systematic review has found no significant difference with immobilisation versus surgery in pain or subjective instability.

Surgery

One systematic review has found no significant difference with surgery versus immobilisation in pain or subjective instability. One systematic review and two RCTs comparing surgery versus functional treatment found conflicting evidence.

UNKNOWN EFFECTIVENESS

Diathermy

One systematic review found insufficient evidence on the effects of diathermy versus placebo in walking ability and reduction in swelling.

Homeopathic ointment

One systematic review of one RCT found limited evidence that homeopathic ointment versus placebo significantly improved outcome on a "composite criteria" of treatment success.

UNLIKELY TO BE BENEFICIAL

Cold pack compression

Two RCTs found no significant difference in symptoms with cold pack placement versus placebo or control. One RCT found significantly less oedema with cold pack placement versus heat or a contrast bath at 3–5 days post injury.

Clin Evid Concise 2003;9:215–216.

Ultrasound

One systematic review found no significant difference with ultrasound versus sham ultrasound in the general improvement of symptoms or the ability to walk or bear weight at 7 days. Three RCTs found conflicting evidence with ultrasound versus other treatments.

DEFINITION Ankle sprain is an injury of the lateral ligament complex of the ankle joint. Such injury can range from mild to severe and is graded according to the following scale on the basis of severity.[1–5] Grade I is a mild stretching of the ligament complex without joint instability. Grade II is a partial rupture of the ligament complex with mild instability of the joint (such as isolated rupture of the anterior talofibular ligament). Grade III involves complete rupture of the ligament complex with instability of the joint.

INCIDENCE/ PREVALENCE Ankle sprain is a common problem in acute medical care occurring at a rate of about one injury/10 000 population a day.[6] Injuries of the lateral ligament complex of the ankle form a quarter of all sports injuries.[6]

AETIOLOGY/ RISK FACTORS The usual mechanism of injury is inversion and adduction (usually referred to as supination) of the plantar flexed foot. Predisposing factors are a history of ankle sprains and specific malalignment, like crus varum and pes cavo-varus.

PROGNOSIS Some sports (e.g. basketball, football [soccer], and volleyball) have a particularly high incidence of ankle injuries. Pain is the most frequent residual problem, often localised on the medial side of the ankle.[4] Other residual complaints include mechanical instability, intermittent swelling, and stiffness. People with more extensive cartilage damage have a higher incidence of residual complaints.[4] Long term cartilage damage can lead to degenerative changes and this is especially true if there is persistent or recurrent instability; every sprain has the potential to add new damage.

Please refer to CD-ROM for full text and references.

Bunions

Search date May 2002

Jill Ferrari

What are the effects of interventions?

LIKELY TO BE BENEFICIAL

Chevron osteotomy plus Akin osteotomy

One small RCT found that chevron osteotomy plus Akin osteotomy(G) versus Akin osteotomy plus distal soft tissue reconstruction(G) significantly improved the hallux abductus angle, intermetatarsal angle, and tibial sesamoid position, but found no significant difference in patient satisfaction, cosmetic appearance, or motion at the toe after a minimum of 1 year.

Chevron osteotomy (compared with no treatment or with orthoses)

One RCT found that chevron osteotomy(G) versus no treatment or orthoses significantly reduced pain intensity, and significantly improved cosmetic appearance, functional status, and footwear problems, but found no significant difference in ability to return to work after 1 year.

Different methods of bone fixation

One RCT found no significant difference with a standard method of fixation versus absorbable pin fixation in clinical outcomes or radiological outcomes after a mean follow up of 11 months. One RCT found that screw fixation followed by early weight bearing in a plaster shoe versus vicryl suture fixation followed by 6 weeks non-weight bearing in a plaster boot significantly reduced both time taken to return to social activities and time taken to return to work but found no significant difference in clinical and radiological outcomes after 6 months.

UNKNOWN EFFECTIVENESS

Chevron osteotomy (compared with proximal osteotomy)

RCTs identified by a systematic review comparing chevron osteotomy versus proximal osteotomy found conflicting results on hallux abductus angle, and found no significant difference in problems with footwear or mobility after a maximum of 38 months.

Chevron osteotomy plus adductor tenotomy

One RCT found no significant difference with chevron osteotomy plus adductor tenotomy versus chevron osteotomy alone in hallux abductus angle, range of motion, pain, satisfaction, problems with footwear, or mobility.

Continuous passive motion

One systematic review found no significant difference between continuous passive motion plus physiotherapy versus physiotherapy alone on joint range of motion or return to normal footwear after 3 months' treatment, but was too small to rule out a clinically important effect.

Early weightbearing

One systematic review has found no significant difference with early versus late weight bearing in numbers of people with non-union at the site of arthrodesis.

Keller's arthroplasty

One systematic review found little good evidence on the effects of Keller's arthroplasty(G) versus other types of operation.

▶

Clin Evid Concise 2003;9:217–219.

Night splints

We found no RCTs examining the use of night splints in the treatment of hallux valgus.

Orthoses to treat hallux valgus in adults

One RCT in adults found that orthoses versus no treatment significantly improved pain intensity after 6 months, but found no significant difference in pain after 12 months.

Slipper cast

One RCT of crepe bandage versus plaster cast slippers after Wilson osteotomy❻ found no significant difference in hallux valgus angle, pain, overall assessment, joint range of movement, or return to normal activities, but was too small to rule out a clinically important effect.

UNLIKELY TO BE BENEFICIAL

Orthoses to prevent hallux valgus in high risk adults

One RCT in men with rheumatoid arthritis found no significant difference with orthoses versus no treatment in the number of people who developed of hallux valgus after 3 years.

LIKELY TO BE INEFFECTIVE OR HARMFUL

Antipronatory orthoses in children

One RCT in children aged 9–10 years found limited evidence that antipronatory orthoses❻ versus no treatment may increase deterioration in metatarsophalangeal joint angles after 3 years.

DEFINITION **Hallux valgus** is a deformity of the great toe whereby the hallux (great toe) moves towards the second toe, overlying it in severe cases. This movement of the hallux is described as abduction (movement away from the midline of the body) and it is usually accompanied by some rotation of the toe so that the nail is facing the midline of the body (valgus rotation). With the deformity, the metatarsal head becomes more prominent and the metatarsal is said to be in an adducted position as it moves towards the midline of the body.[1] Radiological criteria for hallux valgus vary, but a commonly accepted criterion is to measure the angle formed between the metatarsal and the abducted hallux. This is called the metatarsophalangeal joint angle or hallux abductus angle and it is considered abnormal when it is greater than 14.5°.[2] **Bunion** is the lay term used to describe a prominent and often inflamed metatarsal head and overlying bursa. Symptoms include pain, limitation in walking, and problems with wearing normal shoes.

AETIOLOGY/ RISK FACTORS The prevalence of hallux valgus varies in different populations. In a recent study of 6000 UK school children aged 9–10 years, 2.5% had clinical evidence of hallux valgus, and 2% met both clinical and radiological criteria for hallux valgus. An earlier study found hallux valgus in 48% of adults.[2] Differences in prevalence may result from different methods of measurement, varying age groups, or different diagnostic criteria (e.g. metatarsal joint angle > 10° or > 15°).[3]

AETIOLOGY/ RISK FACTORS Nearly all population studies have found that hallux valgus is more common in women. Footwear may contribute to the deformity, but studies comparing people who wear shoes with those who do not have found contradictory results. Hypermobility of the first ray❻ and excessive foot pronation are associated with hallux valgus.[4]

PROGNOSIS We found no studies that looked at progression of hallux valgus. Progression of deformity and symptoms is rapid in some people, others remain asymptomatic. One study found that hallux valgus is often unilateral initially, but usually progresses to bilateral deformity.[2]

Please refer to CD-ROM for full text and references.

Carpal tunnel syndrome

Search date September 2002

Shawn Marshall

What are the effects of treatments?

BENEFICIAL

Local corticosteroid injection (short term)

Two RCTs found local corticosteroid injection (methylprednisolone, hydrocortisone) versus placebo or no treatment significantly improved symptoms after 4–6 weeks. One small RCT found that local betamethasone injection versus betamethasone injection into the deltoid significantly improved symptoms after 1 month. One RCT found no significant difference with local methylprednisolone injection versus oral prednisolone in symptoms after 2 weeks, but found that local methylprednisolone injection versus oral prednisolone significantly improved symptoms after 8 and 12 weeks. One small RCT found that local methylprednisolone injection versus helium neon laser significantly improved symptoms after 20 days, but found no significant difference in symptoms between the two groups after 6 months. One small RCT found no significant difference with local methylprednisolone injection versus non-steroidal anti-inflammatory plus nocturnal neutral angle wrist splints in symptoms after 2 or 8 weeks.

Oral corticosteroids (short term)

One small RCT found that oral prednisone versus placebo significantly improved the mean global symptom score after 2 weeks, but not after 4 or 8 weeks. One small RCT found that oral prednisolone versus placebo significantly improved the mean global symptom score after 2 and 4 weeks. One small RCT found that oral prednisolone versus placebo significantly improved the median global symptom score after 2 and 8 weeks. One RCT found no significant difference with local methylprednisolone injection versus oral prednisolone in symptoms after 2 weeks, but found that local methylprednisolone injection versus oral prednisolone significantly improved symptoms after 8 and 12 weeks.

TRADE OFF BETWEEN BENEFITS AND HARMS

Endoscopic carpal tunnel release versus open carpal tunnel release

We found no RCTs comparing surgery versus placebo. One systematic review and subsequent RCTs found no clear evidence of a difference in symptoms with endoscopic carpal tunnel release versus open carpal tunnel release up to 12 months after the operation. RCTs found conflicting evidence on differences in the time taken to return to work between endoscopic carpal tunnel release versus open carpal tunnel release. Harms resulting from endoscopic carpal tunnel release and open carpal tunnel release vary between RCTs. One systematic review comparing the interventions suggests that endoscopic carpal tunnel release may cause more transient nerve problems whereas open carpal tunnel release may cause more wound problems.

UNKNOWN EFFECTIVENESS

Nerve and tendon gliding exercises

One small RCT found no significant difference with nerve and tendon gliding exercises Ⓖ plus neutral angle wrist splint versus neutral angle wrist splint alone in mean symptom severity score or mean functional status score assessed 8 weeks after the end of the treatment.

▶

Clin Evid Concise 2003;9:220–222.

Pyridoxine

One very small RCT found a similar improvement in symptoms with pyridoxine versus placebo or no treatment after 10 weeks. The RCT may have been too small to detect a clinically important difference between treatments. One small RCT found no significant difference with pyridoxine versus placebo in nocturnal pain, numbness, or tingling after 12 weeks.

Surgery versus placebo or non-surgical intervention

We found no RCTs comparing surgery versus placebo. One very small RCT found limited evidence that surgical section of the anterior carpal ligament versus splinting of the hand, wrist, and arm for 1 month increased the proportion of people with clinical improvement after 1 year.

Therapeutic ultrasound

One RCT found ultrasound versus placebo significantly increased the proportion of wrists with satisfactory improvement or complete remission of symptoms after 6 months. One RCT found no significant difference in mean symptom severity with high intensity or low intensity ultrasound versus placebo after 2 weeks. One RCT found no significant difference in symptom severity scores with ibuprofen plus nocturnal wrist splint versus chiropractic manipulation plus ultrasound plus nocturnal wrist splint after 9 weeks.

Wrist splints

One RCT found a significant improvement in symptoms after 2 and 4 weeks with a nocturnal hand brace versus no treatment. RCTs found no significant difference in symptoms with neutral angle versus 20° extension wrist splinting, or with full time versus night time only neutral angle wrist splinting.

Local corticosteroid injection (long term); oral corticosteroids (long term)

We found no RCTs on the effects of these interventions.

UNLIKELY TO BE BENEFICIAL

Diuretics

One small RCT found no significant difference with trichlormethiazide versus placebo in mean global symptom score after 2 or 4 weeks. One RCT found no significant difference with bendrofluazide versus placebo in the proportion of people with no improvement in symptoms after 4 weeks.

Internal neurolysis in conjunction with open carpal tunnel release

Three RCTs found no significant difference with open carpal tunnel release alone versus open carpal tunnel release plus internal neurolysis in symptoms.

Non-steroidal anti-inflammatory drugs

One small RCT found no significant difference with tenoxicam versus placebo in mean global symptom score after 2 or 4 weeks. One RCT found no significant difference in symptom severity scores with ibuprofen plus nocturnal wrist splint versus chiropractic manipulation plus ultrasound plus nocturnal wrist splint after 9 weeks.

LIKELY TO BE INEFFECTIVE OR HARMFUL

Wrist splinting after carpal tunnel release surgery

Two RCTs in people after carpal tunnel release surgery found no significant difference with wrist splinting versus no splinting in median grip strength or in the number of people who considered themselves "cured". Another RCT found that splinting versus no splinting significantly increased pain at 1 month and the number of days taken to return to work.

Carpal tunnel syndrome

DEFINITION Carpal tunnel syndrome is a neuropathy caused by compression of the median nerve within the carpal tunnel.[1] Classical symptoms of carpal tunnel syndrome include numbness, tingling, burning, or pain in at least two of the three digits supplied by the median nerve (i.e. the thumb, index, and middle fingers).[2] The American Academy of Neurology has described diagnostic criteria**G** that rely on a combination of symptoms and physical examination findings.[3] Other diagnostic criteria include results from electrophysiological studies.[2]

INCIDENCE/ PREVALENCE A general population survey in Rochester, Minnesota, found the age adjusted incidence of carpal tunnel syndrome to be 105 (95% CI 99 to 112) cases per 100 000 person years.[4,5] Age adjusted incidence rates were 52 (95% CI 45 to 59) cases for men and 149 (95% CI 138 to 159) cases for women per 100 000 person years. The study found incidence rates increased from 88 (95% CI 75 to 101) cases per 100 000 person years in 1961–1965 to 125 (95% CI 112 to 138) cases per 100 000 person years in 1976–1980. Incidence rates of carpal tunnel syndrome increased with age for men, whereas for women they peaked between the ages of 45–54 years. A general population survey in the Netherlands found prevalence to be 1% for men and 7% for women.[6] A more comprehensive study in southern Sweden found the general population prevalence for carpal tunnel syndrome was 3% (95% CI 2% to 3%).[7] As in other studies, the overall prevalence in women was higher than in men (male to female ratio 1 : 1.4); however, among older people, the prevalence in women was almost four times that in men (age group 65–74 years: men 1%, 95% CI 0% to 4%; women 5%, 95% CI 3% to 8%).

AETIOLOGY/ RISK FACTORS Most cases of carpal tunnel syndrome have no easily identifiable cause (idiopathic).[4] Secondary causes of carpal tunnel syndrome include the following: space occupying lesions (tumours, hypertrophic synovial tissue, fracture callus, and osteophytes); metabolic and physiological (pregnancy, hypothyroidism, rheumatoid arthritis); infections; neuropathies (associated with diabetes mellitus or alcoholism); and familial disorders.[4] One case control study found that risk factors in the general population included repetitive activities requiring wrist extension or flexion, obesity, very rapid dieting, shorter height, hysterectomy without oopherectomy, and recent menopause.[8]

PROGNOSIS One observational study (carpal tunnel syndrome defined by symptoms and electrophysiological study results) found that 34% of people with idiopathic carpal tunnel syndrome without treatment had complete resolution of symptoms (remission) within 6 months of diagnosis.[9] Remission rates were higher for younger age groups, for women versus men, and for pregnant versus non-pregnant women. A more recent observational study of untreated idiopathic carpal tunnel syndrome also demonstrated that symptoms may spontaneously resolve in some people. The main positive prognostic indicators were short duration of symptoms and young age, whereas bilateral symptoms and a positive Phalen's test were indicators of a poorer prognosis.[10]

Please refer to CD-ROM for full text and references.

Chronic fatigue syndrome

Search date July 2002

Steven Reid, Trudie Chalder, Anthony Cleare, Matthew Hotopf, and Simon Wessely

What are the effects of treatments?

BENEFICIAL

Cognitive behavioural therapy

One systematic review has found that cognitive behavioural therapy versus standard care or relaxation therapy administered by highly skilled therapists in specialist centres improves quality of life and physical functioning. One additional multicentre RCT has found that cognitive behavioural therapy administered by less experienced therapists compared with guided support groups or no intervention may also be effective.

Graded aerobic exercise

RCTs have found that a graded aerobic exercise programme versus flexibity and relaxation training or general advice significantly improves measures of fatigue and physical functioning. One RCT has found a significant improvement in measures of physical functioning, fatigue, mood, and sleep at 1 year with an educational package to encourage graded exercise versus written information only.

UNKNOWN EFFECTIVENESS

Evening primrose oil

One small RCT found no significant difference with evening primrose oil versus placebo in depression scores at 3 months.

Magnesium (intramuscular)

One small RCT found that magnesium injections versus placebo injections significantly improved symptoms at 6 weeks.

Antidepressants; corticosteroids; oral nicotinamide adenine dinucleotide

RCTs found insufficient evidence on the effects of these interventions.

UNLIKELY TO BE BENEFICIAL

Immunotherapy

Small RCTs found that immunoglobulin G versus placebo modestly improved physical functioning and fatigue at 3–6 months, but was associated with considerable adverse effects. Small RCTs found insufficient evidence on the effects of interferon alfa versus placebo.

Prolonged rest

We found no RCTs on the effects of prolonged rest. Indirect observational evidence in healthy volunteers and in people recovering from a viral illness suggests that prolonged rest may perpetuate or worsen fatigue and symptoms.

DEFINITION Chronic fatigue syndrome (CFS) is characterised by severe, disabling fatigue and other symptoms, including musculoskeletal pain, sleep disturbance, impaired concentration, and headaches. Two widely used definitions of CFS, from the US Centers for Disease Control and Prevention[1] and from Oxford, UK,[2] were developed as operational criteria for research Ⓣ. There are two important differences between these definitions. The UK criteria insist upon the presence of mental fatigue, whereas the US criteria include a requirement for several physical symptoms, reflecting the belief that chronic fatigue syndrome has an underlying immunological or infective pathology.

▶

Clin Evid Concise 2003;9:223–224.

Chronic fatigue syndrome

INCIDENCE/ PREVALENCE Community and primary care based studies have reported the prevalence of chronic fatigue syndrome to be 0–3%, depending on the criteria used.[3,4] Systematic population surveys have found similar prevalence of chronic fatigue syndrome in people of different socioeconomic status and in all ethnic groups.[4,5]

AETIOLOGY/ RISK FACTORS The cause of CFS is poorly understood. Women are at higher risk than men (RR 1.3 to 1.7 depending on diagnostic criteria used).[6]

PROGNOSIS Studies have focused on people attending specialist clinics. A systematic review of studies of prognosis (search date 1996) found that children with CFS had better outcomes than adults: 54–94% of children showed definite improvement (after up to 6 years' follow up), whereas 20–50% of adults showed some improvement in the medium term and only 6% returned to premorbid levels of functioning.[7] Despite the considerable burden of morbidity associated with CFS, we found no evidence of increased mortality. The systematic review found that outcome was influenced by the presence of psychiatric disorders (depression and anxiety), and beliefs about causation and treatment.[7]

Please refer to CD-ROM for full text and references.

Fracture prevention in postmenopausal women

Search date September 2002

Olivier Bruyere, John Edwards, and Jean-Yves Reginster

What are the effects of treatments to prevent fractures in postmenopausal women?

BENEFICIAL

Alendronate

One systematic review and one subsequent RCT have found that alendronate versus placebo reduces vertebral and non-vertebral fractures over 1–4 years.

Calcitonin

One large RCT found that calcitonin versus placebo significantly reduced new vertebral fractures over 5 years. One systematic review combined evidence from RCTs in men and women who were taking corticosteroids or had osteoporosis or previous fracture. In this heterogeneous population, it found limited evidence that calcitonin non-significantly reduced vertebral or non-vertebral fracture rates compared with placebo, no treatment, calcium, or calcium plus vitamin D.

Calcium plus vitamin D

One large RCT in elderly women in nursing homes has found that calcium plus vitamin D3 versus placebo reduces non-vertebral fractures over 18 months to 3 years. Two smaller RCTs found no significant difference in vertebral fractures over 2–3 years with calcium plus vitamin D3 versus placebo, but they may have lacked power to exclude a clinically important difference.

Hip protectors

RCTs in elderly residents of nursing home found that hip protectors versus no hip protectors significantly reduced hip fractures over 9–19 months, but found no significant difference in pelvic fractures. One RCT in people aged over 65 years in institutional care found that a multifactorial intervention (including staff education, environmental manipulation**G**, exercise, walking aids, drug regimen reviews, and hip protectors for those considered at higher risk) versus usual care reduced hip fractures over 34 weeks.

LIKELY TO BE BENEFICIAL

Etidronate

One systematic review has found that etidronate versus placebo, calcium, or calcium plus vitamin D reduces vertebral fractures over 2 years. One systematic review has found no significant difference in non-vertebral fractures over 2 years with etidronate versus placebo, calcium, or calcium plus vitamin D.

Pamidronate

One RCT found that pamidronate versus placebo reduced new vertebral fractures after 3 years, but another small RCT found no significant difference with pamidronate versus placebo in vertebral fracture rate.

Risedronate

Two large RCTs in women with previous fractures have found that risedronate versus placebo significantly reduces new vertebral fractures over 3 years. One of the RCTs found that risedronate versus placebo reduced non-vertebral fractures ▶

Clin Evid Concise 2003;9:225–227.

over 3 years, but the other found no significant difference. One large RCT in women aged over 70 years has found that risedronate versus placebo reduces hip fractures over 3 years. Observational evidence suggests that risedronate may be associated with increased pulmonary cancer.

UNKNOWN EFFECTIVENESS

Tiludronate

One RCT in women with low bone mineral density with or without previous fractures found no significant difference with tiludronate versus placebo in vertebral fractures over 3 years, but it may have lacked power to detect a clinically important difference.

Environmental manipulation; exercise

RCTs found insufficient evidence about the effects of these interventions in preventing vertebral and non-vertebral fractures.

UNLIKELY TO BE BENEFICIAL

Calcium alone

One RCT in women with existing fractures found that calcium versus placebo reduced new vertebral or non-vertebral fractures over 3 years, but found no significant difference in new fractures in women without existing fractures. Another RCT found no significant difference with calcium versus placebo in the proportion of women who had one or more new fractures over 2–4 years.

Vitamin D alone

One large RCT identified by a systematic review and one large subsequent RCT found no significant difference with vitamin D3 versus placebo in non-vertebral fractures over 3 years. One systematic review found limited evidence from two small RCTs that calcitriol versus placebo reduced vertebral fractures over 3 years.

LIKELY TO BE INEFFECTIVE OR HARMFUL

Hormone replacement therapy

RCTs found no consistently significant effect of hormone replacement therapy on vertebral fracture. One systematic review and one subsequent RCT found that hormone replacement therapy versus placebo, no treatment, calcium, or calcium plus vitamin D reduced non-vertebral fracture rate. However, another large subsequent RCT found no significant difference in non-vertebral fractures with hormone replacement therapy versus placebo. Another large RCT, comparing oestrogen plus progestin versus placebo in healthy postmenopausal women, was stopped because hormonal therapy increased risks of invasive breast cancer, coronary events, stroke, and pulmonary embolism.

DEFINITION A fracture is a break or disruption of bone or cartilage. Symptoms and signs may include immobility, pain, tenderness, numbness, bruising, joint deformity, joint swelling, limb deformity, and limb shortening.[1] Diagnosis is usually based on a typical clinical picture combined with results from an appropriate imaging technique.

INCIDENCE/ PREVALENCE The lifetime risk of fracture in white women is 20% for the spine, 15% for the wrist, and 18% for the hip.[2]

AETIOLOGY/ RISK FACTORS Fractures usually arise from trauma. Risk factors include those associated with an increased tendency to fall (such as ataxia, drug and alcohol intake, loose carpets), age, osteoporosis, bony metastases, and other bone disorders.

PROGNOSIS Fractures may result in pain, short or long term disability, haemorrhage, thromboembolic disease (see thromboembolism, p 35), shock, and death. Vertebral fractures are associated with pain, physical impairment, muscular atrophy, changes in body shape, loss of physical function, and lower quality of life.[3] About 20% of women die in the first year after a hip fracture, representing an increase in mortality of 12–20% compared with women of similar age and no hip fracture. Half of elderly women who had been independent become partly dependent after hip fracture. A third become totally dependent.

Please refer to CD-ROM for full text and references.

Herniated lumbar disc

Search date April 2002

Jo Jordan, Tamara Shawver Morgan, and James Weinstein

What are the effects of treatments?

LIKELY TO BE BENEFICIAL

Microdiscectomy (as effective as standard discectomy)

We found no RCTs comparing microdiscectomy versus conservative treatment. Three RCTs found no significant difference in clinical outcomes with microdiscectomy versus standard discectomy. One RCT found no significant difference with video-assisted arthroscopic microdiscectomy**G** versus standard discectomy**G** in self reported satisfaction or pain score after about 31 months. The duration of postoperative recovery with standard discectomy was almost twice that with arthroscopic discectomy. We found conflicting evidence on the effects of microdiscectomy versus automated percutaneous discectomy**G**.

Spinal manipulation

One RCT in people with sciatica caused by disc herniation found that spinal manipulation versus a placebo of infrared heat increased self-perceived improvement after 2. A second RCT found no significant difference in improvement between spinal manipulation, manual traction, exercise, and corsets after 1 month. A third RCT found that spinal manipulation versus traction significantly increased the number of people with improved symptoms.

Standard discectomy

One RCT found that standard discectomy versus conservative treatment (physiotherapy) significantly increased self reported improvement at 1 year, but not at 4 and 10 years. Three RCTs found no significant difference in clinical outcomes with standard discectomy versus microdiscectomy.

UNKNOWN EFFECTIVENESS

Advice to stay active

One systematic review of conservative treatments found no RCTs of giving advice to stay active.

Automated percutaneous discectomy

We found no RCTs comparing automated percutaneous discectomy versus either conservative treatment or standard discectomy. We found conflicting evidence on the effects of automated percutaneous discectomy versus microdiscectomy. One RCT found that automated percutaneous discectomy versus microdiscectomy was associated with significantly lower success rates at interim analysis at 6 months, and was terminated prematurely. Another RCT comparing the same interventions found similar investigator rated clinical scores, although participant rated improvement was higher with automated percutaneous discectomy than with microdiscectomy after 2 years. One systematic review found that reoperation rates were higher with automated percutaneous discectomy than with either microdiscectomy or standard discectomy. One RCT in the review found that postoperative recovery was about three times shorter with automated percutaneous discectomy than with microdiscectomy.

Bed rest

One systematic review of conservative therapy found no RCTs of bed rest for symptomatic herniated discs.

Clin Evid Concise 2003;9:228–230.

Epidural corticosteroid injections

One systematic review found limited evidence that epidural steroid injections versus placebo may increase participant perception of global improvement. One subsequent RCT found no significant difference with the addition of epidural steroid injections to conservative treatment in pain, mobility, or return to work at 6 months.

Heat or ice

One systematic review identified no RCTs of heat or ice for sciatica caused by lumbar disc herniation.

Massage

One systematic review identified no RCTs of massage in symptomatic lumbar disc herniation.

Analgesics; antidepressants; laser discectomy; muscle relaxants

We found no systematic reviews or RCTs on these interventions for treatment of symptomatic herniated lumbar disc.

UNLIKELY TO BE BENEFICIAL

Non-steroidal anti-inflammatory drugs

One systematic review found no significant difference between non-steroidal anti-inflammatory drugs versus placebo in participant perception of overall improvement.

DEFINITION Herniated lumbar disc is a displacement of disc material (nucleus pulposus or annulus fibrosis) beyond the intervertebral disc space.[1] The diagnosis can be confirmed by radiological examination; however, magnetic resonance imaging findings of herniated disc are not always accompanied by clinical symptoms.[2,3] This review covers treatment of people who have clinical symptoms relating to confirmed or suspected disc herniation. It does not include treatment of people with spinal cord compression or people with cauda equina syndrome Ⓖ, which often requires emergency intervention. The management of non-specific acute low back pain (see low back pain and sciatica [acute], p 237) and chronic low back pain (see low back pain and sciatica [chronic], p 240) are covered elsewhere.

INCIDENCE/ PREVALENCE The prevalence of symptomatic herniated lumbar disc is around 1–3% in Finland and Italy, depending on age and sex.[4] The highest prevalence is among people aged 30–50 years,[5] with a male : female ratio of 2 : 1.[6] In people aged between 25 and 55 years, about 95% of herniated discs occur at the L4–L5 level; in people over 55 years of age, disc herniation is more common above the L4–L5 level.[7,8]

AETIOLOGY/ RISK FACTORS Radiographical evidence of disc herniation does not necessarily predict low back pain in the future or indicate physical symptoms, because 19–27% of people without symptoms have disc herniation on imaging.[2,9] Risk factors for disc herniation include smoking (OR 1.7, 95% CI 1.0 to 2.5), weight bearing sports, and certain work activities such as repeated lifting (lifting objects < 11.3 kg, < 25 times daily while twisting body, knees not bent, OR 7.2, 95% CI 2.0 to 25.8; lifting objects < 11.3 kg, < 25 times daily while twisting body, knees bent, OR 1.9, 95% CI 0.8 to 4.8). Driving motor vehicles (possibly because of the resonant frequency of the spine being similar to that of certain vehicles) is also associated with increased risk (OR 1.7, 95% CI 0.2 to 2.7, depending on the vehicle model).[6,10,11]

PROGNOSIS The natural history of disc herniation is difficult to determine because most people take some form of treatment for their back pain, and a formal diagnosis is not always made.[6] Clinical improvement is usual in the majority of people, and only about 10% of people still have sufficient pain after 6 weeks to consider surgery. Sequential magnetic resonance images have shown that the herniated portion of the disc tends to regress over time, with partial to complete resolution after 6 months in two thirds of people.[12]

Please refer to CD-ROM for full text and references.

Hip fracture

Search date April 2002

William Gillespie

What are the effects of treatments?

BENEFICIAL

High specification versus standard hospital mattress on operating tables to prevent pressure sores

One systematic review has found that high specification foam mattresses and pressure relieving mattresses on operating tables versus standard hospital mattresses significantly reduce the number of pressure sores.

Perioperative antibiotic prophylaxis

One systematic review has found that multiple dose perioperative and single dose preoperative antibiotic prophylaxis regimens versus control or no antibiotics significantly reduce infection after hip surgery.

Sliding hip screw device for internal fixation of extracapsular fracture

One systematic review found no significant difference with sliding hip screws**G** versus fixed nail plates**G** in mortality, pain at follow up, or impairment of mobility, but found that sliding hip screws significantly reduced the risk of fixation failure. It found limited evidence that a sliding hip screw versus the RAB fixed nail plate**G** significantly increased the risk of leg shortening.

LIKELY TO BE BENEFICIAL

Cyclical compression of the foot or calf to reduce venous thromboembolism

One systematic review has found that cyclical compression devices (foot or calf pumps) significantly reduce deep venous thrombosis, but are associated with non-compliance and skin abrasion.

Geriatric hip fracture programmes in acute orthopaedic units

One systematic review of RCTs and observational studies, and one subsequent RCT in elderly people who have suffered hip fracture, found that geriatric hip fracture programmes versus control programmes significantly increased the number of people able to return to their previous residence, and significantly reduced morbidity whilst in hospital, but had no significant effect on mortality. The systematic review found that geriatric hip fracture programmes also reduced the length of hospital stay. Two additional RCTs found that a geriatrician led geriatric hip fracture programme versus control significantly reduced the incidence of severe delirium.

Nutritional supplementation after fracture

One systematic review in people who had undergone surgery for hip fracture found limited evidence that nutritional supplementation (oral protein and energy feeds) versus control significantly reduced postoperative complications.

Perioperative prophylaxis with antiplatelet agents

One systematic review has found that perioperative antiplatelet prophylaxis versus placebo or no prophylaxis significantly reduces the incidence of pulmonary embolism, but has no significant effect on the incidence of deep venous thrombosis. One subsequent RCT has found that aspirin versus placebo significantly reduces the incidence of both deep venous thrombosis and pulmonary embolism. The systematic review and subsequent RCT both found that antiplatelet treatment versus control significantly increases the risk of bleeding complications.

Perioperative prophylaxis with heparin to reduce venous thromboembolism

One systematic review has found that perioperative prophylaxis with either unfractionated heparin or low molecular weight heparin versus placebo or no treatment significantly reduces the incidence of deep venous thrombosis confirmed by imaging. The systematic review has also found that low molecular weight heparin versus unfractionated heparin significantly reduces deep venous thrombosis confirmed by imaging.

Regional (versus general) anaesthesia for surgery

One systematic review of people after hip fracture surgery found limited evidence that regional versus general anaesthesia significantly reduced the risk of deep venous thrombosis, but had no significant effect on short term mortality.

TRADE OFF BETWEEN BENEFITS AND HARMS

Arthroplasty for intracapsular fracture

One systematic review of randomised and observational studies, and five subsequent RCTs in people with displaced intracapsular fractures, found limited evidence that arthroplasty(G) versus internal fixation(G) significantly reduced the need for re-operation at 12–15 or 24 months after surgery, but significantly increased the number of deep infections and operative blood loss. Two of the subsequent RCTs found that arthroplasty versus internal fixation increased mortality.

Early supported discharge programmes

One systematic review of RCTs and observational studies has found that early supported discharge versus control significantly increases the number of people returning to their previous residence and reduces length of hospital stay, but significantly increases the frequency of readmission to hospital.

Intramedullary fixation with cephalocondylic nail versus extramedullary fixation for extracapsular fracture

One systematic review has found that cephalocondylic nails(G) versus extramedullary fixation significantly reduce length of surgery, the incidence of deep wound sepsis, and operative blood loss. However, the review has also found that cephalocondylic nails significantly increase re-operation rates and the incidence of leg shortening and of external rotation deformity compared with extramedullary fixation.

UNKNOWN EFFECTIVENESS

Arthroplasty for extracapsular fracture

One systematic review in people with unstable extracapsular hip fractures found limited evidence that arthroplasty(G) versus internal fixation(G) using a sliding hip screw(G) did not significantly affect operating times, local wound complications, mortality, or mobility. Arthroplasty significantly increased the number of people who received a blood transfusion.

Different types of implant for intracapsular fracture

One systematic review found insufficient evidence to determine the best implant for internal fixation of intracapsular fractures.

Graduated elastic compression to prevent venous thromboembolism

We found no RCTs in elderly people with hip fracture involving thromboembolism stockings for prevention of thrombotic complications. One systematic review in people undergoing elective total hip replacement has found that graduated elastic compression versus placebo significantly reduces the risk of deep venous thrombosis.

◀ **Nerve blocks for pain control before and after hip fracture**

One systematic review of small RCTs and quasi-randomised trials found that nerve blocks significantly reduced total analgesic intake compared with no nerve block.

Specialised orthopaedic rehabilitation units for elderly people

One systematic review and one subsequent RCT found that rehabilitation in a geriatric outpatient rehabilitation unit versus control significantly increased the number of people able to return to their previous residence, although they found conflicting results on length of hospital stay. The systematic review found that geriatric outpatient rehabilitation units significantly reduced rates of readmission for acute care, but did not significantly reduce mortality or increase quality of life scores.

Systematic home based rehabilitation

One RCT comparing a systematic home based rehabilitation programme versus existing services found no significant difference in recovery to prefracture levels of self care, home management, social activity, balance, or lower extremity strength after 12 months.

UNLIKELY TO BE BENEFICIAL

Conservative (non-surgical) treatment of extracapsular fractures

One systematic review of people with extracapsular hip fractures comparing conservative versus operative treatment found limited evidence that operative treatment significantly reduced the number of people remaining in hospital after 12 weeks. The review found that conservative treatment significantly increased both leg shortening and varus deformity**G**, but found insufficient evidence to determine whether any significant difference exists between treatments in medical complications, mortality, or long term pain.

Preoperative bed traction to the injured limb

One systematic review found no significant difference in analgesic use or ease of fracture reduction with routine preoperative traction versus control. One RCT identified by the review found that skeletal versus skin traction significantly reduced analgesic use.

Short cephalocondylic nail versus sliding hip screw for extracapsular fracture

One systematic review found no significant difference between intramedullary fixation with short cephalocondylic nail versus extramedullary fixation with sliding hip screw for pain at follow up, ability to return to a previous residence, and ability to walk after 3–12 months. The review also found no significant difference between treatments in mortality, wound infection, or fracture non-union, but found that cephalocondylic intramedullary fixation significantly increased intraoperative femoral fractures and re-operation rates.

DEFINITION Hip fracture is a fracture of the femur above a point 5 cm below the distal part of the lesser trochanter.[1] **Intracapsular fractures** occur proximal to the point at which the hip joint capsule attaches to the femur, and can be subdivided into displaced and undisplaced fractures. Undisplaced fractures include impacted or adduction fractures. Displaced intracapsular fractures may be associated with disruption of the blood supply to the head of the femur. Numerous subdivisions and classification methods exist for these fractures. In the most distal part of the proximal femoral segment (below the lesser trochanter), the term "subtrochanteric" is used. **Extracapsular fractures** occur distal to the hip joint capsule. ▶

Hip fracture

INCIDENCE/ PREVALENCE Hip fractures may occur at any age but are most common in elderly people. In industrialised societies, the lifetime risk of hip fracture is about 18% in women and 6% in men.[2] A recent study reported that prevalence increases from about 3/100 women aged 65–74 years to 12.6/100 women aged 85 years and above.[3] The age stratified incidence has also increased in some societies during the past 25 years; not only are people living longer, but the incidence of fracture in each age group may have increased.[4]

AETIOLOGY/ RISK FACTORS Hip fractures are usually sustained through a fall from standing height or less. The pattern of incidence is consistent with two main risk factors: increased risk of falling and loss of skeletal strength from osteoporosis. Both are associated with aging.

PROGNOSIS One in five people die in the first year after a hip fracture,[5] and one in four elderly people require a higher level of long term care after a fracture.[5,6] Those who do return to live in the community after a hip fracture have greater difficulty with activities of daily living than age and sex matched controls.[3]

Please refer to CD-ROM for full text and references.

Leg cramps

Search date February 2002

Gavin Young

What are the effects of treatments for idiopathic leg cramps?

BENEFICIAL

Quinine

One systematic review has found that quinine versus placebo significantly reduces the frequency of nocturnal leg cramp attacks over 4 weeks.

LIKELY TO BE BENEFICIAL

Quinine plus theophylline

One small RCT found limited evidence that quinine plus theophylline versus quinine alone significantly reduced the number of nights affected by leg cramp over 2 weeks.

UNKNOWN EFFECTIVENESS

Analgesics; antiepileptic drugs; compression hosiery

We found no RCTs on the effects of these interventions on idiopathic leg cramps**G**.

UNLIKELY TO BE BENEFICIAL

Vitamin E

One small RCT comparing vitamin E versus placebo found no significant difference in the number of nights disturbed by leg cramps.

What are the effects of treatments for leg cramps in pregnancy?

LIKELY TO BE BENEFICIAL

Magnesium salts

One systematic review of one small RCT found that magnesium tablets (primarily magnesium lactate, magnesium citrate) versus placebo significantly reduced the number of pregnant women with leg cramps after 3 weeks.

UNKNOWN EFFECTIVENESS

Calcium salts

Two RCTs identified by a systematic review comparing calcium versus placebo or no treatment found conflicting results.

Multivitamins and mineral supplements

One systematic review of one small RCT found no significant difference with a multivitamin and mineral tablet versus placebo in the number of pregnant women with cramps in the ninth month of pregnancy.

Sodium chloride

One systematic review found insufficient evidence about the effects of sodium chloride on leg cramps in pregnancy.

DEFINITION Leg cramps are involuntary, localised, and usually painful skeletal muscle contractions, which commonly affect calf muscles. Leg cramps typically occur at night and usually last only seconds to minutes. Leg cramps may be idiopathic or related to a definable process or disease such as renal dialysis, pregnancy, or venous insufficiency.

Leg cramps

INCIDENCE/ PREVALENCE Leg cramps are common and their incidence increases with age. About half of the people attending a general medicine clinic have had leg cramps within 1 month of their visit, and over two thirds of people over 50 years of age have experienced leg cramps.[1]

AETIOLOGY/ RISK FACTORS Very little is known about the causes of leg cramps. Risk factors include exercise, pregnancy, salt depletion, renal dialysis, electrolyte imbalances, peripheral vascular disease (both venous and arterial), peripheral nerve injury, polyneuropathies, motor neuron disease, muscle diseases, and the use of certain drugs. Other causes of calf pain include trauma, deep venous thrombosis (see thromboembolism, p 35), and ruptured Baker's cyst Ⓖ.

PROGNOSIS Leg cramps may cause severe pain and sleep disturbance, both of which are distressing.

Please refer to CD-ROM for full text and references.

Low back pain and sciatica (acute)

Search date June 2002

Maurits van Tulder and Bart Koes

What are the effects of treatments?

BENEFICIAL

Advice to stay active

Two systematic reviews and one subsequent RCT have found that advice to stay active versus advice to rest in bed or bed rest significantly increased the rate of recovery, reduced pain, reduced disability, and reduced time spent off work.

Non-steroidal anti-inflammatory drugs

One systematic review and one additional RCT have found that non-steroidal anti-inflammatory drugs versus placebo significantly increase the proportion of people with overall improvement after 1 week and significantly reduce the proportion of people requiring additional analgesics. One systematic review and additional RCTs have found no significant difference in pain relief with non-steroidal anti-inflammatory drugs versus each other or versus other treatments (paracetamol, opioids, muscle relaxants, and non-drug treatments).

LIKELY TO BE BENEFICIAL

Behavioural therapy

Two RCTs have found that behavioural therapy versus traditional care or electromyographic biofeedback**Ⓖ** reduces acute low back pain and disability.

Multidisciplinary treatment programmes

One systematic review in people with subacute low back pain found limited evidence that multidisciplinary treatment**Ⓖ**, including a workplace visit, versus usual care reduced sick leave.

TRADE OFF BETWEEN BENEFITS AND HARMS

Muscle relaxants

Systematic reviews have found that muscle relaxants versus placebo improve symptoms (including pain and muscle tension)and increase mobility, but found no significant difference in outcomes with muscle relaxants versus each other. Adverse effects in people using muscle relaxants were common and included dependency, drowsiness, and dizziness.

UNKNOWN EFFECTIVENESS

Acupuncture

We found no RCTs of acupuncture**Ⓖ** specifically in people with acute low back pain.

Analgesics (paracatemol, opioids)

We found no placebo controlled RCTs. Systematic reviews have found no consistent difference with analgesics versus non-steroidal anti-inflammatory drugs in reducing pain.

Back schools

One systematic review found limited evidence that back schools versus placebo increased rates of recovery and reduced sick leave in the short term. The review found no significant difference in outcomes with back schools versus physiotherapy, and found that back schools versus McKenzie exercises**Ⓖ** increased pain and sick leave.

▶

Clin Evid Concise 2003;9:237–239.

Epidural steroid injections

One RCT found that epidural steroids versus subcutaneous lidocaine (lignocaine) injections increased the proportion of people who were pain free after 3 months. A second RCT found no significant difference in the proportion of people cured or improved with epidural steroids versus epidural saline versus epidural bupivacaine and versus dry needling.

Lumbar supports

We found no RCTs on the effects of lumbar supports.

Massage

One systematic review found insufficient evidence from one RCT about the effects of massage(G) versus spinal manipulation or electrical stimulation.

Spinal manipulation

Systematic reviews found conflicting evidence on the effects of spinal manipulation.

Traction

RCTs found conflicting evidence on the effects of traction.

Colchicine; electromyographic biofeedback(G); temperature treatments (short wave diathermy, ultrasound, ice, heat); transcutaneous electrical nerve stimulation

We found insufficient evidence on the effects of these interventions.

UNLIKELY TO BE BENEFICIAL

Back exercises

Systematic reviews and additional RCTs have found either no significant difference with back exercises versus conservative or inactive treatments in pain or disability, or have found that back exercises increase pain or disability.

LIKELY TO BE INEFFECTIVE OR HARMFUL

Bed rest

Systematic reviews have found that bed rest could be worse than no treatment, advice to stay active, back exercises, physiotherapy, spinal manipulation, or non-steroidal anti-inflammatory drugs. One systematic review has found that adverse effects of bed rest include joint stiffness, muscle wasting, loss of bone mineral density, pressure sores, and venous thromboembolism.

DEFINITION Low back pain is pain, muscle tension, or stiffness localised below the costal margin and above the inferior gluteal folds, with or without leg pain (sciatica(G)),[1] and is designated as acute when it persists for less than 12 weeks (see definition of low back pain [chronic], p 240).[2] Non-specific low back pain is low back pain not attributed to a recognisable pathology (such as infection, tumour, osteoporosis, rheumatoid arthritis, fracture, or inflammation).[1] This review excludes low back pain or sciatica with symptoms or signs at presentation that suggest a specific underlying condition.

INCIDENCE/ PREVALENCE Over 70% of people in developed countries will experience low back pain at some time in their lives.[3] Each year, 15–45% of adults suffer low back pain, and 1/20 people present to hospital with a new episode. Low back pain is most common between the ages of 35–55 years.[3]

AETIOLOGY/ RISK FACTORS Symptoms, pathology, and radiological appearances are poorly correlated. Pain is non-specific in about 85% of people. About 4% of people with low back pain in primary care have compression fractures and about 1% have a tumour. The prevalence of prolapsed intervertebral disc is about 1–3%.[3] Ankylosing spondylitis and spinal infections are less common.[4] Risk factors for the development of back pain include heavy physical work, frequent bending, twisting, lifting, and prolonged static postures. Psychosocial risk factors include anxiety, depression, and mental stress at work.[3,5]

PROGNOSIS Acute low back pain is usually self limiting (90% of people recover within 6 wks), although 2–7% develop chronic pain. One study found recurrent pain accounted for 75–85% of absenteeism from work.[6]

Please refer to CD-ROM for full text and references.

Low back pain and sciatica (chronic)

Search date June 2002

Maurits van Tulder and Bart Koes

What are the effects of treatments?

BENEFICIAL

Exercise (*v* other treatments)

Systematic reviews and additional RCTs have found that exercise versus other treatments (including usual care) improves pain and functional status. RCTs have found conflicting evidence on the effects of exercise versus inactive treatments.

Intensive multidisciplinary treatment programmes (*v* non-multidisciplinary treatments)

One systematic review has found that intensive multidisciplinary biopsychosocial rehabilitation with functional restoration versus inpatient or outpatient non-multidisciplinary treatments or versus usual care reduces pain and improves function. The review found no significant difference in pain or function with less intensive multidisciplinary treatments versus non-multidisciplinary treatments or usual care.

LIKELY TO BE BENEFICIAL

Analgesics

One RCT found that tramadol versus placebo decreased pain and increased functional status. A second RCT found that paracetamol versus diflunisal increased the number of people who rated the treatment as good or excellent.

Back schools in occupational settings (*v* no treatment)

One systematic review has found that, in occupational settings, back schools versus no treatment improve pain and reduce disability. Systematic reviews and one subsequent RCT found conflicting evidence on the effects of back schools.

Behavioural therapy

Systematic reviews have found that behavioural therapy versus no treatment, placebo, or waiting list control reduces pain and improves functional status and behavioural outcomes. Systematic reviews have found no significant difference with different types of behavioural therapy versus each other in functional status, pain, or behavioural outcomes, and found conflicting results with behavioural therapy versus other treatments in pain, behavioural outcomes, or functional status.

Massage (*v* other treatments)

Systematic reviews and subsequent RCTs have found that massage Ⓖ versus other treatments reduces pain and improves functioning.

Non-steroidal anti-inflammatory drugs

One RCT found that naproxen versus placebo increased pain relief. Systematic reviews and additional RCTs have found no significant differences with non-steroidal anti-inflammatory drugs versus each other for symptom outcomes. Two RCTs found conflicting evidence on the effects of non-steroidal anti-inflammatory drugs versus analgesics.

▶

Clin Evid Concise 2003;9:240–242.

Trigger point and ligamentous injections

One systematic review found limited evidence that steroid plus local anaesthetic injection of trigger points versus local anaesthetic injection alone increased pain relief after 3 months, and that phenol versus saline injection of the lumbar interspinal ligament increased pain relief after 6 months.

UNKNOWN EFFECTIVENESS

Acupuncture

We found conflicting evidence from two systematic reviews and two subsequent RCTs about effects of acupuncture(G) versus placebo or no treatment for clinical outcomes.

Antidepressants

One systematic review and additional RCTs have found that antidepressants versus placebo significantly increase pain relief, but have found no consistent difference in functioning or depression. Additional RCTs have found conflicting results on pain relief with antidepressants versus each other or versus analgesics.

Electromyographic biofeedback

One systematic review found no significant difference in pain relief or functional status with electromyographic biofeedback(G) versus placebo or waiting list control, but found conflicting results on the effects of electromyographic biofeedback versus other treatments.

Epidural steroid injections

One systematic review has found no significant difference with epidural steroid injections versus placebo in pain relief after 6 weeks or 6 months.

Lumbar supports

We found insufficient evidence on the effects of lumbar supports.

Muscle relaxants

We found insufficient evidence about benefits of muscle relaxants. One RCT found that adverse effects in people using muscle relaxants are common and include dependency, drowsiness, and dizziness.

Spinal manipulation

We found four systematic reviews that identified the same 12 RCTs. One of the reviews found that spinal manipulation versus placebo improved outcomes, but the other three reviews found that the results of the RCTs were conflicting.

Transcutaneous electrical nerve stimulation

One systematic review has found no significant difference between transcutaneous electrical nerve stimulation versus sham stimulation for pain relief.

LIKELY TO BE INEFFECTIVE OR HARMFUL

Facet joint injections

One systematic review found no significant difference from two RCTs in pain relief with facet joint injections versus placebo or facet joint nerve blocks.

Traction

One systematic review and two additional RCTs have found no significant difference in pain relief or functional status with traction versus placebo or with traction plus massage versus interferential treatment (electrotherapy).

Low back pain and sciatica (chronic)

DEFINITION Low back pain is pain, muscle tension, or stiffness localised below the costal margin and above the inferior gluteal folds, with or without leg pain (sciatica**G**),[1] and is defined as chronic when it persists for 12 weeks or more (see definition of low back pain [acute], p 238).[2] Non-specific low back pain is low back pain not attributed to a recognisable pathology (such as infection, tumour, osteoporosis, rheumatoid arthritis, fracture, or inflammation).[1] This review excludes low back pain or sciatica with symptoms or signs at presentation that suggest a specific underlying condition.

INCIDENCE/ PREVALENCE See incidence of low back pain (acute), p 238.

AETIOLOGY/ RISK FACTORS See aetiology of low back pain (acute), p 239.

PROGNOSIS See prognosis of low back pain (acute), p 239.

Please refer to CD-ROM for full text and references.

Neck pain

Search date May 2002

Allan Binder

What are the effects of treatments for uncomplicated neck pain without severe neurological deficit?

LIKELY TO BE BENEFICIAL

Manual treatments (mobilisation and manipulation)

Systematic reviews have found that manipulation or mobilisation versus other treatments improve symptoms. One additional and one subsequent RCT have found no significant difference with mobilisation versus manipulation in pain. Rare but serious adverse effects have been reported after manipulation of the cervical spine.

Physical treatments (physiotherapy, pulsed electromagnetic field treatment, exercise)

Systematic reviews and subsequent RCTs have found that pulsed electromagnetic field treatment versus sham treatment, exercise versus stress management, and active physiotherapy versus passive treatment all significantly reduce pain.

UNKNOWN EFFECTIVENESS

Drug treatments (analgesics, non-steroidal anti-inflammatory drugs, antidepressants, or muscle relaxants)

We found insufficient evidence on the effects of analgesics, non-steroidal anti-inflammatory drugs, antidepressants, or muscle relaxants for neck pain, although they are widely used as a preferred treatment. Some are associated with well documented adverse effects.

Multidisciplinary (multimodal) treatment

One systematic review and two subsequent RCTs have found no consistent differences in pain or time off work over 18 months with multimodal cognitive behavioural therapy versus other treatments.

Patient education

Two systematic reviews and one subsequent RCT found insufficient evidence about the effects of patient education (advice or group instruction).

Physical treatments (heat or cold, traction, biofeedback, acupuncture, spray and stretch, laser)

Systematic reviews found insufficient evidence about the effects of these physical treatments.

Soft collars or special pillows

We found no evidence of the effects of soft collars. One RCT found limited evidence that water based pillows versus standard and roll pillows significantly reduced morning pain and improved quality of sleep.

What are the effects of treatments for acute whiplash injury?

LIKELY TO BE BENEFICIAL

Early mobilisation

Systematic reviews and subsequent RCTs found limited evidence that early mobilisation versus immobilisation or versus rest plus a collar significantly reduced pain.

Clin Evid Concise 2003;9:243–245.

Early return to normal activity

Systematic reviews and subsequent RCTs found limited evidence that advice to "act as usual" plus anti-inflammatory drugs versus immobilisation plus 14 days sick leave improved mild subjective symptoms.

Electrotherapy

One RCT found limited evidence that electromagnetic field treatment versus sham treatment significantly reduced pain after 4 weeks but not after 3 months.

Multimodal treatment

One RCT found that multimodal treatment versus physical treatment significantly reduced pain at the end of treatment and after 6 months.

What are the effects of treatments for chronic whiplash injury?

LIKELY TO BE BENEFICIAL

Percutaneous radiofrequency neurotomy for zygapophyseal joint pain

One RCT found limited evidence that percutaneous radiofrequency neurotomy versus a sham procedure significantly increased the number of people who were free from pain after 27 weeks.

UNKNOWN EFFECTIVENESS

Physiotherapy (v multimodal treatment)

A second RCT found no significant difference with physiotherapy alone versus multimodal treatment in disability, pain, or range of movement at the end of treatment or at 3 months.

What are the effects of treatments for neck pain with radiculopathy?

UNKNOWN EFFECTIVENESS

Drug treatments (epidural steroid injections, analgesics, non-steroidal anti-inflammatory drugs, or muscle relaxants)

We found no RCTs about the effects of epidural steroid injections, analgesics, non-steroidal anti-inflammatory drugs, or muscle relaxants.

Surgery versus conservative treatment

One RCT found no significant difference with surgery versus conservative treatment in symptoms after 1 year.

DEFINITION Neck pain can be divided into uncomplicated pain, whiplash, and pain with radiculopathy. Neck pain often occurs in combination with limitation of movement and poorly defined neurological symptoms affecting the upper limbs. The pain can be severe and intractable, and can occur with radiculopathy or myelopathy.

INCIDENCE/ PREVALENCE About two thirds of people will experience neck pain at some time in their lives.[1,2] Prevalence is highest in middle age. In the UK about 15% of hospital based physiotherapy, and in Canada 30% of chiropractic referrals, are for neck pain.[3,4] In the Netherlands neck pain contributes up to 2% of general practitioner consultations.[5]

AETIOLOGY/ RISK FACTORS Most uncomplicated neck pain is associated with poor posture, anxiety and depression, neck strain, occupational injuries, or sporting injuries. With chronic pain, mechanical and degenerative factors (often referred to as cervical spondylosis) are more likely. Some neck pain results from soft tissue trauma, most typically seen in whiplash injuries. Rarely disc prolapse and inflammatory, infective, or malignant conditions affect the cervical spine and present with neck pain with or without neurological features.

PROGNOSIS Neck pain usually resolves within days or weeks but can recur or become chronic. In some industries, neck related disorders account for as much time off work as low back pain (see low back pain and sciatica [acute], p 237).[6] The percentage of people in whom neck pain becomes chronic depends on the cause but is thought to be about 10%:[1] similar to low back pain. Neck pain causes severe disability in 5% of affected people.[2] One systematic review (search date 1996) of the clinical course and prognostic factors of non-specific neck pain identified six observational studies and 17 RCTs.[7] In people who had had pain for at least 6 months, a median of 46% (22–79%) improved with treatment. Whiplash injuries were more likely to cause disability; up to 40% of sufferers reported symptoms even after 15 years' follow up.[8] Factors associated with a poorer outcome after whiplash are not well defined.[9] The incidence of chronic disability following whiplash varies among countries, although reasons for this variation are unclear.[10]

Please refer to CD-ROM for full text and references.

Non-steroidal anti-inflammatory drugs

Search date September 2002

Peter C Gøtzsche

Are there any important differences between available non-steroidal anti-inflammatory drugs (NSAIDs)?

UNKNOWN EFFECTIVENESS

Choice between different NSAIDs

Systematic reviews have found no important differences in benefits among different NSAIDs or doses, but found differences in harms related to choice and dose of NSAID.

UNLIKELY TO BE BENEFICIAL

NSAIDs in increased doses

Systematic reviews have found that benefits of NSAIDs increase towards a maximum value at high doses. Recommended doses are close to creating the maximum benefit. In contrast, three systematic reviews found no ceiling for adverse effects, which increased in an approximately linear fashion with dose.

What are the effects of co-treatments to reduce the risk of gastrointestinal adverse effects of NSAIDs?

LIKELY TO BE BENEFICIAL

H_2 blockers in people who cannot avoid NSAIDs

One systematic review in people who had taken NSAIDs for 3 months has found that double doses of H_2 blockers versus placebo significantly reduce the development of endoscopically diagnosed gastric and duodenal ulcers. One RCT found that omeprazole versus ranitidine in double doses significantly increased remission after 6 months. One RCT with a high withdrawal and exclusion rate found weak evidence that misoprostol versus ranitidine in double doses significantly reduced the number of people with gastric ulcers.

Omeprazole (*v* H_2 blockers) in people in people who cannot avoid NSAIDs

One systematic review in people who had taken NSAIDs for at least 3 months has found that omeprazole versus placebo significantly reduces the incidence of endoscopically diagnosed gastric and duodenal ulcers.

TRADE OFF BETWEEN BENEFITS AND HARMS

Misoprostol in people who cannot avoid NSAIDs

One systematic review in people who had taken NSAIDs for at least 3 months has found that misoprostol versus placebo significantly reduces the development of endoscopically diagnosed gastric and duodenal ulcers. One additional RCT in people with rheumatoid arthritis taking NSAIDs found that misoprostol versus placebo significantly reduced the incidence of serious upper gastrointestinal complications, such as perforation, gastric outlet obstruction, or bleeding over 6 months. Subgroup analysis found a greater absolute effect in people at high risk. RCTs have found that misoprostol versus placebo significantly increases gastrointestinal adverse events, such as diarrhoea and abdominal pain. One RCT found that more people with ulcers who had improved with either omeprazole or misoprostol, and who were then re-randomised to omeprazole or misoprostol and remained in remission with omeprazole versus misoprostol.

Clin Evid Concise 2003;9:246–247.

What are the effects of topical NSAIDs?

BENEFICIAL

Topical NSAIDs in acute and chronic pain conditions

One systematic review in people with acute and chronic pain conditions has found that topical NSAIDs versus placebo significantly reduce pain.

UNKNOWN EFFECTIVENESS

Topical versus systemic NSAIDs or alternative analgesics

One systematic review found no high quality RCTs of topical NSAIDs versus oral forms of the same NSAID, or versus paracetamol.

DEFINITION NSAIDs have anti-inflammatory, analgesic, and antipyretic effects, and inhibit platelet aggregation. The drugs have no documented effect on the course of musculoskeletal diseases such as rheumatoid arthritis and osteoarthritis.

INCIDENCE/ PREVALENCE NSAIDs are widely used. Almost 10% of people in the Netherlands used a non-aspirin NSAID in 1987, and the overall use was 11 defined daily doses(G) per 1000 population per day.[1] In Australia in 1994, overall use was 35 defined daily doses per 1000 population per day, with 36% of the people receiving NSAIDs for osteoarthritis, 42% for sprain and strain or low back pain, and 4% for rheumatoid arthritis; 35% were aged over 60 years.[2]

Please refer to CD-ROM for full text and references.

Osteoarthritis

Search date March 2002

David Scott, Claire Smith, Stefan Lohmander, and Jiri Chard

What are the effects of treatments?

BENEFICIAL

Hip replacement

One systematic review of observational studies has found that hip replacement is effective for at least 10 years.

Knee replacement

Systematic reviews have found that knee replacement is effective in relieving pain and improving function. One RCT found limited evidence that unicompartmental knee operations are more effective than tricompartmental replacement. We found limited evidence that unicompartmental knee operations are more effective than bicompartmental operations.

Systemic analgesics

Systematic reviews in people with osteoarthritis of the hip or knee found limited evidence that simple analgesics, such as paracetamol (acetaminophen), versus placebo reduced pain.

Systemic non-steroidal anti-inflammatory drugs

Systematic reviews in people with osteoarthritis of the hip have found that NSAIDs reduce pain. We found no good evidence that NSAIDs are superior to simple analgesics, such as paracetamol (acetaminophen), or that there are differences between NSAIDs in relieving pain. Serious concerns exist relating to trial quality and commercial bias.

Topical agents

One systematic review and one additional RCT have found that topical agents containing NSAIDs versus placebo significantly reduce pain. One systematic review found that systemic adverse events were no more common than with placebo. RCTs found that capsaicin versus placebo significantly improved pain. We found no RCTs comparing different topical agents or comparing topical agents versus other local treatments such as heat or cold packs.

LIKELY TO BE BENEFICIAL

Analgesic versus non-steroidal anti-inflammatory drugs

RCTs found no good evidence that simple analgesics, such as paracetamol (acetaminophen), are significantly different from NSAIDs in pain relief.

Exercise (pain relief and improved function)

Systematic reviews and subsequent RCTs have found that exercise and physical therapy reduce pain and disability in people with hip or knee osteoarthritis, although many of the trials were limited by poor methods and reporting.

Hip replacement in older people

One systematic review of observational studies found that people over 75 years may have worse outcomes than people age 45–75 years in terms of pain relief and function.

Intra-articular glucocorticoid injections of the knee

One systematic review and one subsequent RCT found limited evidence that intra-articular glucocorticoids versus placebo reduced pain for 1–4 weeks. ▶

Intra-articular hyaluronan injections of the knee

One systematic review and subsequent non-systematic reviews and RCTs found limited evidence that hyaluronan versus placebo reduced pain for 1–6 months.

Knee replacement in older people

We found limited evidence from observational studies suggesting that knee replacement is effective in older people.

Osteotomy

We found no RCTs comparing osteotomy versus conservative treatment. We found limited evidence from two RCTs that osteotomy is as effective as knee replacement.

Physical aids

RCTs in people with knee osteoarthritis found limited evidence that physical aids (joint braces or taping of the joint) may improve disease specific quality of life.

TRADE OFF BETWEEN BENEFITS AND HARMS

Hip replacement in obese people

One systematic review of observational studies suggested that people who weigh over 70 kg may have worse outcomes in terms of pain relief and function after hip replacement. One study found lower rates of long term survival of implant in obese people.

Hip replacement in younger people

One systematic review of observational studies suggested that people under 45 years old may have worse outcomes in terms of pain relief and function after hip replacement. One cohort study found that younger people were at greater risk of revision.

UNKNOWN EFFECTIVENESS

Chondroitin

One systematic review and two subsequent RCTs found limited evidence that chondroitin improved symptoms more than placebo.

Education

We found insufficient evidence to assess the effects of education and behavioural change in people with hip or knee osteoarthritis.

Glucosamine

Systematic reviews and subsequent RCTs found limited evidence that glucosamine versus placebo improved symptoms, but publication bias and poor trial quality makes interpretation of results difficult.

Glucosamine plus chondroitin

We found no RCTs on glucosamine plus chondroitin alone. We found limited evidence in people with mild or moderate osteoarthritis that glucosamine plus chondroitin plus manganese ascorbate versus placebo significantly improved disease severity scores.

Knee replacement in obese people

We found limited and conflicting evidence from observational studies on the effects of obesity on outcomes after knee replacement.

Other intra-articular injections of the knee

We found limited evidence on other intra-articular treatments such as radioactive isotopes, glycosaminoglycan poly sulphuric acid, orgotein and morphine.

LIKELY TO BE INEFFECTIVE OR HARMFUL

Systemic analgesics in people with existing liver damage

Observational evidence suggests that lower doses of paracetamol (acetominophen) may cause liver damage in people with liver disease.

Systemic non-steroidal anti-inflammatory drugs in older people and people at risk of renal disease or peptic ulceration

One RCT found that NSAIDs increased the risk of renal or gastrointestinal damage in older people with osteoarthritis, particularly those with intercurrent disease.

DEFINITION Osteoarthritis is a heterogeneous condition for which the prevalence, risk factors, clinical manifestations, and prognosis vary according to the joints affected. It most commonly affects hands, knees, hips, and spinal apophyseal joints. It is usually defined by pathological or radiological criteria rather than clinical features, and is characterised by focal areas of damage to the cartilage surfaces of synovial joints, associated with remodelling of the underlying bone and mild synovitis. When severe, there is characteristic joint space narrowing and osteophyte formation, with visible subchondral bone changes on radiography.

INCIDENCE/ PREVALENCE Osteoarthritis is common and an important cause of pain and disability in older adults.[1,2] Radiographic features are practically universal in at least some joints in people aged over 60 years, but significant clinical disease probably affects 10–20% of people. Knee disease is about twice as prevalent as hip disease in people aged over 60 years (about 10% *v* 5%).[3,4]

AETIOLOGY/ RISK FACTORS The main initiating factors are abnormalities in joint shape or injury. Genetic factors are probably implicated.

PROGNOSIS The natural history of osteoarthritis is poorly understood. Only a minority of people with clinical disease of the hip or knee joint progress to requiring surgery.

Please refer to CD-ROM for full text and references.

Plantar heel pain and fasciitis

Search date May 2002

Fay Crawford

What are the effects of treatments?

TRADE OFF BETWEEN BENEFITS AND HARMS

Corticosteroid injection plus local anaesthesia versus local anaesthetic injection alone (short term)

One RCT found a significant reduction in pain with prednisolone plus lidocaine injection versus lidocaine alone after 1 month. Observational studies have found a high rate of plantar fascia rupture and other complications associated with corticosteroid injections, which may lead to chronic disability in some people.

UNKNOWN EFFECTIVENESS

Casted orthoses (custom made insoles⊕)

We found no RCTs about the effects of casted orthoses versus placebo or no treatment. One systematic review and subsequent RCTs found limited and conflicting evidence about the effects of orthoses versus heel pads or other physical supports.

Corticosteroid injection plus local anaesthesia versus pads (short term)

One RCT found a significant improvement in pain with triamcinolone plus lidocaine injection versus heel pad after 1 month. One small RCT found no significant difference in pain with triamcinolone plus lidocaine injection versus heel pad at 1, 2, or 12 weeks. One RCT found no significant difference in pain with dexamethasone plus local anaesthetic injection plus oral etodolac versus heel pads plus paracetemol at 3 months.

Corticosteroid injection alone or plus local anaesthetic injection versus placebo (short term)

We found no RCTs of corticosteroid injections alone versus placebo that assessed short term outcomes. One systematic review identified no RCTs comparing corticosteroid injection plus local anaesthesia versus placebo.

Extracorporeal shock wave therapy

One small RCT found limited evidence that extracorporeal shock wave therapy⊕ versus sham treatment improved pain at 6 weeks. Two RCTs found a non-significant reduction in pain with extracorporeal shock wave therapy versus sham treatment after 2 months and 12 weeks, respectively. One RCT found limited evidence of a significant improvement in pain with high dose versus low dose extracorporeal shock wave therapy.

Heel pads and heel cups

We found no RCTs about the effects of heel pads⊕ versus placebo or no treatment. One systematic review and subsequent RCTs found limited and conflicting evidence about the effects of heel pads and heel cups versus other treatment modalities.

Lasers

One small RCT identified by a systematic review found no significant difference in pain with laser treatment versus placebo.

Local anaesthetic injection

We found no RCTs on the effects of local anaesthesia versus placebo or no treatment. One RCT found a significant reduction in pain with prednisolone plus lidocaine injection versus lidocaine alone after 1 month; the difference was not significant after 3 or 6 months.

Night splints

One RCT found no significant difference with a night splint versus no splint in pain after 3 months.

Surgery

One systematic review identified no RCTs of surgery for heel pain.

Ultrasound

One systematic review of one small RCT found no significant difference in pain with ultrasound versus sham ultrasound.

LIKELY TO BE INEFFECTIVE OR HARMFUL

Corticosteroid injection alone or plus local anaesthetic injection versus placebo (medium to long term)

One small RCT found no significant reduction in pain with hydrocortisone injection versus placebo assessed 6–18 months after the injection. One systematic review identified no RCTs comparing corticosteroid plus local anaesthetic injection versus placebo. Observational studies have found a high rate of plantar fascia rupture and other complications associated with corticosteroid injections, which may lead to chronic disability in some people.

Corticosteroid injection plus local anaesthesia versus local anaesthetic injection alone (medium to long term)

One RCT found no significant difference in pain with prednisolone plus lidocaine (lignocaine) injection versus lidocaine alone after 3 or 6 months. Observational studies have found a high rate of plantar fascia rupture and other complications associated with corticosteroid injections, which may lead to chronic disability in some people.

Corticosteroid injection plus local anaesthesia versus pads (medium to long term)

One RCT found no significant difference in pain with triamcinolone plus lidocaine injection versus heel pad**G** after 24 weeks. One RCT found no significant difference in pain with dexamethasone plus local anaesthetic injection plus oral etodolac versus heel pads plus paracetemol at 3 months. Observational studies have found a high rate of plantar fascia rupture and other complications associated with corticosteroid injections, which may lead to chronic disability in some people.

DEFINITION Plantar heel pain is soreness or tenderness of the heel. It often radiates from the central part of the heel pad or the medial tubercle of the calcaneum, but may extend along the plantar fascia into the medial longitudinal arch of the foot. Severity may range from an irritation at the origin of the plantar fascia, which is noticeable on rising after rest, to an incapacitating pain. This review excludes clinically evident underlying disorders, for example, infection, calcaneal fracture, and calcaneal nerve entrapment, which can be distinguished by their characteristic history and signs. (A calcaneal fracture may present after trauma, whereas calcaneal nerve entrapment gives rise to shooting pains and feelings of "pins and needles" on the medial aspect of the heel.)

Plantar heel pain and fasciitis

INCIDENCE/ PREVALENCE The incidence and prevalence of plantar heel pain is uncertain. Plantar heel pain primarily affects those in mid to late life.[1]

AETIOLOGY/ RISK FACTORS Unknown.

PROGNOSIS One systematic review (search date 1997) found that almost all of the included trials reported an improvement in discomfort regardless of the intervention received (including placebo), suggesting that the condition is at least partially self limiting.[1] A telephone survey of 100 people treated conservatively (average follow up 47 months) found that 82 people had resolution of symptoms, 15 had continued symptoms but no limitations of activity or work, and three had continued symptoms that limited activity or changed work status.[2] Thirty one people said that they would have seriously considered surgical treatment at the time medical attention was sought. The three people still with limitation had bilateral symptoms but no other clear risk factors.

Please refer to CD-ROM for full text and references.

Raynaud's phenomenon (primary)

Search date June 2002

Janet Pope

What are the effects of treatments? New

TRADE OFF BETWEEN BENEFITS AND HARMS

Nifedipine

Six RCTs found that nifedipine significantly reduced the frequency and severity of attacks over 4–12 weeks compared with placebo🅣, and was rated by participants as more effective than placebo in improving overall symptoms. The RCTs found that nifedipine was associated with higher rates of adverse effects compared with placebo, including flushing, headache, oedema, and tachycardia.

UNKNOWN EFFECTIVENESS

Nicardipine

We found inconclusive evidence from two RCTs about the effects of nicardipine compared with placebo.

Prazosin

One small crossover RCT found no clear evidence of benefit from prazosin. It found that prasozin significantly reduced the number and duration of attacks over 6 weeks after crossover compared with placebo, but found no significant difference in the severity of attacks.

Amlodopine; diltiazem; moxisylyte (thymoxamine)

We found no good RCTs of these interventions.

Inositol nicotinate; naftidrofuryl oxalate

RCTs provided insufficient evidence to assess these interventions.

DEFINITION Raynaud's phenomenon is episodic vasospasm of the peripheral arteries causing pallor followed by cyanosis and redness with pain and sometimes paraesthesia, and, rarely, ulceration of the fingers and toes (and in some cases of the ears or nose). Primary or idiopathic Raynaud's phenomenon (Raynaud's disease) occurs without an underlying disease. Secondary Raynaud's phenomenon (Raynaud's syndrome) occurs in association with an underlying disease — usually connective tissue disorders such as scleroderma, systemic lupus erythematosus, rheumatoid arthritis, or polymyositis. This review excludes secondary Raynaud's phenomenon.

INCIDENCE/ PREVALENCE The prevalence of primary Raynaud's phenomenon varies by gender, country, and exposure to workplace vibration. One large US cohort study (4182 people) found symptoms in 9.6% of women and 8.1% of men, of whom 81% had primary Raynaud's phenomenon.[1] Smaller cohort studies in Spain have estimated the prevalence of Raynaud's phenomenon to be 3.7–4.0%, of which 90% is primary Raynaud's phenomenon.[2,3] One cohort study in Japan (332 men, 731 women) found symptoms of primary Raynaud's phenomenon in 3.4% of women and 3.0% of men.[4]

AETIOLOGY/ RISK FACTORS The aetiology of primary Raynaud's phenomenon is unknown.[5] There is evidence for genetic predisposition,[6,7] most likely in those people with early onset Raynaud's phenomenon (aged < 40 years).[8] One prospective observational study (424 people with Raynaud's phenomenon) found that 73% of sufferers first developed symptoms before age 40 years.[8] Women are more at risk than ▶

men (OR 3.0, 95% CI 1.2 to 7.8, in 1 US case control study [235 people]).[9] The other known risk factor is occupational exposure to vibration from tools (symptoms developed in about 8% with exposure *v* 2.7% with no exposure in 2 cohorts from Japan).[10,11] People who are obese may be less at risk.[9] Symptoms are often worsened by cold or emotion.

PROGNOSIS Attacks may last from several minutes to a few hours. One systematic review (search date 1996, 10 prospective observational studies, 639 people with primary Raynaud's phenomenon) found that only 13% of long term sufferers later manifested an underlying disorder such as scleroderma.[12]

Please refer to CD-ROM for full text and references.

Rheumatoid arthritis

Search date July 2002

Paul Emery and Maria Suarez-Almazor

What are the effects of treatments?

BENEFICIAL

Antimalarials

One systematic review has found that hydroxychloroquine reduces disease activity and joint inflammation compared with placebo in people with rheumatoid arthritis. We found insufficient evidence about effects on functional status. One systematic review found no consistent difference in effectiveness between antimalarials and other disease modifying antirheumatic drugs (DMARDs).

Early intervention with DMARDs

One systematic review and one additional RCT found that early DMARDs (oral gold, im gold, hydroxychloroquine, methotrexate, minocycline) significantly improved radiological progression, swollen joint counts, and quality of life scores at 12–60 months compared with delayed treatment.

Methotrexate

One systematic review has found that methotrexate reduces joint inflammation and radiological progression and improves functional status compared with placebo in people with rheumatoid arthritis. One systematic review and subsequent RCTs have found no consistent differences in efficacy between methotrexate versus leflunomide, parenteral gold, or etanercept.

Minocycline

RCTs have found that minocycline improves control of disease activity compared with placebo. We found no RCTs comparing minocycline versus other DMARDs.

Short term low dose oral corticosteroids

One systematic review has found that low dose oral corticosteroids for several weeks significantly reduces disease activity and joint inflammation compared with placebo.

Sulfasalazine

Systematic reviews have found that sulfasalazine versus placebo for 6 months significantly reduces disease activity and joint inflammation. We found inadequate evidence on radiological progression and functional status. One systematic review found no consistent differences between sulfasalazine and other DMARDs. Another systematic review of observational studies and RCTs found that over 5 years people were less likely to continue sulfasalazine than methotrexate.

LIKELY TO BE BENEFICIAL

Auranofin (less effective than other DMARDs)

One systematic review has found that auranofin (oral gold) versus placebo reduces disease activity and joint inflammation, but found no evidence on radiological progression or long term functional status. Limited evidence from RCTs suggests that auranofin is less effective than DMARDs.

Clin Evid Concise 2003;9:256–258.

Leflunomide (long term safety unclear)

One systematic review has found that leflunomide versus placebo reduces disease activity and joint inflammation, improves functional status and health related quality of life, and decreases radiological progression. We found no good evidence on long term adverse effects. We found no consistent evidence of a difference in clinical efficacy between leflunomide and methotrexate or sulfasalazine.

Treatment with several DMARDs combined

One systematic review and subsequent RCTs have found that combining certain DMARDs is more effective than using individual drugs alone. However, the balance between benefit and harm varies among combinations.

Tumour necrosis factor antagonists (long term safety unclear)

RCTs have found that tumour necrosis factor antibodies (etanercept and infliximab) significantly improve symptoms, and reduce long term disease activity and joint inflammation compared with placebo. One RCT found no significant difference between etanercept and methotrexate for quality of life at 1 year. Short term toxicity is relatively low, but long term safety is less clear.

TRADE OFF BETWEEN BENEFITS AND HARMS

Azathioprine

One systematic review has found that azathioprine versus placebo reduces disease activity in the short term (16 wks to 6 months). We found no evidence on radiological progression or long term functional status. A high level of toxicity limits the usefulness of azathioprine.

Ciclosporin

One systematic review has found that ciclosporin for a minimum of 4 months significantly reduces disease activity and joint inflammation, improves functional status, and may decrease the rate of radiological progression compared with methotrexate. One RCT found no significant difference betwen parenteral gold versus ciclosporin for radiological joint damage or self assessment of change in disease activity at 36 months. A very high frequency of toxicity limits the usefulness of ciclosporin.

Cyclophosphamide

One systematic review has found that cyclophosphamide significantly reduces disease activity and joint inflammation compared with placebo at 6 months. It may also reduce the rate of radiological progression, but evidence was limited. We found no evidence of its effect on long term functional status. Severe toxicity limits its usefulness.

Long term low dose oral corticosteroids

One systematic review and one subsequent RCT have found that low dose oral corticosteroids for at least 3 months significantly reduce pain, joint inflammation, and functional status compared with placebo. However, long term use is associated with considerable adverse effects.

Parenteral gold

One systematic review has found that parenteral gold reduces disease activity and joint inflammation, and slows radiological progression compared with placebo in people with rheumatoid arthritis. We found no evidence on long term functional status. One systematic review and one RCT both indicate increased withdrawals because of toxicity. RCTs found no significant differences in clinical efficacy between parenteral gold versus methotrexate or ciclosporin at 1–3 years.

Penicillamine

One systematic review has found that penicillamine reduces disease activity and joint inflammation compared with placebo at 4–6 months. We found no evidence about effects of penicillamine on radiological progression or long term functional status. One systematic review has found no consistent difference between penicillamine versus other DMARDs. Common and potentially serious adverse effects limit the usefulness of penicillamine.

DEFINITION Rheumatoid arthritis is a chronic inflammatory disorder. It is characterised by a chronic polyarthritis that primarily affects the peripheral joints and related periarticular tissues. It usually starts as an insidious symmetric polyarthritis, often with non-specific systemic symptoms. Diagnostic criteria include arthritis lasting longer than 6 weeks (although evidence suggests that 12 wks is more specific), positive rheumatoid factor, and radiological damage.[1]

INCIDENCE/ PREVALENCE Prevalence ranges from 0.5–1.5% of the population in industrialised countries.[2,3] Rheumatoid arthritis occurs more frequently in women than men (ratio 2.5 : 1).[2,3] The annual incidence in women was recently estimated at 36/100 000 and in men at 14/100 000.[3]

AETIOLOGY/ RISK FACTORS The evidence suggests that the cause is multifactorial in people with genetic susceptibility.[4]

PROGNOSIS The course of rheumatoid arthritis is variable and unpredictable. Some people experience flares and remissions, and others a progressive course. Over years, structural damage occurs, leading to articular deformities and functional impairment. About half of people will be unable to work within 10 years.[5] Rheumatoid arthritis shortens life expectancy.[6]

Please refer to CD-ROM for full text and references.

Shoulder pain

Search date October 2002

Cathy Speed and Brian Hazleman

What are the effects of treatments?

Shoulder pain is not a specific diagnosis. Well designed, double blind RCTs of specific interventions in specific shoulder disorders are needed.
Systematic reviews have found RCTs mostly with poor methods, and pronounced heterogeneity of study populations and outcome measures.
We found insufficient evidence on the effects of most interventions in people with non-specific shoulder pain.

UNKNOWN EFFECTIVENESS

Arthroscopic laser subacromial decompression
One systematic review found no RCTs on arthroscopic laser subacromial decompression.

Electrical stimulation
One RCT found no significant difference in pain between electrical stimulation versus control. However, the study may have lacked power to detect clinically important differences.

Extracorporeal shock wave therapy
We found mixed results from three RCTs. The first RCT found that one or two sessions of high energy extracorporeal shock wave therapy versus placebo improved pain and function in people with calcific tendinitis. However, two further RCTs in people with rotator cuff tendinosis found no significant difference for extracorporeal shock wave therapy versus sham treatment for pain or function at 3–6 months.

Intra-articular corticosteroid injection
One small RCT found no significant difference for intra-articular triamcinolone versus saline in pain score, change in mobility, or function at 3 weeks. One small RCT found no significant difference for intra-articular methylprednisolone plus lidocaine (lignocaine) versus lidocaine alone in pain or shoulder motion at 24 weeks. The RCTs were small and may have lacked power to detect clinically important differences.

Intra-articular guanethidine
We found no systematic review or RCTs of intra-articular guanethidine in people with non-arthritic shoulder pain.

Laser treatment
We found mixed results from four small RCTs that compared laser treatment versus placebo in shoulder pain. Two short term RCTs found that laser improved recovery rate and pain compared with placebo at 2–4 weeks. However, two longer term RCTs found no significant difference in pain or recovery rate at 8–12 weeks.

Multidisciplinary biopsychosocial rehabilitation
One systematic review found no good quality RCTs of multidisciplinary biopsychosocial rehabilitation Ⓖ in people with shoulder pain.

Oral non-steroidal anti-inflammatory drugs
We found insufficient evidence from one systematic review and one additional RCT to draw firm conclusions about effects of oral non-steroidal anti-inflammatory drugs versus placebo in people with non-specific shoulder pain. ▶

Clin Evid Concise 2003;9:259–261.

Phonophoresis©

We found no RCTs solely in people with shoulder pain.

Physiotherapy (exercises and manual treatments)

One systematic review has found insufficient evidence about effects of physiotherapy alone versus no treatment or advice to exercise in people with shoulder pain.

Subacromial corticosteroid injection

We found no RCTs comparing subacromial injection of steroids versus placebo. We found insufficient evidence from two small RCTs to compare clinical effects of corticosteroid plus lidocaine versus lidocaine alone in people with rotator cuff tendinitis. One small RCT found limited evidence that intra-articular plus subacromial corticosteroid injections versus intra-articular and subacromial lidocaine alone increased remission rates at 4 weeks.

Surgery/forced manipulation

We found no placebo-controlled RCTs. One small RCT found that forced manipulation plus intra-articular hydrocortisone injection versus intra-articular hydrocortisone injection alone increased recovery rate at 3 months.

Transdermal glyceryl trinitrate

We found no reliable RCTs.

Ice; paracetamol or opiates; topical or intra-articular non-steroidal anti-inflammatory drugs

We found no RCTs about these interventions.

UNLIKELY TO BE BENEFICIAL

Oral corticosteroids

Two small RCTs found no evidence of reduced pain or improved abduction with oral corticosteroids versus placebo or versus no treatment at 4–8 months. Adverse effect of corticosteroids are well documented (see rheumatoid arthritis, p 256 and asthma, p 304).

Ultrasound

One systematic review and two subsequent RCTs found no clinically important difference in pain, abduction or quality of life with ultrasound versus sham treatment or no treatment.

DEFINITION Shoulder pain arises in or around the shoulder from the glenohumeral, acromioclavicular, sternoclavicular, "subacromial", and scapulothoracic articulations, and surrounding soft tissues. Regardless of the disorder, pain is the most common reason for consulting a practitioner. In adhesive capsulitis (frozen shoulder), pain is associated with pronounced restriction of movement. For most shoulder disorders, diagnosis is based on clinical features, with imaging studies playing a role in some people. Post-stroke shoulder pain is not addressed in this topic.

INCIDENCE/ PREVALENCE Each year in primary care in the UK, about 1% of adults aged over 45 years present with a new episode of shoulder pain.[1] Prevalence is uncertain, with estimates from 4–20%.[2–6] One community survey (392 people) found a 1 month prevalence of shoulder pain of 34%.[7] A second community survey (644 people aged $\geq$ 70 years) reported a point prevalence of 21%, with a higher frequency in women than men (25% *v* 17%).[8] Seventy per cent of cases involved the rotator cuff. One survey of 134 people in a community based rheumatology clinic found that 65% of cases were rotator cuff lesions; 11% were caused by localised tenderness in the pericapsular musculature; 10% acromioclavicular joint pain; 3% glenohumeral joint arthritis; and 5%

were referred pain from the neck.[9] One survey found that in adults, the annual incidence of frozen shoulder was about 2%, with those aged 40–70 years most commonly affected.[10] The age distribution of specific shoulder disorders in the community is unknown.

AETIOLOGY/ RISK FACTORS Rotator cuff disorders are associated with excessive overloading, instability of the glenohumeral and acromioclavicular joints, muscle imbalance, adverse anatomical features (narrow coracoacromial arch and a hooked acromion), cuff degeneration with aging, ischaemia, and musculoskeletal diseases that result in wasting of the cuff muscles.[11–14] Risk factors for frozen shoulder include female sex, older age, shoulder trauma, surgery, diabetes, cardiorespiratory disorders, cerebrovascular events, thyroid disease, and hemiplegia.[10,15,16] Arthritis of the glenohumeral joint can occur in numerous forms, including primary and secondary osteoarthritis, rheumatoid arthritis, and crystal arthritides.[11]

PROGNOSIS One survey in an elderly community found that most people with shoulder pain were still affected 3 years after the initial survey.[17] One prospective cohort study of 122 people in primary care found that 25% of people with shoulder pain reported previous episodes and 49% reported full recovery at 18 months' follow up.[18]

Please refer to CD-ROM for full text and references.

Tennis elbow

Search date August 2002

Willem Assendelft, Sally Green, Rachelle Buchbinder, Peter Struijs, and Nynke Smidt

What are the effects of treatments for tennis elbow (lateral epicondylitis)?

BENEFICIAL

Topical non-steroidal anti-inflammatory drugs for short term pain relief

One systematic review has found that topical non-steroidal anti-inflammatory drugs versus placebo significantly improve pain in the short term. Minor adverse effects have been reported. We found no RCTs comparing oral versus topical non-steroidal anti-inflammatory drugs.

LIKELY TO BE BENEFICIAL

Oral non-steroidal anti-inflammatory drugs

One systematic review found limited evidence of a short term improvement in pain and function with an oral non-steroidal inflammatory drug versus placebo. The review found limited evidence that fewer people receiving an oral non-steroidal anti-inflammatory drug versus a corticosteroid injection had self perceived improvement at 4 weeks, but found that an oral non-steroidal anti-inflammatory drug significantly reduced pain at 26 weeks.

TRADE OFF BETWEEN BENEFITS AND HARMS

Corticosteroid injections

We found one systematic review and two subsequent RCTs of corticosteroid injections, which found limited evidence of a short term improvement in symptoms with steroid injections versus placebo, a local anaesthetic, elbow strapping, or physiotherapy. It found no good evidence on long term effects of corticosteroids versus placebo or local anaesthetic. It found no evidence of a difference with corticosteroid injection versus mobilisation plus massage or elbow strapping in overall improvement at 1 year. However, one RCT identified by the review found significantly greater improvement in symptoms with physiotherapy versus an injection at 26 and 52 weeks. The review found limited evidence of greater self perceived improvement at 4 weeks with a corticosteroid injection versus an oral non-steroidal anti-inflammatory drug (NSAID), but found greater improvement in pain at 26 weeks with an oral non-steroidal anti-inflammatory drug.

UNKNOWN EFFECTIVENESS

Acupuncture

One systematic review and one subsequent RCT found insufficient evidence to assess the effects of acupuncture (either needle or laser).

Exercise and mobilisation

One systematic review found limited evidence of a better outcome with exercise versus ultrasound plus friction massage at 8 weeks.

Extra-corporeal shock wave therapy

One systematic review found conflicting evidence from two RCTs of the effects on symptoms of extra-corporeal shock wave therapy versus sham treatment.

Clin Evid Concise 2003;9:262–263.

Non-steroidal anti-inflammatory drugs for longer term pain relief

We found insufficient evidence to assess the longer term effects of oral or topical non-steroidal anti-inflammatory drugs.

Orthoses

One systematic review found insufficient evidence about the effects of orthoses (braces).

Surgery

One systematic review found no RCTs of surgical treatment for tennis elbow.

DEFINITION Tennis elbow has many analogous terms, including lateral elbow pain, lateral epicondylitis, rowing elbow, tendonitis of the common extensor origin, and peritendonitis of the elbow. Tennis elbow is characterised by pain and tenderness over the lateral epicondyle of the humerus and pain on resisted dorsi-flexion of the wrist, middle finger or both. For the purposes of this review, tennis elbow was restricted to lateral elbow pain, or lateral epicondylitis.

INCIDENCE/PREVALENCE Lateral elbow pain is common (population prevalence 1–3%).[1] Peak incidence is 40–50 years and for women of 42–46 years of age the incidence increases to 10%.[2,3] The incidence of lateral elbow pain in general practice is 4–7/1000 people a year.[3–5]

AETIOLOGY/RISK FACTORS Tennis elbow is considered to be an overload injury, typically after minor and often unrecognised trauma of the extensor muscles of the forearm. Despite the title tennis elbow, tennis is a direct cause in only 5% of those with epicondylitis.[6]

PROGNOSIS Although lateral elbow pain is generally self limiting, in a minority of people symptoms persist for 18 months to 2 years and in some cases for much longer.[7] The cost is therefore high, both in terms of lost productivity, and healthcare use. In a general practice trial of an expectant waiting policy 80% of the people with elbow pain of already greater than 4 weeks' duration were recovered after 1 year.[8]

Please refer to CD-ROM for full text and references.

Bell's palsy

Search date March 2002

Rodrigo Salinas

What are the effects of treatments?

UNKNOWN EFFECTIVENESS

Antiviral treatment

Two systematic reviews found no RCTs of aciclovir versus placebo. One RCT found limited evidence that aciclovir plus prednisone versus prednisone alone significantly decreased the number of people with incomplete recovery of facial function after 4 months.

Corticosteroids

One systematic review found no clear evidence that corticosteroid versus control improved the recovery of facial motor function or cosmetically disabling sequelae after 6 months.

Facial nerve decompression surgery

One systematic review identified no RCTs of facial nerve decompression.

DEFINITION Bell's palsy is an acute, unilateral paresis or paralysis of the face in a pattern consistent with peripheral nerve dysfunction, without detectable causes.[1] Additional symptoms may include pain in or behind the ear, numbness in the affected side of the face, hyperacusis, and disturbed taste on the ipsilateral anterior part of the tongue.[2–5]

INCIDENCE/ PREVALENCE The incidence is about 23/100 000 people a year, or about 1/60–70 people in a lifetime.[6] Bell's palsy affects men and women more or less equally, with a peak incidence between the ages of 10 and 40 years. It occurs with equal frequency on the right and left sides of the face.[7]

AETIOLOGY/ RISK FACTORS The cause is unclear. Viral infection, vascular ischaemia, autoimmune inflammatory disorders, and heredity have been proposed as underlying causes.[2,8,9] A viral cause has gained popularity since the isolation of the herpes simplex virus 1 genome from facial nerve endoneurial fluid in people with Bell's palsy.[10]

PROGNOSIS More than two thirds of people with Bell's palsy achieve full spontaneous recovery. The largest series of people with Bell's palsy who received no specific treatment (1011 people) found the first signs of improvement within 3 weeks of onset in 85% of people.[11] For the other 15%, some improvement occurred 3–6 months later. The same series found that 71% of people recovered normal function of the face, 13% had insignificant sequelae, and the remaining 16% had permanently diminished function, with contracture and synkinesis Ⓖ. These figures are roughly similar to those of other series of people receiving no specific treatment for Bell's palsy.[7,8,12]

Please refer to CD-ROM for full text and references.

Epilepsy

Search date July 2002

Anthony Marson and Sridharan Ramaratnam

What are the effects of treatments?

BENEFICIAL

Addition of second line drugs for drug resistant partial epilepsy

Systematic reviews in people with drug resistant partial epilepsy have found that adding gabapentin, levetiracetam, lamotrigine, oxcarbazepine, tiagabine, topiramate, vigabatrin, or zonisamide versus adding placebo to usual treatment significantly reduces seizure frequency. Adding second line drugs versus adding placebo increases the frequency of adverse effects. We found no good evidence from RCTs on which to make a choice among drugs.

Antiepileptic monotherapy in generalised epilepsy

We found no placebo controlled trials of the main antiepileptic drugs (carbamazepine, phenobarbital [phenobarbitone], phenytoin, sodium valproate), but widespread consensus holds that these drugs are effective. Systematic reviews have found no good evidence on which to base a choice among these drugs in terms of seizure control.

Antiepileptic monotherapy in partial epilepsy

We found no placebo controlled trials of the main antiepileptic drugs (carbamazepine, phenobarbital, phenytoin, sodium valproate), but widespread consensus holds that these drugs are effective. Systematic reviews have found no good evidence on which to base a choice among these drugs in terms of seizure control. One systematic review has found that phenobarbital versus phenytoin is more likely to be withdrawn, presumably because of adverse effects.

LIKELY TO BE BENEFICIAL

Educational programmes

One RCT found that a two day education programme significantly reduced seizure frequency at 6 months compared with waiting list control, although it found no significant difference for health related quality of life. Two RCTs found that an educational package versus control improved knowledge and understanding of epilepsy, adjustment to epilepsy and psychosocial functioning.

TRADE OFF BETWEEN BENEFITS AND HARMS

Antiepileptic drugs after a single seizure

RCTs have found that immediate treatment of single seizures with antiepileptic drugs versus no treatment reduces seizure frequency at 2 years. We found no evidence that treatment alters long term prognosis. Long term antiepileptic drug treatment is potentially harmful.

Antiepileptic drug withdrawal for people in remission

One systematic review of observational studies and one RCT have found that antiepileptic drug withdrawal for people in remission is associated with a higher risk of seizure recurrence than continued treatment. Clinical predictors of relapse after drug withdrawal include age, seizure type, number of antiepileptic drugs being taken, whether seizures have occurred since antiepileptic drugs were started, and the period of remission before drug withdrawal.

▶

Clin Evid Concise 2003;9:265–266.

UNKNOWN EFFECTIVENESS

Cognitive behavioural therapy

Two small RCTs found no significant difference with cognitive behavioural therapy(G) versus control in seizure frequency or psychosocial function. Another small RCT found that cognitive behavioural treatment versus control treatment significantly improved a depression score in people with epilepsy plus depressed mood.

Family counselling

One small RCT with weak methods found that family counselling versus no treatment significantly improved perceived acceptance by the family, emotional adjustment, interpersonal adjustment, adjustment to seizures, and overall psychosocial function. The RCT gave no information on seizure reduction.

Relaxation plus behavioural modification therapy

RCTs found insufficient evidence about the effects of combined relaxation and behavioural modification on seizures. One RCT found that relaxation plus behavioural therapy versus control significantly improved anxiety and adjustment.

Biofeedback; relaxation therapy(G); yoga

Systematic reviews have found insufficient evidence on the effects of these interventions.

DEFINITION Epilepsy is a group of disorders rather than a single disease. Seizures can be classified by type as partial (categorised as simple partial(G), complex partial(G), and secondary generalised tonic clonic seizures), or generalised (categorised as generalised tonic clonic, absence, myoclonic, tonic, and atonic seizures(G)).[1]

INCIDENCE/ PREVALENCE Epilepsy is common, with an estimated prevalence in the developed world of 5–10/1000, and an annual incidence of 50/100 000 people.[2] About 3% of people will be given a diagnosis of epilepsy at some time in their lives.[3]

AETIOLOGY/ RISK FACTORS Epilepsy can also be classified by cause.[1] Idiopathic generalised epilepsies (such as juvenile myoclonic epilepsy or childhood absence epilepsy) are largely genetic. Symptomatic epilepsies result from a known cerebral abnormality — for example, temporal lobe epilepsy may result from a congenital defect, mesial temporal sclerosis, or a tumour. Cryptogenic epilepsies are those that cannot be classified as idiopathic or symptomatic and in which no causative factor has been identified, but is suspected.

PROGNOSIS For most people with epilepsy the prognosis is good. About 70% go into remission, defined as being seizure free for 5 years on or off treatment. This leaves 20–30% who develop chronic epilepsy, often treated with multiple antiepileptic drugs.[4] About 60% of untreated people suffer no further seizures in the 2 years after their first seizure.[5]

Please refer to CD-ROM for full text and references.

Essential tremor

Search date September 2002

Joaquim Ferreira and Cristina Sampaio

What are the effects of drug treatments in people with essential tremor of the hand?

LIKELY TO BE BENEFICIAL

Propranolol (evidence for short term only)

Small RCTs have found that propranolol versus placebo significantly improves short term clinical scores, tremor amplitude, and symptom severity for up to 6 weeks.

TRADE OFF BETWEEN BENEFITS AND HARMS

Botulinum A toxin–haemagglutinin complex (evidence for short term only)

RCTs comparing botulinum A toxin–haemagglutinin complex versus placebo found short term improvement of clinical rating scales, but no consistent improvement of motor task performance or functional disability. Hand weakness, which is dose dependent and transient, is a frequent adverse effect.

Phenobarbital (evidence for short term only)

One small RCT found limited evidence that phenobarbital (phenobarbitone) versus placebo significantly improved tremor scores at 5 weeks. However, two further RCTs found no significant difference between phenobarbital and placebo. Phenobarbital is associated with depression and cognitive and behavioural effects.

Primidone (evidence for short term only)

Three small, short term RCTs found limited evidence that primidone versus placebo improved tremor and functional ability. We found no long term RCTs. Primidone is associated with depression and cognitive and behavioural adverse effects.

Topiramate (evidence for short term only) *New*

One RCT found that topiramate improved observer rated tremor score but was associated with more adverse effects compared with placebo. The clinical importance of the difference in tremor score is uncertain.

UNKNOWN EFFECTIVENESS

All treatment options (long term)

We found no RCTs that reported the long term effects of drug treatments for essential tremor.

β Blockers other than propranolol (atenolol, sotalol)

Small RCTs found weak evidence that sotalol or atenolol versus placebo significantly improved symptoms and self evaluated measures of tremor at 5 days to 4 weeks. However, we were unable to draw reliable conclusions about effects.

Benzodiazepines

Two small short term RCTs found weak evidence that alprazolam may improve tremor and function compared with placebo. However, we were unable to draw reliable conclusions about effects. We found insufficient evidence to compare effects of clonazepam versus placebo. Adverse effects with benzodiazepines, including sedation and cognitive and behavioural effects, have been well described for other conditions (see panic disorder, p 208).

Calcium channel blockers (nicardipine, nimodipine)

Poor quality RCTs found insufficient evidence about the effects of dihydropyridine calcium channel blockers versus placebo.

▶

Carbonic anhydrase inhibitors

Two RCTs found no evidence of benefit with carbonic anhydrase inhibitors compared with placebo.

Clonidine

One RCT found no significant difference between clonidine and placebo for clinical improvement. However, the study may have lacked power to detect clinically important differences.

Flunarizine

One small RCT found weak evidence that flunarizine versus placebo may improve symptoms after 1 month of treatment.

Gabapentin

Small crossover RCTs found insufficient evidence about the effects of gabapentin versus placebo.

Isoniazid

One RCT found no significant difference with isoniazid versus placebo in clinical score. However, the study may have lacked power to detect clinically important differences.

DEFINITION Tremor is a rhythmic, mechanical oscillation of at least one body region. The term essential tremor is used when there is either a persistent bilateral tremor of hands and forearms, or an isolated tremor of the head without abnormal posturing, and when there is no evidence that the tremor arises from another identifiable or separately named cause. The diagnosis is not made if there are abnormal neurological signs, known causes of enhanced physiological tremor, a history or signs of psychogenic tremor, sudden change in severity, primary orthostatic tremor, isolated voice tremor, isolated position specific or task specific tremors, and isolated tongue, chin, or leg tremor.[1]

INCIDENCE/PREVALENCE Essential tremor is one of the most common movement disorders throughout the world, with a prevalence of 0.4–3.9% in the general population.[2]

AETIOLOGY/RISK FACTORS Essential tremor is sometimes inherited with an autosomal dominant pattern. About 40% of people with essential tremor have no family history. Alcohol ingestion provides symptomatic benefit in 50–70% of people.[3]

PROGNOSIS Essential tremor is a persistent and progressive condition. It usually begins during young adulthood and the severity of the tremor increases slowly. Only a small proportion of people with essential tremor seek medical advice, but the proportion in different surveys varies from 0.5–11%.[2] Most people with essential tremor are only mildly affected. However, most of the people who seek medical care are disabled to some extent, and most are socially handicapped by the tremor.[4] A quarter of people receiving medical care for the tremor change jobs or retire because of essential tremor induced disability.[3,5]

Please refer to CD-ROM for full text and references.

Headache (chronic tension type)

Search date June 2002

Peter J Goadsby

What are the effects of treatments?

BENEFICIAL

Amitriptyline (only short term evidence)

One systematic review of small, brief RCTs has found that amitriptyline versus placebo reduces duration and frequency of chronic tension-type headache (CTTH).

LIKELY TO BE BENEFICIAL

Cognitive beahvioural therapy

One systematic review of three small RCTs and one subsequent RCT found limited evidence that cognitive behavioural therapy reduced symptoms at 6 months compared with no treatment.

UNKNOWN EFFECTIVENESS

Acupuncture

Two systematic reviews and one small RCT found insufficient evidence from heterogeneous RCTs that acupuncture was more effective than placebo in people with episodic or chronic tension-type headache. Many of the RCTs were of poor quality. Some of the RCTs may have lacked power to exclude a clinically important effect.

Botulinum toxin; relaxation⊖ and electromyographic biofeedback therapy⊖; serotonin reuptake inhibitors; tricyclic antidepressants other than amitriptyline

We found insufficient evidence about the effects of these interventions.

LIKELY TO BE INEFFECTIVE OR HARMFUL

Benzodiazepines

Two RCTs found insufficient evidence about the effects of benzodiazepines compared with placebo or other treatments. Benzodiazepines are commonly associated with adverse effects if taken regularly.

Regular acute pain relief medication

We found no RCTs. We found insufficient evidence from one non-systematic review of observational studies about benefits of common analgesics in people with chronic tension type headache. It found that sustained frequent use of some analgesics was associated with chronic headache and reduced effectiveness of prophylactic treatment.

DEFINITION The 1988 International Headache Society criteria for CTTH are headaches on 15 or more days a month (180 days/year) for at least 6 months; pain that is bilateral, pressing, or tightening in quality, of mild or moderate intensity, that does not prohibit activities, and that is not aggravated by routine physical activity; presence of no more than one additional clinical feature (nausea, photophobia, or phonophobia) and no vomiting.[1] CTTH is distinguished from chronic daily headache, which is simply a descriptive term for any headache type occurring for 15 days or more a month that may be due to CTTH as well as migraine or analgesic associated headache.[2] In contrast to CTTH, episodic tension-type headache can last for 30 minutes to 7 days and occurs for fewer ▶

than 180 days a year. Terms based on assumed mechanisms (muscle contraction headache, tension headache) are not operationally defined, and old studies that used these terms may have included people with many different types of headache. The greatest obstacle to the study of tension-type headache is the lack of any single proven specific or reliable, clinical, or biological defining characteristic of the disorder.

INCIDENCE/ PREVALENCE The prevalence of chronic daily headache from a survey of the general population in the USA was 4.1%. Half of sufferers met the International Headache Society criteria for CTTH.[3] In a survey of 2500 undergraduate students in the USA, the prevalence of CTTH was 2%.[4] The prevalence of CTTH was 2.5% in a Danish population based survey of 975 individuals.[5]

AETIOLOGY/ RISK FACTORS Tension-type headache is more prevalent in women (65% of cases in one survey).[6] Symptoms begin before the age of 10 years in 15% of people with CTTH. Prevalence declines with age.[7] There is a family history of some form of headache in 40% of people with CTTH.[8]

PROGNOSIS The prevalence of CTTH declines with age.[7]

Please refer to CD-ROM for full text and references.

Migraine headache

Search date April 2002

Luis Morillo

What are the effects of drug treatment?

BENEFICIAL

Eletriptan

One systematic review found that eletriptan versus placebo significantly increased headache relief**G**. One subsequent RCT found that eletriptan versus placebo or versus sumatriptan significantly increased headache relief.

Naratriptan

Three RCTs have found that naratriptan versus placebo significantly increases headache relief at 4 hours. One RCT comparing naratriptan versus sumatriptan found no significant difference in headache recurrence**G**.

Rizatriptan

One systematic review has found that rizatriptan versus placebo significantly improves headache relief. Two additional RCTs found rizatriptan versus placebo significantly increased headache relief.

Salicylates (oral or iv lysine-acetylsalicylate [L-ASA] alone or in combination with metoclopramide; aspirin alone or in combination with metoclopramide; aspirin in combination with paracetamol and caffeine)

Three RCTs have found that oral or intravenous L-ASA (alone or in combination with metoclopramide) versus placebo significantly increases the proportion of people with headache relief. Two RCTs found that effervescent aspirin (alone or in combination with metoclopramide) versus placebo significantly increased headache relief. One large RCT found that aspirin plus paracetamol plus caffeine versus placebo significantly increased headache relief. One RCT found no significant difference between aspirin versus paracetamol plus codeine in headache relief, although both were significantly superior to placebo. One RCT found no significant difference with aspirin plus metoclopramide versus sumatriptan in headache relief. One small crossover RCT found limited evidence that acetylsalicylic acid versus placebo significantly reduced the duration of attack and headache intensity.

Sumatriptan

RCTs have found that subcutaneous, oral, or intranasal sumatriptan versus placebo significantly increases headache relief. One RCT found no significant difference with sumatriptan versus aspirin plus metoclopramide in headache relief. One RCT found no significant difference with sumatriptan versus tolfenamic acid in headache relief. One RCT found that sumatriptan versus ergotamine plus caffeine was significantly more effective for headache relief or reducing the need for rescue medication. One RCT comparing sumatriptan versus naratriptan found no significant difference in headache recurrence. One RCT found no significant difference between sumatriptan versus zolmitriptan in headache relief.

Zolmitriptan

Two large RCTs have found that oral zolmitriptan versus placebo significantly increases headache relief. One RCT found no significant difference between zolmitriptan versus sumatriptan in headache relief.

▶

Clin Evid Concise 2003;9:271–273.

LIKELY TO BE BENEFICIAL

Diclofenac

Three RCTs found that diclofenac versus placebo significantly improved outcome (measured by treatment success, headache relief, and headache pain, respectively). One RCT found that intramuscular diclofenac versus intramuscular paracetamol significantly increased the number of people with partial relief of overall migraine symptoms within 35 minutes.

Ergotamine derivatives

One systematic review found three RCTs in which ergotamine or ergotamine plus caffeine versus placebo significantly improved headache relief, and one RCT which found no significant difference with ergotamine plus caffeine versus placebo. One additional RCT found that ergotamine plus caffeine versus sumatriptan was significantly less effective for headache relief or reducing the need for rescue medication**G**. Another additional RCT found no difference between ergotamine alone versus ergotamine plus metoclopramide in headache intensity**G**. One RCT found a significantly higher migraine intensity with ergotamine plus caffeine plus cyclizine versus naproxen. One RCT found a significantly higher migraine intensity with ergotamine versus naproxen, but another found no significant difference with ergotamine versus naproxen in pain relief after 1 hour. One overview of harms suggested that ergotamine versus placebo increased nausea and vomiting.

Ibuprofen

Three RCTs found that ibuprofen versus placebo significantly improved outcome (measured by headache relief, migraine index, and severity of attacks, respectively). One RCT found that ibuprofen arginine versus placebo significantly increased the number of people who achieved "considerable" or "complete" relief.

Naproxen

One crossover RCT found limited evidence that naproxen versus placebo significantly reduced headache intensity. One crossover RCT found limited evidence that naproxen versus placebo significantly reduced overall pain intensity. One RCT found that naproxen versus ergotamine plus caffeine plus cyclizine significantly reduced migraine intensity. One RCT found that naproxen versus ergotamine significantly reduced migraine intensity, but another RCT found no significant difference with naproxen versus ergotamine in pain relief after 1 hour.

Tolfenamic acid

One RCT found limited evidence that tolfenamic acid versus placebo significantly increased the proportion of people with headache relief, and found no significant difference between tolfenamic acid versus sumatriptan. One small crossover RCT found limited evidence tolfenamic acid versus placebo significantly reduced the duration of attack and headache intensity. One RCT found no significant difference between tolfenamic acid versus paracetamol in headache intensity. One crossover RCT found that tolfenamic acid (alone or in combination with either metoclopramide or caffeine) versus placebo significantly reduced headache intensity.

DEFINITION Migraine is a primary headache disorder manifesting as recurring attacks, usually lasting for 4–72 hours, and involving pain of moderate to severe intensity, often with nausea, and sometimes vomiting, and/or sensitivity to light, sound, and other sensory stimuli. The 1988 International Headache Society**G** criteria include separate criteria for migraine with and without aura.[1]

INCIDENCE/ PREVALENCE Migraine is common worldwide. Prevalence has been reported to be between 5% and 25% in women and 2% and 10% in men. Overall, the highest incidence for migraine without aura has been reported between the ages of

10 and 11 years at 10/1000 person years. The peak incidence of migraine without aura in males is between ages 10 and 11 years (10/1000 person years) and in females between ages 14 and 17 years (19/1000 person years). The incidence of migraine with aura peaks in males around age 5 years (7/1000 person years) and in females around age 12–13 years (14/1000 person years).[2]

AETIOLOGY/ RISK FACTORS Data arising from independent representative samples from Canada,[3,4] the USA,[5,6] several countries in Latin America,[7] several countries in Europe,[8–11] Hong Kong,[12] and Japan[13] demonstrate a female to male predominance and a peak in middle aged women. Migraine risk has been reported to be 50% more likely in people with a family history of migraine.[14]

PROGNOSIS Acute migraine is self limited and only rarely results in permanent neurological complications. Chronic recurrent migraine may cause disability through pain, and may affect daily functioning and quality of life. Female prevalence of migraine with or without aura has a declining trend after age 45–50 years.

Please refer to CD-ROM for full text and references.

Multiple sclerosis

Search date July 2002

Mike Boggild and Helen Ford

What are the effects of interventions aimed at reducing relapse rates and disability?

LIKELY TO BE BENEFICIAL

Interferon beta

Two RCTs in people experiencing a first demyelinating event found that interferon beta-1a significantly decreased the risk of conversion to clinically definite multiple sclerosis over 2–3 years compared with placebo. One systematic review in people with active relapsing remitting multiple sclerosis found that, compared with placebo, interferon beta-1a/b significantly reduced exacerbations and disease progression over 2 years, although if sensitivity analysis assumed all people lost to follow up had relapse or disease progression (worst case scenario) the effects were no longer significant. One subsequent RCT in people with relapsing remitting multiple sclerosis found that interferon beta-1b significantly reduced the proportion of people with relapse over 2 years compared with interferon beta-1a. We found conflicting evidence from two RCTs about the effects of interferon beta on disease progression in people with secondary progressive multiple sclerosis.

UNKNOWN EFFECTIVENESS

Azathioprine

One systematic review in people with relapsing and remitting or progressive multiple sclerosis comparing azathiopine versus placebo or no treatment found a modest reduction in relapse rates over 2 years, but no evidence of a difference in disability.

Glatiramer acetate

We found insufficient evidence to assess the effects of glatiramer acetate. One RCT in people with relapsing and remitting multiple sclerosis found that, compared with placebo, glatiramer acetate reduced relapse rates over 2 years, but found no effect on disability. We found no good quality RCTs in people with secondary progressive multiple sclerosis.

Intravenous immunoglobulin

One RCT in people with relapsing and remitting multiple sclerosis found limited evidence from baseline comparisons that intravenous immunoglobulin may reduce disability over 2 years compared with placebo. We found no good quality RCTs in people with secondary progressive multiple sclerosis.

Methotrexate

One small RCT in people with progressive multiple sclerosis found limited evidence that low dose, weekly methotrexate may delay progression compared with placebo.

Mitoxantrone

One small RCT in people with active multiple sclerosis found limited evidence that mitoxantrone plus methylprednisolone reduced annual clinical relapse rates compared with methylprednisolone alone.

Clin Evid Concise 2003;9:274–276.

What are the effects of treatments for acute relapse?

LIKELY TO BE BENEFICIAL

Corticosteroids (methylprednisolone or corticotrophin)

One systematic review in people with multiple sclerosis requiring treatment for acute exacerbations has found that corticosteroids (methylprednisolone or corticotrophin) versus placebo reduces the proportion of people whose symptoms are worse or unimproved within the first 5 weeks of treatment. The optimal dose, route, and duration of treatment are unclear.

UNKNOWN EFFECTIVENESS

Plasma exchange

One small RCT provided insufficient evidence to assess plasma exchange in people with acute relapses of multiple sclerosis.

What are the effects of treatments for fatigue?

UNKNOWN EFFECTIVENESS

Amantadine

One systematic review of poor quality RCTs found modest evidence suggesting that amantadine may reduce fatigue in multiple sclerosis compared with placebo.

Behaviour modification

We found no RCTs on the effects of behavioural modification treatment in people with multiple sclerosis related fatigue.

Exercise

Two RCTs found insufficient evidence about the effects of exercise in people with multiple sclerosis related fatigue.

UNLIKELY TO BE BENEFICIAL

Pemoline

One systematic review found no significant difference in the self reporting of fatigue with pemoline compared with placebo.

What are the effects of treatments for spasticity?

UNKNOWN EFFECTIVENESS

Botulinum toxin (for focal hip adductor spasticity)

One small RCT comparing three different doses of botulinum toxin versus placebo found limited evidence of improvement in hip adductor spasticity at 4 weeks.

Intrathecal baclofen

One small crossover RCT provided insufficient evidence to assess intrathecal baclofen.

Oral drug treatments

Two RCTs found limited evidence that tizanidine reduced spasticity in people with multiple sclerosis compared with placebo, but found no evidence of improved mobility. RCTs provided insufficient evidence to assess other oral drug treatments.

Physiotherapy

Two small RCTs provide no clear evidence of benefit from physiotherapy. One found limited evidence that twice weekly hospital or home based physiotherapy for 8 weeks briefly improved mobility compared with no physiotherapy. The other, in people with progressive multiple sclerosis, found no significant difference between early versus delayed physiotherapy in mobility or activities of daily living.

What are the effects of multidisciplinary care?

UNKNOWN EFFECTIVENESS

Inpatient rehabilitation

Two small RCTs provided insufficient evidence to assess the effectiveness of inpatient rehabilitation. Both RCTs found short term benefit, but no reduction in neurological impairment. Longer term effects are uncertain.

Outpatient rehabilitation

One small RCT provided insufficient evidence to assess the effectiveness of outpatient rehabilitation.

DEFINITION Multiple sclerosis is a chronic inflammatory disease of the central nervous system. Diagnosis requires evidence of lesions that are separated in both time and space, and the exclusion of other inflammatory, structural, or hereditary conditions that might give a similar clinical picture. The disease takes three main forms: relapsing and remitting multiple sclerosis, characterised by episodes of neurological dysfunction interspersed with periods of stability; primary progressive multiple sclerosis, where progressive neurological disability occurs from the outset; and secondary progressive multiple sclerosis, where progressive neurological disability occurs later in the course of the disease.

INCIDENCE/ PREVALENCE Prevalence varies with geography and racial group; it is highest in white populations in temperate regions.[1] In Europe and North America, prevalence is 1/800 people, with an annual incidence of 2–10/100 000, making multiple sclerosis the most common cause of neurological disability in young adults. Age of onset is broad, peaking between 20 and 40 years.[2]

AETIOLOGY/ RISK FACTORS The cause remains unclear, although current evidence suggests that multiple sclerosis is an autoimmune disorder of the central nervous system resulting from an environmental stimulus in genetically susceptible individuals. Multiple sclerosis is currently regarded as a single disorder with clinical variants, but there is some evidence that it may consist of several related disorders with distinct immunological, pathological, and genetic features.[1,3]

PROGNOSIS In 90% of people, early disease is relapsing and remitting. Although some people follow a relatively benign course over many years, most develop secondary progressive disease, usually 6–10 years after onset. In 10% of people, initial disease is primary progressive. Apart from a minority of people with "aggressive" multiple sclerosis, life expectancy is not greatly affected and the disease course is often of more than 30 years' duration.

Please refer to CD-ROM for full text and references.

Parkinson's disease

Search date April 2002

Carl Clarke and A Peter Moore

What are the effects of treatments?

LIKELY TO BE BENEFICIAL

Dopamine agonists versus levodopa* in people with early disease

One systematic review and one subsequent RCT have found that dopamine agonist monotherapy versus levodopa monotherapy reduces the incidence of dyskinesias**G** and fluctuations in motor response**G**. One systematic review and subsequent RCTs have found that dopamine agonist treatment plus levodopa versus levodopa alone reduces dyskinesia. However, some of the RCTs found that levodopa alone versus dopamine agonist plus levodopa improved motor impairments and disability.

Selegiline in people with early disease

RCTs have found that selegiline versus placebo significantly improves symptoms, but one of the RCTs found increased mortality in people treated with selegiline. One large RCT found that selegiline versus placebo delayed the need for levodopa for 9 months.

TRADE OFF BETWEEN BENEFITS AND HARMS

Dopamine agonists plus levodopa in people with a fluctuating response to levodopa*

Systematic reviews in people with later stage disease taking levodopa have found that adjuvant dopamine agonists reduce "off time"**G**, improve motor impairments and activities of daily living, and reduce levodopa dose, but increase dopaminergic adverse effects**G** and dyskinesias.

Levodopa* in people with early disease

Experience suggests that levodopa improves motor function, but that dyskinesias and fluctuations in motor response are related to long term levodopa treatment and are irreversible.

Pallidal surgery in people with later disease

One systematic review found limited evidence that unilateral pallidotomy**G** versus medical treatment improved motor examination and activities of daily living. One RCT found insufficient evidence to assess the effects of pallidotomy versus deep brain stimulation**G**. We found no systematic review or RCTs comparing pallidal deep brain stimulation versus medical treatment. One small RCT found insufficient evidence to assess the effects of pallidal deep brain stimulation versus subthalamic deep brain stimulation. There is a high incidence of adverse effects with pallidotomy.

UNKNOWN EFFECTIVENESS

Subthalamic surgery in people with later disease

One systematic review found no RCTs comparing subthalamic surgery versus medical treatment. One small RCT comparing subthalamic deep brain stimulation versus pallidal deep brain stimulation found no significant difference in motor scores.

Thalamic surgery in people with later disease

One systematic review identified no RCTs comparing thalamic surgery versus medical treatment. One RCT found that thalamic deep brain stimulation versus ▶

thalamotomy improved functional status and caused fewer adverse effects. Case series found that thalamotomy was associated with permanent complications, including speech disturbance, apraxia, and death in 14–23% of people.

Occupational therapy in people with later disease; physiotherapy in people with later disease; speech and language therapy for speech disturbance in people with later disease; swallowing therapy for dysphagia in people with later disease

Systematic reviews of poor quality RCTs found insufficient evidence of the effects of these interventions.

UNLIKELY TO BE BENEFICIAL

Modified release levodopa (*v* immediate release levodopa*) in people with early disease

RCTs found no significant difference with modified versus immediate release levodopa in motor complications or disease control after 5 years.

*We have used the term "levodopa" to refer to a combination of levadopa and a peripheral decarboxylase inhibitor.

DEFINITION Idiopathic Parkinson's disease is an age related neurodegenerative disorder and the most common cause of the parkinsonian syndrome: a combination of asymmetric bradykinesia, hypokinesia, and rigidity, sometimes combined with rest tremor and postural changes. Clinical diagnostic criteria have a sensitivity of 80% and specificity of 30% compared with the gold standard of diagnosis at autopsy.[1] The primary pathology is progressive loss of cells producing the neurotransmitter dopamine from the substantia nigra in the brainstem. Treatment aims to replace or compensate for the lost dopamine. A good response to treatment supports, but does not confirm, the diagnosis. Several other catecholaminergic neurotransmitter systems are also affected in Parkinson's disease.

INCIDENCE/ PREVALENCE Parkinson's disease occurs worldwide with equal incidence in both sexes. In 5–10% of people who develop Parkinson's disease it appears before the age of 40 years (young onset), with a mean age of onset of about 65 years. Overall age adjusted prevalence is 1% worldwide and 1.6% in Europe, rising from 0.6% at age 60–64 years to 3.5% at age 85–89 years.[2,3]

AETIOLOGY/ RISK FACTORS The cause is unknown. Parkinson's disease may represent different conditions with a final common pathway. People may be affected differently by a combination of genetic and environmental factors (viruses, toxins, 1-methyl-4-phenyl-1,2,3,6-tetrahydropyridine, well water, vitamin E, and smoking).[4–7] First degree relatives of affected people may have twice the risk of developing Parkinson's disease (17% chance of developing the condition in their lifetime) compared with people in the general population.[8–10] However, purely genetic varieties probably affect a small minority of people with Parkinson's disease.[11,12]. The parkin gene on chromosome 6 may be associated with Parkinson's disease in families with at least one member with young onset Parkinson's disease, and multiple genetic factors, including the tau gene on chromosome 17q21, may be involved in idiopathic late onset disease.[13,14]

PROGNOSIS Parkinson's disease is currently incurable. Disability is progressive and associated with increased mortality (RR of death compared with matched control populations ranges from 1.6 to 3).[15] Treatment can reduce symptoms and slow progression but rarely achieves complete control. The question of whether treatment reduces mortality remains controversial.[16] Levodopa seemed to reduce mortality in the UK for 5 years after its introduction, before a "catch up" effect was noted and overall mortality rose towards previous levels. This suggested a limited prolongation of life.[17] An Australian cohort study followed

130 people treated for 10 years.[18] The standardised mortality ratio was 1.58 ($P < 0.001$). At 10 years, 25% had been admitted to a nursing home and only four were still employed. The mean duration of disease until death was 9.1 years. In a similar Italian cohort study over 8 years, the relative risk of death for affected people versus healthy controls was 2.3 (95% CI 1.60 to 3.39).[19] Age at initial census date was the main predictor of outcome (for people aged < 75 years, the RR of death was 1.80, 95% CI 1.04 to 3.11; for people aged > 75 years: the RR of death was 5.61, 95% CI 2.13 to 14.8).

Please refer to CD-ROM for full text and references.

Trigeminal neuralgia

Search date July 2002

Joanna M Zakrzewska

What are the effects of treatments?

LIKELY TO BE BENEFICIAL

Carbamazepine

One systematic review of three crossover RCTs has found that carbamazepine versus placebo increases pain relief at 5–14 days. The review found that carbamazepine versus placebo increases drowsiness, dizziness, constipation, and ataxia.

TRADE OFF BETWEEN BENEFITS AND HARMS

Pimozide

One RCT found that pimozide versus carbamazepine significantly reduced pain over 8 weeks but increased adverse effects, including hand tremors, memory impairment, and involuntary movements. Cardiac toxicity and sudden death have been reported with pimozide.

UNKNOWN EFFECTIVENESS

Baclofen

We found insufficient evidence f on the effects of baclofen versus placebo or versus other active drugs.

Combined streptomycin and lidocaine nerve block

Small poor quality RCTs found insufficient evidence about the effects of nerve block with streptomycin plus lidocaine versus nerve block with lidocaine alone.

Lamotrigine

One systematic review found insufficient evidence about effects of lamotrigine versus placebo in people with trigeminal neuralgia.

Other drugs (phenytoin, clonazepam, sodium valproate, gabapentin, mexiletine, oxcarbazepine, topiramate)

We found no RCTs about the effects of these drugs.

Tizanidine

One small RCT found insufficient evidence about the effects of tizanidine.

Cryotherapy⊙ of peripheral nerves; peripheral acupuncture; peripheral alcohol injection; peripheral injection of phenol; peripheral neurectomy; peripheral radiofrequency thermocoagulation; peripheral laser treatment⊙

We found no RCTs about the effects of these interventions.

UNLIKELY TO BE BENEFICIAL

Proparacaine

One RCT found no significant difference in pain at 30 days with a single application of proparacaine hydrochloride versus placebo eye drops to the eye on the same side as the pain.

Clin Evid Concise 2003;9:280–281.

LIKELY TO BE INEFFECTIVE OR HARMFUL

Tocainide

One systematic review found no RCTs that reported precrossover results. The use of tocainide is limited by considerable harms. The RCT reported a death attributed to haematological effects of tocainide.

DEFINITION Trigeminal neuralgia is a characteristic pain in the distribution of one or more branches of the fifth cranial nerve. The diagnosis is made on the history alone, based on characteristic features of the pain. It occurs in paroxysms that last a few seconds to 2 minutes. The frequency of paroxysms is highly variable: from hundreds of attacks a day to long periods of remission that can last years. The pain is severe and described as intense, sharp, superficial, stabbing, burning, or like an electric shock. In any individual, the pain has the same character in different attacks. It is often triggered by touch in a specific area or by eating, talking, washing the face, or cleaning the teeth. Between paroxysms the person is asymptomatic. Other causes of facial pain may need to be excluded.[1] In trigeminal neuralgia the neurological examination is usually normal.[2,3]

INCIDENCE/ PREVALENCE Most evidence about the incidence and prevalence of trigeminal neuralgia is from the USA.[4] The annual incidence (when age adjusted to 1980 age distribution of the USA) is 5.9/100 000 women and 3.4/100 000 men. The incidence tends to be slightly higher in women at all ages. The incidence increases with age. In men aged over 80 years the incidence is 45.2/ 100 000.[5] Other published surveys are small. One questionnaire survey of neurological disease in a single French village found one person with trigeminal neuralgia among 993 people.[6]

AETIOLOGY/ RISK FACTORS The cause of trigeminal neuralgia remains unclear.[7] It is more common in people with multiple sclerosis (RR 20.0, 95% CI 4.1 to 59.0).[5] Hypertension is a risk factor in women (RR 2.1, 95% CI 1.2 to 3.4) but the evidence is less clear for men (RR 1.53, 95% CI 0.30 to 4.50).[5] A study in the USA found that people with trigeminal neuralgia smoked less, consumed less alcohol, had fewer tonsillectomies, and were less likely than matched controls to be Jewish or an immigrant.[8]

PROGNOSIS One study found no reduction of 10 year survival with trigeminal neuralgia.[9] We found no evidence about the natural history of trigeminal neuralgia. The illness is characterised by recurrences and remissions. Many people have periods of remission with no pain for months or years.[3] Anecdotal reports suggest that in many people it becomes more severe and less responsive to treatment with time.[10] Most people with trigeminal neuralgia are initially managed medically, and a proportion eventually have a surgical procedure.[5] We found no good evidence about the proportion of people who require surgical treatment for pain control.

Please refer to CD-ROM for full text and references.

Aphthous ulcers (recurrent)

Search date April 2002

Stephen Porter and Crispian Scully

What are the effects of treatments?

LIKELY TO BE BENEFICIAL

Chlorhexidine (but no effect on recurrence rates)

RCTs found that chlorhexidine gluconate mouth rinses versus control preparations increased the number of ulcer free days and reduced the severity of each episode of ulceration, but did not affect the incidence of recurrent ulceration.

UNKNOWN EFFECTIVENESS

Topical corticosteroids

Nine small RCTs found no consistent difference in the incidence of new ulcers with topical corticosteroids versus control preparations. They found weak evidence that topical corticosteroids may reduce the duration of ulcers and hasten pain relief.

UNLIKELY TO BE BENEFICIAL

Hexitidine

One RCT found no significant difference in the incidence or duration of ulceration with hexitidine mouthwash versus a control mouthwash.

DEFINITION Recurrent aphthous ulcers are superficial and rounded, with painful mouth ulcers usually occurring in recurrent bouts at intervals of a few days to a few months.[1]

INCIDENCE/ PREVALENCE The point prevalence of recurrent aphthous ulcers in Swedish adults has been reported as 2%.[1] Prevalence may be 5–10% in some groups of children. Up to 66% of young adults give a history consistent with recurrent aphthous ulceration.[1]

AETIOLOGY/ RISK FACTORS The causes of aphthous ulcers remain unknown. Associations with haematinic deficiency, infections, gluten sensitive enteropathy, food sensitivities, and psychological stress have rarely been confirmed. Similar ulcers are seen in Behçet's syndrome.

PROGNOSIS About 80% of people with recurrent aphthous ulcers develop a few ulcers smaller than 1 cm in diameter that heal within 5–14 days without scarring (the pattern known as minor aphthous ulceration). The episodes recur typically after an interval of 1–4 months. One in 10 sufferers has a more severe form (major aphthous ulceration) with lesions larger than 1 cm that may recur after a shorter interval and can cause scarring. Likewise, 1/10 people with such recurrent ulceration may have multiple minute ulcers (herpetiform ulceration).

Please refer to CD-ROM for full text and references.

Burning mouth syndrome

Search date October 2002

John Buchanan and Joanna Zakrzewska

What are the effects of treatments?

LIKELY TO BE BENEFICIAL

Cognitive behavioural therapy

One small RCT found that cognitive behavioural therapy in people with resistant burning mouth syndrome versus no cognitive behavioural therapy significantly reduced symptom intensity after 6 months.

UNKNOWN EFFECTIVENESS

Antidepressants; benzydamine hydrochloride; dietary supplementation; hormone replacement therapy in postmenopausal women

We found insufficient evidence on the effects of these interventions.

DEFINITION Burning mouth syndrome is a psychogenic or idiopathic burning discomfort or pain affecting people with clinically normal oral mucosa in whom a medical or dental cause has been excluded.[1–3] Terms previously used to describe what is now called burning mouth syndrome include glossodynia, glossopyrosis, stomatodynia, stomatopyrosis, sore tongue, and oral dysaesthesia.[4] A survey of 669 men and 758 women randomly selected from 48 500 people aged between 20 and 69 years found that people with burning mouth also have subjective dryness (66%), take some form of medication (64%), report other systemic illnesses (57%), and have altered taste (11%).[5] Many studies of people with symptoms of burning mouth do not distinguish those with burning mouth syndrome (i.e. idiopathic disease) from those with other conditions (such as vitamin B deficiency), making results unreliable.

INCIDENCE/ PREVALENCE Burning mouth syndrome mainly affects women,[6–8] particularly after the menopause when its prevalence may be 18–33%.[9] One recent study in Sweden found a prevalence of 4% for the symptom of burning mouth without clinical abnormality of the oral mucosa (11/669 [2%] men, mean age 59 years; 42/758 [6%] women, mean age 57 years), with the highest prevalence (12%) in women aged 60–69 years.[5] Reported prevalence in general populations varies from 1%[10] to 15%.[6] Incidence and prevalence vary according to diagnostic criteria,[4] and many studies included people with the symptom of burning mouth rather than with burning mouth syndrome as defined above.

AETIOLOGY/ RISK FACTORS The cause is unknown, and we found no good aetiological studies. Hormonal disturbances associated with the menopause[7–9] and psychogenic factors (including anxiety, depression, stress, life events, personality disorders, and phobia of cancer) are possible causal factors.[11–13] Local and systemic factors (such as infections, allergies, ill fitting dentures,[12] hypersensitivity reactions,[14] and hormone and vitamin deficiencies[15–17]) may cause the symptom of burning mouth and should be excluded before diagnosing burning mouth syndrome.

PROGNOSIS We found no prospective cohort studies or other reliable evidence describing the natural history of burning mouth syndrome.[18] We found anecdotal reports of at least partial spontaneous remission in about half of people with burning mouth syndrome within 6–7 years.[12]

Please refer to CD-ROM for full text and references.

Candidiasis (oropharyngeal)

Search date June 2002

Caroline Pankhurst

What are the effects of preventive interventions?

BENEFICIAL

Antifungal prophylaxis in people with advanced HIV disease

RCTs have found that daily or weekly antifungal prophylaxis with fluconazole, itraconazole, or nystatin versus placebo significantly reduces the incidence of oropharyngeal candidiasis.

Antifungal prophylaxis in people with cancer and neutropenia

One systematic review in people with cancer and immunosuppression found that antifungal prophylaxis significantly reduced the number of episodes of oropharyngeal candidiasis compared with placebo. Another systematic review in people receiving chemotherapy for cancer found that antifungal prophylaxis drugs that arefully or partially absorbed from the gastrointestinal tract significantly reduced oral candidiasis compared with placebo or no treatment. It found no significant difference with unabsorbed drugs versus placebo or no treatment.

LIKELY TO BE BENEFICIAL

Antifungal prophylaxis in immunocompromised infants and children

One large RCT in immunocompromised infants and children has found that fluconazole versus oral polyenes significantly reduces the incidence of oropharyngeal candidiasis.

UNKNOWN EFFECTIVENESS

Chlorhexidine oral rinse in neutropenic adults undergoing treatment for cancer

Two RCTs found conflicting evidence about chlorhexidine oral rinse versus placebo or nystatin.

Continuous prophylaxis versus intermittent treatment in people with HIV infection and acute episodes of oropharyngeal candidiasis (in preventing antifungal resistance)

One RCT found no significant difference with continuous antifungal prophylaxis with fluconazole versus intermittent treatment with fluconazole in the emergence of antifungal resistance.

Preventive interventions in people with diabetes

We found no systematic review or RCTs.

What are the effects of treatments?

BENEFICIAL

Antifungal treatment in immunocompetent and immunocompromised infants and children

In immunocompetent infants, two RCTs have found that miconazole gel versus nystatin suspension or gel significantly increased the rate of clinical cure of oropharyngeal candidiasis. In immunocompromised infants and children, one RCT found that fluconazole versus nystatin significantly increased clinical cure of oropharyngeal candidiasis after 2 weeks.

Clin Evid Concise 2003;9:284–286.

Oral suspension of systemic azoles in people with HIV infection

RCTs have found that topical preparations of itraconazole, fluconazole, or clotrimazole are effective for treatment oropharyngeal candidiasis in people with HIV infection. One RCT found that fluconazole versus topical nystatin significantly reduced symptoms and signs of oropharyngeal candidiasis after 14 days.

UNKNOWN EFFECTIVENESS

Antifungal treatment for denture stomatitis

RCTs found conflicting evidence about the effects of antifungal agents versus placebo in clinical improvement or cure of denture stomatitis. Co-interventions included professional cleaning of the dentures at the start of the study, combined with advice on denture hygiene and advice not to wear the dentures while asleep at night, which may explain the high clinical cure rate in the placebo groups. Three RCTs comparing different antifungal drugs found no significant difference in clinical cure rates. Two RCTs comparing miconazole dental lacquer versus miconazole gel applied to the denture found no significant difference in palatal erythema.

Antifungal treatment in people undergoing chemotherapy and/or radiotherapy treatment for cancer

One systematic review of one small RCT found limited evidence that ketoconazole versus placebo significantly reduced the proportion of people with oral candidiasis after 14 days. The same systematic review of one small RCT found no significant difference with clotrimazole versus placebo in cure rates. It found no significant difference in cure rates among different absorbed drugs, or between absorbed versus non-absorbed drugs, although there was significant trial heterogeneity.

Denture hygiene

Two RCTs found insufficient evidence about the effects of mouth rinses or disinfectants versus placebo in preventing or treating denture stomatitis. One small RCT using acrylic dentures comparing microwave plus scrubbing plus topical antifungal versus soaking in chlorhexidine plus scrubbing plus topical antifungal found a non-significant decrease in the proportion of dentures recolonised with *Candida albicans* after 3 months. Microwave treatment is not suitable for all dentures.

Treatments in people with diabetes mellitus

We found no RCTs assessing treatments for oral candidiasis in people with diabetes mellitus.

DEFINITION Oropharyngeal candidiasis is an opportunistic mucosal infection caused, in the majority of cases, by *Candida albicans*. The four main types of oropharyngeal candidiasis are: (1) pseudomembranous (thrush), comprising white discrete plaques on an erythematous background, located on the buccal mucosa, throat, tongue, or gingivae; (2) erythematous, comprising smooth red patches on the hard or soft palate, dorsum of tongue, or buccal mucosa; (3) hyperplastic, comprising white, firmly adherent patches or plaques, usually bilateral on the buccal mucosa; and (4) denture induced stomatitis, presenting as either a smooth or granular erythema confined to the denture bearing area of the hard palate and often associated with an angular cheilitis.[1] Symptoms vary, ranging from none to a sore, painful mouth with a burning tongue and altered taste, which can impair speech, nutritional intake, and quality of life.

INCIDENCE/ PREVALENCE Candida species are commensals in the gastrointestinal tract. Transmission occurs directly between infected people or on fomites (objects that can harbour pathogenic organisms). Candida is found in the mouth of 31–60% of healthy people.[2] Denture stomatitis associated with candida is prevalent in 65% of denture wearers.[2] Oropharyngeal candidiasis affects 15–60% of people with haematological or oncological malignancies during periods of immunosuppression.[3] Oropharyngeal candidiasis occurs in 7–48% of people with HIV infection and in over 90% of those with advanced disease. In severely immunosuppressed people, relapse rates are high (30–50%) and usually occur within 14 days of treatment cessation.[4]

AETIOLOGY/ RISK FACTORS Risk factors associated with symptomatic oropharyngeal candidiasis include local or systemic immunosuppression, haematological disorders, broad spectrum antibiotic use, inhaled or systemic steroids, xerostomia, diabetes, and wearing dentures, obturators, or orthodontic appliances.[1,5] The same strain may persist for months or years in the absence of infection. In people with HIV infection, there is no direct correlation between the number of organisms and the presence of clinical disease. Symptomatic oropharyngeal candidiasis associated with *in vitro* resistance to fluconazole occurs in 5% of people with advanced HIV disease.[6] Resistance to azole antifungals is associated with severe immunosuppression (≤ 50 CD4 cells/mm^3), more episodes treated with antifungal drugs, and longer median duration of systemic azole treatment.[7]

PROGNOSIS Untreated candidiasis persists for months or years unless associated risk factors are treated or eliminated. In neonates, spontaneous cure of oropharyngeal candidiasis usually occurs after 3–8 weeks.

Please refer to CD-ROM for full text and references.

Impacted wisdom teeth

Search date June 2002

Stephen Worrall

What are the effects of prophylactic removal of impacted wisdom teeth?

LIKELY TO BE INEFFECTIVE OR HARMFUL

Extraction of asymptomatic impacted wisdom teeth

We found limited evidence that the harms of removing asymptomatic impacted wisdom teeth outweigh the benefits.

DEFINITION Wisdom teeth are third molars that develop in almost all adults by about the age of 20 years. In some people, the teeth become partially or completely impacted below the gumline because of lack of space, obstruction, or abnormal position. Impacted wisdom teeth may be diagnosed because of pain and swelling or incidentally by routine dental radiography.

INCIDENCE/ PREVALENCE Third molar impaction is common. Over 72% of Swedish people aged 20–30 years have at least one impacted lower third molar.[1] The surgical removal of impacted third molars (symptomatic and asymptomatic) is the most common procedure performed by oral and maxillofacial surgeons. It is performed on about 4/1000 people per year in England and Wales, making it one of the top 10 inpatient and day case procedures.[2–4] Up to 90% of people on oral and maxillofacial surgery hospital waiting lists are awaiting removal of wisdom teeth.[3]

AETIOLOGY/ RISK FACTORS Impacted wisdom teeth are partly a by-product of improved oral hygiene and changes in diet. Less gum disease and dental caries, and less wear and tear on teeth because of a more refined diet, have increased the likelihood of retaining teeth into adult life, leaving less room for wisdom teeth.

PROGNOSIS Impacted wisdom teeth can cause pain, swelling, and infection, as well as destroying adjacent teeth and bone. The removal of diseased and symptomatic wisdom teeth alleviates pain and suffering and improves oral health and function. We found no good evidence on what happens without treatment in people with asymptomatic impacted wisdom teeth.

Please refer to CD-ROM for full text and references.

Postoperative pulmonary infections

Search date March 2002

Andrew Smith

What are the effects of interventions to reduce postoperative pulmonary infections?

BENEFICIAL

Chest physiotherapy (incentive spirometry and deep breathing exercises)

One systematic review and one subsequent RCT have found that deep breathing exercises significantly reduce postoperative pulmonary infections. The review also found that incentive spirometry versus control significantly reduces pulmonary complications.

Epidural anaesthesia

Two systematic reviews have found that epidural anaesthesia versus general anaesthesia followed by systemic opioid analgesia significantly reduces postoperative pulmonary infection. Neither review provided information on adverse effects. Three subsequent and one additional RCT found inconsistent results.

LIKELY TO BE BENEFICIAL

Chest physiotherapy (intermittent positive pressure breathing)

One RCT has found that intermittent positive pressure breathing versus control significantly reduces postoperative pulmonary complications.

UNKNOWN EFFECTIVENESS

Advice to stop smoking preoperatively

We found no RCTs of the effects of preoperative advice to stop cigarette smoking on postoperative pulmonary infection. Two observational studies found that stopping smoking reduced the risk of postoperative pulmonary complications.

DEFINITION A working diagnosis of postoperative pulmonary infection may be based on three or more new findings from: cough, phlegm, shortness of breath, chest pain, temperature above 38°C, and pulse rate above 100/min.[1] In this topic, the diagnosis of pneumonia implies consolidation observed on a chest x ray.[2]

INCIDENCE/ PREVALENCE Reported morbidity for chest complications depends on how carefully they are investigated. One study found blood gas and chest radiograph abnormalities in about 50% of people after open cholecystectomy.[3] However, less than 20% of these had abnormal clinical signs and only 10% had a clinically significant chest infection. Another study estimated the incidence of pneumonia as 20%.[4] Another used a similarly strict definition and found 23%.[5]

AETIOLOGY/ RISK FACTORS Risk factors include increasing age (> 50 years), cigarette smoking, obesity, thoracic or upper abdominal operations, and pre-existing lung disease.[6] One multivariate analysis did not confirm the association with cigarette smoking but ▶

suggested that longer preoperative hospital stay and higher grading on the American Society of Anesthesiologists' physical status scale (> 2) increased the risk of postoperative pulmonary complications.[5] Depression of the immune system may also contribute.[7]

PROGNOSIS In one large systematic review (search date 1997, 141 RCTs, 9559 people), 10% of people with postoperative pneumonia died.[8] If systemic sepsis ensues, mortality is likely to be substantial.[9] Pneumonia delays recovery from surgery and poor tissue oxygenation may contribute to delayed wound healing.

Please refer to CD-ROM for full text and references.

Acute organophosphorus poisoning

Search date July 2002

Michael Eddleston, Surjit Singh, and Nick Buckley

What are the effects of treatments for acute organophosphorus poisoning?

LIKELY TO BE BENEFICIAL

Atropine*

Consensus supports atropine treatment. Many case series have found that it reverses the early muscarinic effects of acute organophosphorus poisoning. We found no RCTs comparing atropine versus placebo, but such an RCT would now be considered unethical.

Glycopyrronium bromide (glycopyrrolate)*

We found one small RCT of glycopyrronium bromide versus atropine, but it was not big enough to find a clinically important difference.

Intravenous benzodiazepines*

Consensus supports benzodiazepines for organphosporus induced seizures. We found no RCTs comparing a benzodiazepine versus placebo or another anticonvulsant. It would be unethical to conduct an RCT comparing benzodiazepine versus placebo.

Washing the poisoned person*

Washing the poisoned person with warm water and soap, and removing contaminated clothes after dermal and mucocutaneous exposure appears important and widely recommended, but this intervention has not been assessed in an RCT.

*Based on consensus, RCTs would be considered unethical.

UNKNOWN EFFECTIVENESS

Gastric lavage

We found no RCTs assessing the role of gastric lavage in acute organophosphorus poisoning. In locations where the procedure cannot be performed in sedated and intubated patients, the risk of harm is likely to surpass its potential benefits.

Oximes

One systematic review found insufficient evidence about the effects of oximes in acute organophosphorus poisoning.

α_2 Adrenergic receptor agonists (clonidine); activated charcoal (single or multiple dose); milk or other home remedies soon after ingestion; N-methyl-D-aspartate receptor antagonists; sodium bicarbonate

We found insufficient evidence about the effects of these interventions.

LIKELY TO BE INEFFECTIVE OR HARMFUL

Ipecacuanha (ipecac)

We found no RCTs on the effects of ipecacuanha in acute organophosphorus poisoning. The significant risk of harm, although not quantified, probably outweighs potential benefits.

Acute organophosphorus poisoning

DEFINITION Acute organophosphorus poisoning occurs following dermal, respiratory, or oral exposure to either low volatility pesticides (e.g. chlorpyrifos, dimethoate) or high volatility nerve gases (e.g. sarin, tabun). Acetylcholinesterase(G) inhibition at synapses results in accumulation of acetylcholine and over-activation of acetylcholine receptors at the neuromuscular junction and in the autonomic and central nervous systems.[1] Early clinical features mainly involve the parasympathetic system: bradycardia, bronchorrhoea, miosis, salivation, lachrymation, defecation, urination, and hypotension. Features of neuromuscular junction (muscle weakness and fasciculation) and central nervous system (seizures, coma) involvement are also common at this stage. An intermediate syndrome has been described (cranial nerve palsies and proximal muscle weakness with preserved distal muscle power after resolution of early cholinergic symptoms), but its definition, pathophysiology, and incidence are still unclear. A late motor or motor/sensory peripheral neuropathy may also develop after recovery from acute poisoning with some organophosphorus compounds.[1]

INCIDENCE/ PREVALENCE Most cases occur in the developing world following occupational or deliberate exposure to organophosphorus pesticides.[2] Although data are sparse, organophosphates appear to be the most important cause of death from deliberate self poisoning worldwide.[3] In Sri Lanka, at least 17 000 cases of organophosphorus or carbamate poisoning occurred in 1999, resulting in 1700 deaths. More than 80% were intentional.[4] Case fatality rates across the developing world are commonly greater than 20%.[3] In central America, occupational poisoning is more common than intentional poisoning and deaths are fewer.[5] Extrapolating from limited data, the World Health Organization has estimated that each year more than 200 000 people worldwide die from pesticide poisoning,[6] but, these figures are old and widely contested.[2] Most deaths occur in Asia, and organophosphorus pesticides probably represent at least 50% of cases.[3] Deaths from organophosphorus nerve gases occurred in Iran during the Iran–Iraq war.[7] Military or terrorist action with these chemical weapons remains possible. Twelve people died in the Tokyo attack and thousands probably died in Iran after military or terrorist exposure.

AETIOLOGY/ RISK FACTORS The widespread accessibility of pesticides in rural parts of the developing world makes them easy options for acts of self harm.[3] Occupational exposure is due to insufficient or inappropriate protective equipment in the use of toxic compunds.[2]

PROGNOSIS There are no validated scoring systems for categorising severity or predicting outcome, although many have been proposed. The highly variable natural history and difficulty in determining ingested dose make predicting outcome for an individual inaccurate and potentially hazardous, because people admitted in good condition can deteriorate rapidly and require intubation and mechanical ventilation. Prognosis in acute self poisoning is likely to depend on dose and toxicity of the ingested organophosphorus (e.g. neurotoxicity potential, half life, rate of aging(G), whether activation to the toxic compound is required [propoison(G)], and whether dimethylated or diethylated).[8,9] Prognosis in occupational exposure is better because the dose is normally smaller and the route is dermal.

Please refer to CD-ROM for full text and references.

Paracetamol (acetaminophen) poisoning

Search date March 2002

Nick Buckley and Michael Eddleston

What are the effects of treatments?

BENEFICIAL

Acetylcysteine

One small RCT in people with established paracetamol induced liver failure found that acetylcysteine versus placebo significantly reduced mortality at day 21. One observational study found that people given early treatment with acetylcysteine were less likely to develop liver damage than untreated historical controls.

LIKELY TO BE BENEFICIAL

Methionine

One small RCT found that methionine versus supportive care reduced the risk of hepatotoxicity, but it was too small to rule out a clinically important effect on mortality.

UNKNOWN EFFECTIVENESS

Activated charcoal (single or multiple dose); gastric lavage; ipecacuanha

We found no evidence from systematic reviews, RCTs, or cohort studies on the effects of these interventions on mortality, liver failure, or hepatotoxicity.

DEFINITION Paracetamol poisoning occurs as a result of either accidental or intentional overdose with paracetamol (acetaminophen).

INCIDENCE/PREVALENCE Paracetamol is the most common drug used for self poisoning in the UK.[1] It is also a common means of self poisoning in the rest of Europe, North America, and Australasia. An estimated 41 200 cases of poisoning with products containing paracetamol occurred in 1989–1990 in England and Wales, with a mortality of 0.40% (95% CI 0.38% to 0.46%). Overdoses owing to paracetamol alone result in an estimated 150–200 deaths and 15–20 liver transplants each year in England and Wales.

AETIOLOGY/RISK FACTORS Most cases in the UK are impulsive acts of self harm in young people.[1,2] In one study of 80 people who had overdosed with paracetamol, 42 had obtained the tablets for the specific purpose of taking an overdose and 33 had obtained them less than 1 hour before the act.[2]

PROGNOSIS People with blood paracetamol concentrations above the standard treatment line (defined in the UK as a line joining 200 mg/L at 4 h and 30 mg/L at 15 h on a semilogarithmic plot) have a poor prognosis without treatment Ⓕ.[4,5] In one study of 57 untreated people with blood concentrations above this line, 33 developed severe liver damage and three died.[4] People with a history of chronic alcohol misuse, use of enzyme inducing drugs, eating disorders, or multiple paracetamol overdoses may be at risk of liver damage with blood concentrations below this line.[6] In the USA, a lower line is used as an indication for treatment but we found no data relating this line to prognostic outcomes.[7] **Dose effect:** The dose ingested also indicates the risk of hepatotoxicity. People ingesting less than 125 mg/kg had no significant hepatotoxicity with a sharp dose dependent rise for higher doses.[8] The threshold for toxicity after acute ingestion may be higher in children, where a single dose of less than 200 mg/kg has not been reported to lead to death and rarely causes hepatotoxicity.[9]

Please refer to CD-ROM for full text and references.

Clin Evid Concise 2003;9:292.

Nausea and vomiting in early pregnancy

Search date October 2002

David Jewell

What are the effects of treatment for nausea and vomiting in early pregnancy?

LIKELY TO BE BENEFICIAL

Antihistamines (H1 antagonists)

Systematic reviews have found limited evidence that antihistamines reduce the number of women suffering nausea and vomiting, with no evidence of teratogenicity.

Cyanocobalamin (vitamin B_{12})

One systematic review has found that cyanocobalamin**G** significantly reduces vomiting episodes compared with placebo.

Ginger

One RCT found that ginger reduced nausea and vomiting in early pregnancy.

Pyridoxine (vitamin B_6)

Systematic reviews have found limited evidence that pyridoxine reduces nausea score but no evidence on the effect on vomiting.

UNKNOWN EFFECTIVENESS

Acupuncture *New*

One RCT found limited evidence that acupuncture improved nausea scores, retching, and wellbeing compared with no acupuncture, without increasing adverse effects. A significant improvement was found with traditional acupuncture, PC6 acupuncture**G** and sham acupuncture compared with no treatment after 3 weeks.

Dietary interventions (excluding ginger)

We found insufficient evidence to assess the effects of dietary interventions (excluding ginger).

P6 acupressure

One systematic review, including small RCTs, has found limited evidence that P6 acupressure**G** significantly reduces self reported morning sickness. One subsequent RCT found that P6 acupressure reduced duration, but not intensity, of nausea and vomiting.

Phenothiazines

One systematic review has found limited evidence that phenothiazines reduce the number of women with nausea and vomiting.

What are the effects of treatments for hyperemesis gravidarum?

UNKNOWN EFFECTIVENESS

Corticosteroids

Systematic reviews have found insufficient evidence to assess the effects of methylprednisolone in hyperemesis. One RCT found insufficient evidence on the effects of oral prednisolone.

▶

Clin Evid Concise 2003;9:293–294.

Nausea and vomiting in early pregnancy

Diazepam

One systematic review has found insufficient evidence on the effects of diazepam in pregnancy.

Dietary interventions (excluding ginger)

We found insufficient evidence to assess the effects of dietary interventions.

Ginger

One systematic review has found insufficient evidence to assess the effects of ginger in hyperemesis gravidarum.

Ondansetron

We found insufficient evidence to assess the effects of ondansetron in hyperemesis gravidarum.

DEFINITION The severity of nausea and vomiting in early pregnancy varies greatly among women. Hyperemesis gravidarum is persistent vomiting that is severe enough to cause fluid and electrolyte disturbance. It usually requires hospital admission.

INCIDENCE/ PREVALENCE Nausea and vomiting are the most common symptoms experienced in the first trimester of pregnancy, affecting 70–85% of women.[1–3] Only 17% of women report that nausea and vomiting are confined to the morning and 13% are affected beyond 20 weeks' gestation.[2] Hyperemesis is much less common, with an incidence of 3.5/1000 deliveries.[4]

AETIOLOGY/ RISK FACTORS The causes of nausea and vomiting in pregnancy are unknown. One theory, that they are caused by the rise in human chorionic gonadotrophin concentration, is compatible with the natural history of the condition, its severity in pregnancies affected by hydatidiform mole Ⓖ, and its good prognosis (see below).[4] The aetiology of hyperemesis gravidarum is also uncertain. Again, endocrine and psychological factors are suspected, but evidence is inconclusive.[4]

PROGNOSIS One systematic review (search date 1988, 11 studies) found that nausea and vomiting were associated with a reduced risk of miscarriage (6 studies, 14 564 women, OR 0.36, 95% CI 0.32 to 0.42), but found no association with perinatal mortality.[5] Nausea and vomiting and hyperemesis usually improve over the course of pregnancy, but one observational study found that 13% of women reported nausea and vomiting to persist beyond 20 weeks' gestation.[2]

Please refer to CD-ROM for full text and references.

Perineal care

Search date April 2002

Chris Kettle and Clinical Evidence freelance writers

What are the effects of intrapartum interventions on rates of perineal trauma and of different methods and materials used for primary repair of perineal trauma?

BENEFICIAL

Absorbable synthetic material for perineal repair of first and second degree tears and episiotomies (reduces short term pain)

One systematic review has found that absorbable synthetic suture materials versus catgut sutures significantly reduce analgesia use within 10 days of birth. There was no significant difference between absorbable synthetic suture materials versus catgut sutures in perineal pain or dyspareunia 3 months after birth. One large RCT included in the systematic review found that absorbable synthetic sutures versus catgut sutures significantly reduced dyspareunia at 12 months.

Continuous subcutaneous technique of perineal skin closure of first and second degree tears and episiotomies (reduces short term pain)

One systematic review has found that continuous subcutaneous suture versus interrupted, transcutaneous suture of perineal skin significantly reduces pain in the 10 days after birth.

Restrictive use of episiotomy (reduces risk of posterior trauma)

One systematic review has found that restricting episiotomy to specific fetal and maternal indications significantly reduces rates of posterior perineal trauma, need for suturing, and healing complications, but increases the rates of anterior vaginal and labial trauma.

LIKELY TO BE BENEFICIAL

Continuous support during labour (reduces instrumental delivery)

One systematic review has found that providing continuous support**G** for women during childbirth versus usual care significantly reduces the rate of instrumental delivery or episiotomy but found no significant difference in the risk of perineal trauma.

Non-suturing of perineal skin in first and second degree tears and episiotomies (reduces dyspareunia)

One large RCT has found no significant difference between leaving the perineal skin unsutured versus conventional suturing in pain 10 days after birth, but found that non-suturing significantly reduced dyspareunia 3 months after birth.

TRADE OFF BETWEEN BENEFITS AND HARMS

"Hands poised" versus "hands on" method of delivery (increases pain, no significant difference in rate of perineal trauma and reduces episiotomy rate)

One RCT found that the "hands poised" method (not touching the baby's head or supporting the mother's perineum) versus the conventional "hands on" method (applying pressure to the baby's head during delivery and supporting the mother's perineum) significantly increased perineal pain at day 10 but reduced episiotomy rates. However, it found no evidence of an effect on the overall risk of perineal trauma or third/fourth degree tears.

Clin Evid Concise 2003;9:295–297.

Upright versus supine or lateral position during delivery

One systematic review comparing any upright position versus supine or lateral positions for delivery found that an upright position marginally but reduced. This was offset by a significant increase in second degree tears.

Vacuum extractor (less perineal trauma than with forceps but newborns have increased risk of cephalhaematoma)

One systematic review has found that the use of the vacuum extractor versus forceps delivery significantly reduces the rate of perineal trauma, but increases the incidence of neonatal cephalhaematoma and retinal haemorrhage.

UNKNOWN EFFECTIVENESS

Different methods and materials for repair of third and fourth degree tears

We found no RCTs on the best method or material for repairing third and fourth degree tears and major vaginal lacerations.

Non-suturing of perineal muscle in second degree tears and episiotomies

One small RCT found no significant difference with non-suturing versus suturing of first and second degree tears in burning sensation or soreness 2–3 days after birth or in healing 2–3 days or 8 weeks after birth.

Passive descent in the second stage of labour

One RCT comparing passive fetal descent versus immediate active pushing found no significant difference in perineal trauma.

Sustained breath holding (Valsalva) method of pushing

One systematic review of two poor quality controlled trials found no significant difference in the extent or rate of perineal trauma when sustained breath holding (Valsalva) versus spontaneous exhalatory methods of pushing were used during the second stage of labour. One additional RCT comparing passive fetal descent**G** with immediate active pushing also found no significant differences in the rates of perineal trauma.

UNLIKELY TO BE BENEFICIAL

Midline episiotomy incision (associated with higher risk of third/fourth degree tears compared with mediolateral incision)

We found no evidence that midline episiotomy incision versus mediolateral incision improved perineal pain or wound dehiscence. Limited evidence from one quasi randomised trial suggests that midline incision versus mediolateral incision may increase the risk of third and fourth degree tears.

LIKELY TO BE INEFFECTIVE OR HARMFUL

Epidural anaesthesia (increases instrumental delivery, which is associated with increased rates of perineal trauma)

One systematic review found no direct evidence about the effect of epidural versus other forms of anaesthesia on rates of perineal trauma. However, RCTs found that epidural anaesthesia maintained beyond the first stage of labour versus epidural restricted to the first stage of labour significantly increased the risk of instrumental delivery, which in turn is associated with an increased risk of perineal trauma.

Perineal care

DEFINITION Perineal trauma is any damage to the genitalia during childbirth that occurs spontaneously or intentionally by surgical incision (episiotomy). Anterior perineal trauma is injury to the labia, anterior vagina, urethra, or clitoris, and is usually associated with little morbidity. Posterior perineal trauma is any injury to the posterior vaginal wall, perineal muscles, or anal sphincter. Depending on severity, posterior perineal trauma is associated with increased morbidity. First degree spontaneous tears involve only skin; second degree involve perineal muscles; third degree partially or completely disrupt the anal sphincter; and fourth degree tears completely disrupt the external and internal anal sphincter and epithelium.[1]

INCIDENCE/ PREVALENCE Over 85% of women having a vaginal birth sustain some form of perineal trauma,[2] and 60–70% receive stitches — equivalent to 400 000 women per year in the UK in 1997.[2,3] There are wide variations in rates of episiotomy: 8% in the Netherlands, 26–67% in the UK, 50% in the USA, and 99% in east European countries.[4–8] Sutured spontaneous tears are reported in about a third of women in the USA[4] and the UK,[6] but this is probably an underestimate because of inconsistency of reporting and classification of perineal trauma. The incidence of anal sphincter tears varies between 0.5% in the UK, 2.5% in Denmark, and 7% in Canada.[9]

AETIOLOGY/ RISK FACTORS Perineal trauma occurs during spontaneous or assisted vaginal delivery and is usually more extensive after the first vaginal delivery.[1] Associated risk factors include parity, size of baby, mode of delivery, malpresentation, and malposition of the fetus. Other maternal factors that may contribute to the extent and degree of trauma are ethnicity, age, tissue type, and nutritional state.[10] Clinicians' practices or preferences in terms of intrapartum interventions may influence the severity and rate of perineal trauma.

PROGNOSIS Perineal trauma affects women's physical, psychological, and social wellbeing in the immediate postnatal period as well as the long term. It can also disrupt breast feeding, family life, and sexual relations. In the UK, about 23–42% of women will continue to have pain and discomfort for 10–12 days after birth, and 7–10% of women will continue to have long term pain (3–18 months after delivery);[2,3,11] 23% of women will experience superficial dyspareunia at 3 months; 3–10% will report faecal incontinence;[12,13] and up to 24% will have urinary problems.[2,3] Complications depend on severity of perineal trauma and on effectiveness of treatment.

Please refer to CD-ROM for full text and references.

Pre-eclampsia and hypertension

Search date August 2002

Lelia Duley

What are the effects of preventive interventions?

BENEFICIAL

Antiplatelet drugs

One systematic review has found that, in women considered at risk of pre-eclampsia, antiplatelet drugs (mainly aspirin) versus placebo or no treatment significantly reduces the risk of pre-eclampsia, death of the baby and delivery before 37 weeks, with no significant difference in other important outcomes. One small subsequent RCT found similar results. The systematic review found no evidence that aspirin versus placebo increased the risk of bleeding in mother or baby.

Calcium supplementation (in high risk women or those with low intake)

One systematic review has found that calcium supplementation (mainly 2 g daily) versus placebo reduces the risk of pre-eclampsia and hypertension and reduces the risk of having a baby with birthweight under 2500 g. There was no significant effect on the risk of stillbirth or perinatal death before discharge from hospital, caesarean section, or preterm delivery.

UNKNOWN EFFECTIVENESS

Magnesium supplementation

One systematic review found insufficient evidence about the effects of magnesium supplements on the risk of pre-eclampsia or its complications.

Other pharmacological interventions

Two RCTs comparing atenolol or glyceryl trinitrate patches versus placebo were too small to draw reliable conclusions.

Salt restriction

Limited evidence from one systematic review found no significant difference in the risk of pre-eclampsia with a low salt diet versus a normal diet.

Vitamin C and E

One RCT in high risk women found limited evidence that vitamins C and E versus placebo significantly reduced the risk of pre-eclampsia. However, we were unable to draw reliable conclusions about effects. We found insufficient evidence about effects on other clinical outcomes.

Evening primrose oil; fish oil

We found six RCTs of evening primrose and fish oil, which were too small to draw reliable conclusions.

What are the effects of treatments?

BENEFICIAL

Magnesium sulphate for eclampsia (better than other anticonvulsants)

Systematic reviews have found that magnesium sulphate versus phenytoin, diazepam, or lytic cocktail significantly reduces further fits in women with eclampsia. All reviews found trends towards reduced maternal mortality with magnesium sulphate, although the benefit was not significant.

Clin Evid Concise 2003;9:298–300.

Prophylactic magnesium sulphate in severe pre-eclampsia

One systematic review and one large RCT have found that prophylactic magnesium sulphate halves the risk of eclampsia compared with placebo in women with severe pre-eclampisa. The trials found no evidence of a difference between magnesium sulphate and placebo for rate of stillbirth or perinatal mortality in babies born to women with severe pre-eclampsia. A quarter of women reported mild adverse effects, mainly flushing.

LIKELY TO BE BENEFICIAL

Antihypertensive drugs for very high blood pressure (although insufficient evidence on best choice of agent)

One systematic review and one subsequent RCT in women with blood pressures high enough to merit immediate treatment found no evidence of a difference in the control of blood pressure by various antihypertensive drugs. The studies were too small to draw any further conclusions about the relative effects of different agents.

UNKNOWN EFFECTIVENESS

Aggressive versus expectant management for severe early onset pre-eclampsia

One systematic review based on two small RCTs found no evidence that aggressive management significantly reduced stillbirth or perinatal death rates compared with expectant management in babies born to mothers with severe early onset pre-eclampsia. However, it found that aggressive management increased rates of admission to neonatal intensive care and increased the risk of necrotising enterocolitis and respiratory distress in the baby compared with expectant management. We found insufficient evidence about effects of aggressive versus expectant management in the mother.

Antihypertensive drugs for mild to moderate hypertension

Two systematic reviews have found that antihypertensive agents versus placebo, no antihypertensive drug, or another antihypertensive drug significantly reduce the chance of developing severe hypertension, but found no clear effect on pre-eclampsia and perinatal death. Systematic reviews found that angiotensin converting enzyme inhibitors used in pregnancy were associated with fetal renal failure, and that β blockers increased the risk of the baby being small for its gestational age.

Antioxidants in severe pre-eclampsia

One RCT found insufficient evidence about the effects of a combination of vitamin E, vitamin C, and allopurinol versus placebo.

Bed rest for proteinuric hypertension

One systematic review found insufficient evidence about the effects of bed rest in hospital versus normal ambulation in hospital.

Bed rest/hospital admission

We found insufficient evidence about hospital admission, bed rest, or day care versus outpatient care or normal activities in hospital.

Choice of analgesia during labour with severe pre-eclampsia

One RCT found that epidural analgesia during labour versus intravenous patient controlled analgesia significantly reduced mean pain scores, but the clinical importance of the difference was unclear.

Hospital admission for non-proteinuric hypertension

One systematic review found no significant difference in any major outcome with hospital admission versus outpatient clinic assessment.

Plasma volume expansion in severe pre-eclampsia

One systematic review found insufficient evidence about the effects of plasma volume expansion versus no expansion.

Prophylactic diazepam in severe pre-eclampsia

One systematic review found insufficient evidence to compare prophylactic diazepam versus no anticonvulsant treatment in women with severe pre-eclampsia.

DEFINITION Hypertension during pregnancy may be associated with one of several conditions. **Pregnancy induced hypertension** is a rise in blood pressure, without proteinuria, during the second half of pregnancy. **Pre-eclampsia** is a multisystem disorder, unique to pregnancy, which is usually associated with raised blood pressure and proteinuria. It rarely presents before 20 weeks' gestation. **Eclampsia** is one or more convulsions in association with the syndrome of pre-eclampsia. **Pre-existing hypertension** is known hypertension before pregnancy or raised blood pressure before 20 weeks' gestation. It may be essential hypertension or, less commonly, secondary to underlying disease.[1]

INCIDENCE/ PREVALENCE Pregnancy induced hypertension affects 10% of pregnancies and pre-eclampsia complicates 2–8%.[2] Eclampsia occurs in about 1/2000 deliveries in developed countries.[3] In developing countries, estimates of the incidence of eclampsia vary from 1/100 to 1/1700.[4,5]

AETIOLOGY/ RISK FACTORS The cause of pre-eclampsia is unknown. It is likely to be multifactorial and may result from deficient placental implantation during the first half of pregnancy.[6] Pre-eclampsia is more common among women likely to have a large placenta, such as those with multiple pregnancy, and among women with medical conditions associated with microvascular disease, such as diabetes, hypertension, and collagen vascular disease.[7,8] Other risk factors include genetic susceptibility, increased parity, and older maternal age.[9] Cigarette smoking seems to be associated with a lower risk of pre-eclampsia, but this potential benefit is outweighed by an increase in adverse outcomes such as low birth weight, placental abruption, and perinatal death.[10]

PROGNOSIS The outcome of pregnancy in women with pregnancy induced hypertension alone is at least as good as that for normotensive pregnancies.[7,11] However, once pre-eclampsia develops, morbidity and mortality rise for both mother and child. For example, perinatal mortality for women with severe pre-eclampsia is double that for normotensive women.[7] Perinatal outcome is worse with early gestational hypertension.[7,9,11] Perinatal mortality also increases in women with severe essential hypertension.[12]

Please refer to CD-ROM for full text and references.

Preterm birth

Search date May 2002

Bridgette Byrne and John J Morrison

What are the effects of treatments?

BENEFICIAL

Antenatal corticosteroids

One systematic review in women with anticipated preterm delivery has found that antenatal treatment with corticosteroids versus placebo or no treatment significantly reduces the risk of respiratory distress syndrome, neonatal mortality, and intraventricular haemorrhage in preterm infants.

LIKELY TO BE BENEFICIAL

Antibiotic treatment for premature rupture of the membranes (prolongs gestation and may reduce infection, but unknown effect on perinatal mortality)

One systematic review in women with preterm premature rupture of membranes has found that antibiotics versus placebo significantly prolong pregnancy and reduce the risk of neonatal morbidity, such as neonatal infection, requirement for treatment with oxygen, and abnormal cerebral ultrasound. It found that co-amoxiclav (amoxicillin plus clavulanic acid) was associated with a significant increase in the incidence of neonatal necrotising enterocolitis.

Prophylactic cervical cerclage for women at risk of cervical incompetence

One large RCT has found that, in women presumed to have cervical incompetence, prophylactic cervical cerclage versus no cerclage significantly reduces preterm birth (< 33 wks' gestation), but significantly increases the risk of puerperal. It found that 24 women would need to undergo cerclage to prevent one additional preterm delivery. A second RCT in women with cervix changes detected by ultrasound found that cerclage plus bed rest versus bed rest alone significantly reduced deliveries before 34. A third RCT found no significant difference in preterm birth with cerclage plus bed rest versus bed rest alone when midtrimester cervical change has been detected by transvaginal ultrasound.

TRADE OFF BETWEEN BENEFITS AND HARMS

Tocolytic treatment in threatened preterm labour

One systematic review has found that atosiban, β mimetics, indomethacin, and ethanol versus placebo or no tocolytic significantly prolong pregnancy for women with threatened preterm labour, but do not significantly reduce perinatal mortality or neonatal morbidity. One subsequent RCT found that atobisan versus placebo significantly prolonged pregnancy for up to 7 days. The systematic review found no significant difference with magnesium sulphate versus placebo or no tocolytic in prolongation of pregnancy or reduction of perinatal mortality or neonatal morbidity. The review has found that tocolytics versus placebo significantly increase maternal adverse effects, such as chest pain, nausea and vomiting, and breathlessness. One systematic review found that calcium channel versus other tocolytics (mainly β mimetics) significantly reduced deliveries within 48 hours, withdrawals owing to maternal adverse effects, and neonatal morbidity.

UNKNOWN EFFECTIVENESS

Amnioinfusion for preterm rupture of the membranes

One systematic review found insufficient evidence about the effects of amnioinfusion.

Clin Evid Concise 2003;9:301–303.

UNLIKELY TO BE BENEFICIAL

Enhanced antenatal care programmes for socially deprived population groups/high risk groups

RCTs carried out in a range of countries found no significant difference with enhanced antenatal care versus usual care in reducing the risk of preterm delivery.

Elective versus selective caesarean delivery in preterm labour

One systematic review found limited evidence that elective versus selective caesarean delivery in women with preterm labour increases the risk of maternal morbidity, without clear evidence of benefit in neonatal morbidity or mortality.

LIKELY TO BE INEFFECTIVE OR HARMFUL

Antibiotic treatment for preterm labour with intact membranes

One systematic review of women during preterm labour with intact membranes has found that antibiotics versus placebo or no antibiotics significantly prolong pregnancy, and reduce the incidence of maternal infection and necrotising enterocolitis. One large subsequent RCT has found no significant difference in length of pregnancy or neonatal outcomes. The review found that antibiotics versus placebo or no treatment significantly increased perinatal mortality, but the subsequent RCT found no significant difference in perinatal mortality.

Thyrotropin releasing hormone before preterm delivery

One systematic review in women at risk of preterm birth has found no significant difference with thyrotropin releasing hormone plus corticosteroids versus corticosteroids alone in improving neonatal outcomes. Thyrotropin releasing hormone plus corticosteroids versus corticosteroids alone significantly increased maternal and fetal adverse events.

DEFINITION Preterm or premature birth is defined by the World Health Organization as delivery of an infant before 37 completed weeks of gestation.[1] There is no set lower limit to this definition, but 23–24 weeks' gestation is widely accepted,[1] which approximates to an average fetal weight of 500 g.

INCIDENCE/ PREVALENCE Preterm birth occurs in about 5–10% of all births in developed countries,[2–4] but in recent years the incidence seems to have increased in some countries, particularly the USA.[5] We found little reliable evidence for less developed countries that used the exact definition of premature birth. The rate in northwestern Ethiopia has been reported to vary between 11–22% depending on the age group studied, being highest in teenagers.[6]

AETIOLOGY/ RISK FACTORS About 30% of preterm births are unexplained and spontaneous.[4,7,8] The two strongest risk factors for idiopathic preterm labour**Ⓖ** are low socioeconomic status and previous preterm delivery. Multiple pregnancy accounts for about another 30% of cases.[4,7] Other known risk factors include genital tract infection, preterm premature rupture of the membranes**Ⓖ**, antepartum haemorrhage, cervical incompetence, and congenital uterine abnormalities, which ▶

collectively account for about 20–25% of cases. The remaining cases (15–20%) are attributed to elective preterm delivery secondary to hypertensive disorders of pregnancy, intrauterine fetal growth restriction, congenital abnormalities, and medical disorders of pregnancy.[4,5,7,8]

PROGNOSIS Preterm labour usually results in preterm birth. One systematic review (search date not stated) of tocolysis versus placebo found that about 27% of preterm labours spontaneously resolved, and about 70% progressed to preterm delivery.[9] Observational studies have found that one preterm birth significantly raises the risk of another in a subsequent pregnancy.[10]

Please refer to CD-ROM for full text and references.

Asthma

Search date September 2002

J Mark FitzGerald and Clinical Evidence freelance writers

What are the effects of treatments for chronic and acute asthma?

BENEFICIAL

Adding inhaled long acting β_2 agonists to inhaled corticosteroids in poorly controlled mild to moderate, persistent asthma (for symptom control)

RCTs have found that, in people with asthma that is poorly controlled with inhaled corticosteroids, adding regular long acting inhaled β_2 agonists significantly improves symptoms and lung function compared with adding placebo or a leukotriene antagonist. One systematic review and one additional RCT have found that adding regular doses of long acting inhaled β_2 agonists significantly improves lung function and symptoms and reduces rescue medication compared with increasing the dose of inhaled corticosteroids. However, one further RCT found that increasing inhaled corticosteroid dose reduced exacerbations compared with adding long acting inhaled β_2 agonists.

Inhaled corticosteroids for acute asthma (better than placebo)

One systematic review has found that inhaled corticosteroids versus placebo given in the emergency department significantly reduces hospital admission rates in adults. One systematic review found no significant difference in relapse rates for oral versus inhaled steroids at 7–10 days.

Inhaled plus oral corticosteroid for acute asthma (as effective as oral corticosteroid alone)

One systematic review found no significant difference in relapse rates for inhaled plus oral corticosteroid versus oral corticosteroids up to 24 days.

Inhaled short acting β_2 agonists as needed for symptom relief (as effective as regular use) in adults with mild or to moderate, persistent asthma

One systematic review and one subsequent RCT have found no significant difference between regular and as needed inhaled short acting β_2 agonists for clinically important outcomes.

Ipratropium bromide added to β_2 agonists for acute exacerbations

Two systematic reviews and one subsequent RCT have found that ipratropium bromide plus salbutamol**G** versus salbutamol alone improves lung function and is likely to reduce hospital admission in people with severe acute asthma.

Low dose, inhaled corticosteroids in mild, persistent asthmaa

Systematic reviews and RCTs have found that, in people with mild, persistent asthma, low doses of inhaled corticosteroids significantly improve symptoms and lung function compared with placebo or regular inhaled β_2 agonists.

Short courses of oral systemic corticosteroids for acute exacerbations

Two systematic reviews and one subsequent RCT have found that early treatment with systemic corticosteroids reduces admission and relapse rates compared with placebo in people with acute asthma. One systematic review found no significant difference between oral and inhaled steroids for relapse rates at 7–10 days in adults with acute asthma.

Clin Evid Concise 2003;9:304–306.

Spacer devices for delivering inhaled medications from pressurised metered dose inhalers in acute asthma (as good as nebulisers)

One systematic review in people with acute, but not life threatening exacerbations of asthma found no significant difference with β_2 agonists delivered by spacer device/holding chamber versus nebulisers in rates of hospital admission, time spent in the emergency department, peak expiratory flow rate, or forced expiratory volume in 1 second**G**.

LIKELY TO BE BENEFICIAL

Adding leukotriene antagonists in people with mild to moderate, persistent asthma (*v* no added treatment)

RCTs in people taking β_2 agonists alone have found that leukotriene antagonists versus placebo significantly reduce asthma symptoms and β_2 agonist use. One systematic review and subsequent RCTs have found that adding leukotriene antagonists increased exacerbations, reduced lung function and were less effective for symptom control compared with inhaled corticosteroids. Two RCTs have found that an inhaled corticosteroid plus a long acting β_2 agonist significantly improved symptoms, lung function, and exacerbations compared with a leukotriene antagonist at 12 weeks.

Education about acute asthma

One systematic review and one subsequent RCT found that education to facilitate self management of asthma in adults versus usual care significantly reduced hospital admission, unscheduled visits to the doctor, and days off work. However, a second subsequent RCT found no significant effect of asthma education for quality of life or social functioning at 6 months.

Magnesium sulphate for people with severe acute asthma

One systematic review and three subsequent RCTs found no significant difference between intravenous magnesium sulphate and placebo for hospital admission rates. However, we found limited evidence from one systematic review and two subsequent RCTs that intravenous magnesium versus placebo improved lung function compared with placebo in people with severe acute asthma.

Mechanical ventilation for people with severe acute asthma*

We found no RCTs comparing mechanical ventilation with or without inhaled β_2 agonists versus no mechanical ventilation in people with severe acute asthma. Evidence from cohort studies support its use, although observational studies suggest that ventilation is associated with a high level of morbidity.

Oxygen supplementation for acute asthma*

We found no systematic review or RCTs of oxygen in acute asthma. However, consensus opinion and pathophysiology suggest that its role is vital in acute asthma.

Specialist versus generalist care for acute exacerbations

One systematic review found limited evidence that specialist versus generalist care improved outcomes in adults and children.

*Highly likely to be effective. RCTs unlikely to be conducted.

UNLIKELY TO BE BENEFICIAL

Continuous versus intermittent nebulised short acting β_2 agonists for acute asthma

One systematic review and one RCT have found no significant difference between continuous and intermittent nebulised short acting β_2 agonists for hospital admission rates in adults.

Intravenous versus nebulised delivery of short acting β_2 agonists for acute asthma

One systematic review found that intravenous delivery of short acting β_2 agonists was no more effective than nebulised delivery in improving peak expiratory flow rate**G** at 60 minutes.

UNKNOWN EFFECTIVENESS

Adding leukotriene antagonists plus inhaled corticosteroids in people with mild to moderate, persistent asthma

One systematic review in people taking inhaled corticosteroids found no significant difference between leukotriene antagonists and placebo for exacerbation rates at 4–16 weeks. We found limited evidence from two RCTs that, in people with asthma that is poorly controlled with inhaled corticosteroids, adding a leukotriene antagonist was less effective for symptoms and lung function compared with adding a long acting β_2 agonist.

Helium–oxygen mixture for acute asthma

One systematic review found no significant difference for helium–oxygen mixture versus air or oxygen in pulmonary function tests at 60 minutes in adults and children with acute asthma.

DEFINITION Chronic asthma is characterised by variable airflow obstruction and airway hyperresponsiveness. Symptoms include dyspnoea, cough, chest tightness, and wheezing. The normal diurnal variation**G** of peak expiratory flow rate is increased in people with asthma**T**. Chronic asthma is defined here as asthma requiring maintenance treatment. Asthma is classified differently in the USA and UK**T**. Where necessary, the text specifies the system of classification used.[1,2] Acute asthma is defined here as an exacerbation of underlying asthma requiring urgent treatment.

INCIDENCE/ PREVALENCE Reported prevalence of asthma is increasing worldwide. About 10% of people have suffered an attack of asthma.[3–5] Epidemiological studies have also found marked variations in prevalence in different countries.[6,7]

AETIOLOGY/ RISK FACTORS Most people with asthma are atopic. Exposure to certain stimuli initiates inflammation and structural changes in airways causing airway hyperresponsiveness and variable airflow obstruction, which in turn cause most asthma symptoms. There are a large number of such stimuli; the more important include environmental allergens, occupational sensitising agents, and respiratory viral infections.[8,9]

PROGNOSIS **Chronic asthma:** In people with mild asthma, prognosis is good and progression to severe disease is rare. However, as a group, people with asthma lose lung function faster than those without asthma, although less quickly than people without asthma who smoke.[10] People with chronic asthma can improve with treatment. However, for reasons not clearly understood, some people (possibly up to 5%) have severe disease that responds poorly to treatment. These people are most at risk of morbidity and death from asthma. **Acute asthma:** About 10–20% of people presenting to the emergency department with asthma are admitted to hospital. Of these, fewer than 10% receive mechanical ventilation,[11,12] although previous ventilation is associated with a 19-fold increased risk of ventilation for a subsequent episode.[13] It is unusual for people to die unless they have suffered respiratory arrest before reaching hospital.[14] One prospective study of 939 people discharged from emergency care found that 17% (95% CI 14% to 20%) relapsed by 2 weeks.[15]

Please refer to CD-ROM for full text and references.

Bronchiectasis

Search date October 2002

Clinical Evidence freelance writers

What are the effects of pharmacological treatments in people with bronchiectasis but without cystic fibrosis? New

UNKNOWN EFFECTIVENESS

Bromhexine

One systematic review found insufficient evidence to compare the effects of bromhexine versus placebo.

Inhaled steroids

One systematic review found insufficient evidence from two small RCTs about the effects of inhaled steroids versus placebo in people with bronchiectasis not due to a specific congenital disease.

Long acting β_2 agonists

One systematic review found no RCTs comparing long acting β_2 agonists versus placebo or other treatments in people with non-cystic fibrosis bronchiectasis.

Oral steroids

One systematic review found no RCTs comparing oral steroids versus placebo, no steroids, or other treatments in people with non-cystic fibrosis bronchiectasis.

Recombinant human deoxyribonuclease

One systematic review found insufficient evidence to compare the effects of recombinant human deoxyribonuclease versus those of placebo

DEFINITION Bronchiectasis is defined as irreversible widening of medium sized airways (bronchi) in the lung. It is characterised by inflammation, destruction of bronchial walls, and chronic bacterial infection. The condition may be limited to a single lobe or lung segment, or it may affect one or both lungs more diffusely. Clinically, the condition manifests as chronic cough and chronic overproduction of sputum (up to about 500 mL daily), which is often purulent.[1] People with severe bronchiectasis may have life threatening haemoptysis and may develop features of chronic obstructive airways disease, such as wheezing, chronic respiratory failure, pulmonary hypertension, and right sided heart failure.

INCIDENCE/ PREVALENCE We found few reliable data. Incidence has declined over the past 50 years and prevalence is low in higher income countries. Prevalence is much higher in poorer countries and is a major cause of morbidity and mortality.

AETIOLOGY/ RISK FACTORS Bronchiectasis is most commonly a long term complication of previous lower respiratory infections such as measles pneumonitis, pertussis, and tuberculosis. Foreign body inhalation and allergic, autoimmune, and chemical lung damage also predispose to the condition.[2] Underlying congenital disorders such as cystic fibrosis, cilial dysmotility syndromes, α_1 antitrypsin deficiency, and congenital immunodeficiencies may also predispose to bronchiectasis and may be of greater aetiological importance than respiratory infection in higher income countries. Cystic fibrosis is the most common congenital cause.

Clin Evid Concise 2003;9:307–308.

PROGNOSIS Bronchiectasis is a chronic condition with frequent relapses of varying severity. Long term prognosis is variable. Data on morbidity and mortality are sparse.[3] Bronchiectasis frequently coexists with other respiratory disease, making it difficult to distinguish prognosis for bronchiectasis alone.

Please refer to CD-ROM for full text and references.

Chronic obstructive pulmonary disease

Topic search date October 2002

Huib Kerstjens and Dirkje Postma

What are the effects of maintenance drug treatment in stable chronic obsructive pulmonary disease?

We found no evidence about effects of most interventions on progression of chronic obstructive pulmonary disease (measured by decline in lung function). However, we found good evidence from RCTs that inhaled corticosteroids do not prevent progression.

BENEFICIAL

Inhaled anticholinergics

RCTs have found that inhaled anticholinergics versus placebo significantly improve forced expiratory volume in 1 second (FEV_1)Ⓖ, exercise capacity, and symptoms. One large RCT found that adding ipratropium to a smoking cessation programme had no significant impact on decline in FEV_1 over 5 years. One RCT found that inhaled tiotropium (a long acting anticholinergic drug) reduced exacerbation and admission rates compared with placebo at 1 year.

Inhaled anticholinergics plus β_2 agonists

RCTs have found that combining a β_2 agonist with an anticholinergic drug for 2–12 weeks modestly but significantly improves FEV_1 compared with either drug alone. One RCT found that, when combined with an anticholinergic drug, a long acting β_2 agonist improved FEV_1 and peak expiratory flowⒼ rate significantly more than a short acting β_2 agonist.

Inhaled β_2 agonists

RCTs found that inhaled β_2 agonists improve FEV_1Ⓖ and symptoms compared with placebo after 1 week to 6 months' treatment.

LIKELY TO BE BENEFICIAL

Inhaled anticholinergics versus β_2 agonists

RCTs have found that 3 months of a short acting inhaled anticholinergic significantly improved FEV_1 compared with short acting β_2 agonists. One RCT found that 6 months of a long acting inhaled anticholinergic significantly improved FEV_1 and quality of life compared with a long acting inhaled β_2 agonist. RCTs have found inconsistent evidence about effects of short acting inhaled anticholinergics versus long acting β_2 agonists over 3 months.

Long term domiciliary oxygen

RCTs found limited evidence that domiciliary oxygen versus no oxygen improved survival over 2 years in people with chronic obstructive pulmonary disease and hypoxaemia.

Mucolytics*

We found evidence from two systematic reviews that mucolytics versus placebo for 3–24 months may reduce the frequency and duration of exacerbations in people with chronic bronchitis. However, it is not clear whether these effects are generalisable to people with chronic obstructive pulmonary disease.

*Extrapolated from studies of different types of pulmonary disease, including chronic obstructive pulmonary disease.

▶

Clin Evid Concise 2003;9:309–311.

Chronic obstructive pulmonary disease

TRADE OFF BETWEEN BENEFITS AND HARMS

Inhaled corticosteroids

RCTs have found no significant difference between inhaled corticosteroids and placebo in lung function (FEV_1) over 10 days to 10 weeks. However, large RCTs lasting at least 6 months suggested that inhaled steroids increased FEV_1 during the first 3–6 months of use, but we found evidence of no effect on subsequent decline in lung function. One systematic review found that long term inhaled steroids versus placebo reduced the frequency of exacerbations. Long term inhaled steroids may predispose to adverse effects, including osteoporosis, skin bruising, and oral candidiasis.

Theophyllines

One systematic review has found a slight but significant improvement in FEV_1 with theophyllines compared with placebo after 3 months. One large RCT has found that theophyllines significantly improve FEV_1 compared with placebo after 12 months of treatment. The usefulness of these drugs is limited by adverse effects and the need for monitoring of blood concentrations.

UNKNOWN EFFECTIVENESS

α_1 Antitrypsin infusion

One RCT in people with α_1 antitrypsin deficiency and moderate emphysema found no significant difference with α_1 antitrypsin infusion versus placebo in the decline in FEV_1 after 1 year.

Antibiotics

Two poor quality RCTs found no significant difference with antibiotics in frequency of exacerbations or decline in lung function over 5 years compared with placebo.

Deoxyribonuclease

We found no RCTs comparing long term effects of deoxyribonuclease versus placebo.

UNLIKELY TO BE BENEFICIAL

Oral corticosteroids

We found no evidence on long term benefits. One systematic review has found that oral corticosteroids for 2–4 weeks significantly improve lung function compared with placebo. Long term oral corticosteroids are associated with serious adverse effects, including osteoporosis and diabetes.

Oral versus inhaled corticosteroids

Three RCTs provided insufficient evidence about effects of oral versus inhaled corticosteroids over 2 weeks. Systemic corticosteroids are associated with serious adverse effects, including osteoporosis and diabetes.

DEFINITION Chronic obstructive pulmonary disease is characterised by chronic bronchitis or emphysema. Emphysema is abnormal permanent enlargement of the air spaces distal to the terminal bronchioles, accompanied by destruction of their walls and without obvious fibrosis. Chronic bronchitis is chronic cough or mucus production for at least 3 months in at least two successive years when other causes of chronic cough have been excluded.[1]

INCIDENCE/ PREVALENCE Chronic obstructive pulmonary disease mainly affects middle aged and elderly people. It is one of the leading causes of morbidity and mortality worldwide. In the USA, it affects about 14 million people and is the fourth leading cause of death. Both morbidity and mortality are rising. Estimated prevalence in the USA has risen by 41% since 1982, and age adjusted death rates rose by 71%

between 1966 and 1985. All cause age adjusted mortality declined over the same period by 22% and mortality from cardiovascular diseases by 45%.[1] In the UK, physician diagnosed prevalence was 2% in men and 1% in women between 1990 and 1997.[2]

AETIOLOGY/ RISK FACTORS Chronic obstructive pulmonary disease is largely preventable. The main cause is exposure to cigarette smoke. The disease is rare in lifelong non-smokers (estimated incidence 5% in 3 large representative US surveys from 1971–1984), in whom "passive" exposure to environmental tobacco smoke has been proposed as a cause.[3,4] Other proposed causes include airway hyperresponsiveness, air pollution, and allergy.[5–7]

PROGNOSIS Airway obstruction is usually progressive in those who continue to smoke, resulting in early disability and shortened survival. Smoking cessation reverts the rate of decline in lung function to that of non-smokers.[8] Many people will need medication for the rest of their lives, with increased doses and additional drugs during exacerbations.

Please refer to CD-ROM for full text and references.

Community acquired pneumonia

Search date April 2002

Mark Loeb

What are the effects of treatments?

BENEFICIAL

Antibiotics (amoxicillin, cephalosporins, macrolides, penicillin, quinolones) in hospital

RCTs evaluating different oral antibiotics in people admitted to hospital found cure or improvement in 73–96% of people, regardless of the antibiotic taken. RCTs found no significant difference in cure with cephalosporins versus penicillin or quinolones versus amoxicillin or versus cephalosporins. However, most trials were small and were designed to show equivalence between treatments rather than superiority of one over another.

Antibiotics (amoxicillin, cephalosporins, macrolides, penicillin, quinolones) in outpatient settings

One systematic review evaluating different oral antibiotics in outpatient settings has found clinical cure or improvement in over 90% of people, regardless of antibiotic taken. Another systematic review found that azithromycin versus other macrolides, cephalosporins, or penicillin significantly reduced clinical failures over 6–21 days. A third systematic review found no significant difference in clinical cure or improvement with quinolones versus amoxicillin, cephalosporins, or macrolides. Most trials were designed to show equivalence between treatments rather than superiority of one over another.

LIKELY TO BE BENEFICIAL

Prompt versus delayed administration of antibiotics in people severely ill with community acquired pneumonia

Retrospective studies found that prompt administration of antibiotics significantly improved survival. It would probably be unethical to perform an RCT of delayed antibiotic treatment.

UNKNOWN EFFECTIVENESS

Bottle blowing

One unblinded RCT in people receiving antibiotics and usual medical care found that bottle blowing physiotherapy plus early mobilisation plus encouragement to regularly sit up and take deep breaths versus early mobilisation alone significantly reduced mean hospital stay.

Guidelines for treating pneumonia (for clinical outcomes)

One systematic review found no significant difference with the use of guidelines (incorporating early switch from intravenous to oral antibiotics and early discharge strategies, or both) versus usual care in improving clinical outcomes in community acquired pneumonia.

Specific combinations of antibiotics in intensive care settings

We found no RCTs comparing one combination of antibiotics versus another in intensive care units.

Clin Evid Concise 2003;9:312–314.

UNLIKELY TO BE BENEFICIAL

Intravenous versus oral antibiotics in immunocompetent people in hospital without life threatening illness

Two RCTs found that in immunocompetent people admitted to hospital who were not suffering life threatening illness, intravenous versus oral co-amoxiclav (amoxicillin plus clavulanic acid) or cefuroxime did not increase cure rates or reduce mortality. Intravenous antibiotics increased the length of hospital stay.

What are the effects of preventive interventions?

BENEFICIAL

Pneumococcal vaccine in immunocompetent adults

One systematic review in immunocompetent people has found that over one winter season, pneumococcal vaccination versus no vaccination significantly reduces pneumococcal pneumonia.

LIKELY TO BE BENEFICIAL

Influenza vaccine in elderly people

One RCT in people aged 60 years or over found that influenza vaccine versus placebo significantly reduced the incidence of influenza at 5 months.

UNKNOWN EFFECTIVENESS

Pneumococcal vaccine in chronically ill, immunosuppressed, or elderly people

One systematic review found no significant difference with pneumococcal vaccination versus no vaccination in the incidence of pneumonia in elderly people or people likely to have an impaired immune system.

DEFINITION Community acquired pneumonia is pneumonia contracted in the community rather than in hospital. It is defined by clinical symptoms and signs with radiological confirmation.

INCIDENCE/PREVALENCE In the northern hemisphere, community acquired pneumonia affects about 12/1000 people a year, particularly during winter and at the extremes of age (incidence: < 1 year old 30–50/1000 people a year; 15–45 years 1–5/1000 people a year; 60–70 years 10–20/1000 people a year; 71–85 years 50/1000 people a year).[1–6]

AETIOLOGY/RISK FACTORS Over 100 microorganisms have been implicated in community acquired pneumonia, but most cases are caused by *Streptococcus pneumoniae* Ⓣ.[4–7] Smoking is probably an important risk factor.[8]

PROGNOSIS Severity varies from mild to life threatening illness within days of the onset of symptoms. One systematic review (search date 1995, 33 148 people) of prognosis studies for community acquired pneumonia found overall mortality to be 13.7%, ranging from 5.1% for ambulant people to 36.5% for people requiring intensive care.[9] The following prognostic factors were significantly ▶

associated with mortality: male sex (OR 1.3, 95% CI 1.2 to 1.4); pleuritic chest pain (OR 0.5, 95% CI 0.3 to 0.8, i.e. lower mortality); hypothermia (OR 5.0, 95% CI 2.4 to 10.4); systolic hypotension (OR 4.8, 95% CI 2.8 to 8.3); tachypnoea (OR 2.9, 95% CI 1.7 to 4.9); diabetes mellitus (OR 1.3, 95% CI 1.1 to 1.5); neoplastic disease (OR 2.8, 95% CI 2.4 to 3.1); neurological disease (OR 4.6, 95% CI 2.3 to 8.9); bacteraemia (OR 2.8, 95% CI 2.3 to 3.6); leucopenia (OR 2.5, 95% CI 1.6 to 3.7); and multilobar radiographic pulmonary infiltrates (OR 3.1, 95% CI 1.9 to 5.1).

Please refer to CD-ROM for full text and references.

Lung cancer

Search date May 2002

Alan Neville

What are the effects of treatments for non-small cell lung cancer?

BENEFICIAL

Palliative chemotherapy with cisplatin or docetaxel containing regimens in stage 4 non-small cell lung cancer

Systematic reviews in people with stage 4 non-small cell lung cancer have found that chemotherapy regimens containing cisplatin plus best supportive care versus supportive care alone significantly increase survival at 1 year. Limited evidence from RCTs suggests that chemotherapy plus best supportive care versus best supportive care alone may improve quality of life.

Thoracic irradiation plus chemotherapy versus irradiation alone in unresected stage 3 non-small cell lung cancer

Systematic reviews and one subsequent RCT in people with unresectable stage 3 non-small cell lung cancer have found that adding chemotherapy to thoracic irradiation versus irradiation alone significantly improves survival at 2–5 years. Another subsequent RCT has found no significant difference in median survival with radical radiotherapy plus chemotherapy versus radiotherapy alone.

UNKNOWN EFFECTIVENESS

Hyperfractionated radiation treatment versus conventional radiotherapy in unresectable stage 3 non-small cell lung cancer

One systematic review in people with stage 3 non-small cell lung cancer has found no significant difference with standard hyperfractionation versus conventional radiotherapy in survival at 2 years. One RCT in people with stage 3 non-small cell lung cancer found that continuous, hyperfractionated, accelerated radiotherapy(G) versus conventional radiotherapy significantly increased survival at 2 years.

Newer single drug or combined drug regimens in stage 4 non-small cell lung cancer (not clearly better than cisplatin or docetaxel based regimens)

One systematic review and subsequent RCTs in people with stage 3 and 4 non-small cell lung cancer found conflicting evidence on the effects of single versus combined chemotherapy. One RCT in people with stage 3 and 4 non-small cell lung cancer found no significant difference in survival at 1 year with first line platinum based versus non-platinum based chemotherapy.

Preoperative chemotherapy in people with resectable stage 3 non-small cell lung cancer

One systematic review of two small RCTs in people with technically resectable stage 3A non-small cell lung cancer found that preoperative chemotherapy versus no preoperative chemotherapy significantly improved survival at 2 years. One additional RCT found that preoperative chemotherapy versus no preoperative chemotherapy improved survival at 4 years compared with no preoperative chemotherapy in people with resectable stages 1 to 3 non-small cell lung cancer, but the result was not significant.

UNLIKELY TO BE BENEFICIAL

Postoperative chemotherapy in people with resected stage 1–3 non-small cell lung cancer

Systematic reviews and one subsequent RCT in people with completely resected stage 2 and 3 non-small cell lung cancer have found no significant difference in survival at 5 years with postoperative cisplatin based chemotherapy versus surgery with or without concomitant radiotherapy. One systematic review has found that postoperative alkylating agents increase mortality compared with no chemotherapy.

What are the effects of treatments for small cell lung cancer?

BENEFICIAL

Chemotherapy plus thoracic irradiation versus chemotherapy alone in limited stage small cell lung cancer

Two systematic reviews in people with limited stage small cell lung cancer have found that adding thoracic irradiation to chemotherapy versus chemotherapy alone significantly improves survival at 3 years. However, one of these reviews has found that chemotherapy plus thoracic irradiation significantly increases deaths related to treatment.

LIKELY TO BE BENEFICIAL

Prophylactic cranial irradiation for people in complete remission with limited or extensive stage small cell lung cancer

One systematic review in people in with small cell lung cancer in complete remission has found that prophylactic cranial irradiation versus no irradiation significantly improves survival at 3 years and reduces the risk of developing brain metastases. Long term cognitive dysfunction following cranial irradiation has been described, but longer follow up studies are needed to assess its significance and importance.

LIKELY TO BE INEFFECTIVE OR HARMFUL

Dose intensive chemotherapy versus standard chemotherapy

Two RCTs found that dose intensification versus standard chemotherapy significantly increased deaths related to toxicity, and did not improve progression free survival. One RCT in people with limited disease found that early dose intensification of chemotherapy alternating with radiotherapy versus no early intensification of chemotherapy significantly increased survival at 2 years. One RCT found that cisplatin plus irinotecan versus cisplatin plus etoposide may improve survival over 2 years. Two RCTs found conflicting evidence about the effects of dose intensification plus growth factor support.

Oral etoposide in extensive stage small cell lung cancer

RCTs in people with extensive stage small cell lung cancer have found that oral etoposide improves survival at 1 year significantly less than combination chemotherapy. One RCT found that etoposide versus combination chemotherapy caused less nausea and vomiting in the short term but found no evidence that etoposide offers significantly better quality of life overall.

DEFINITION Lung cancer (bronchogenic carcinoma) is an epithelial cancer arising from the bronchial surface epithelium or bronchial mucous glands❶.

INCIDENCE/ PREVALENCE Lung cancer is the leading cause of cancer death in both men and women, affecting about 100 000 men and 80 000 women annually in the USA, and about 40 000 men and women in the UK. Small cell lung cancer constitutes about 20–25% of all lung cancers, the remainder being non-small cell lung cancers, of which adenocarcinoma is now the most prevalent form.[1]

AETIOLOGY/ RISK FACTORS Smoking remains the major preventable risk factor, accounting for about 80–90% of all cases.

PROGNOSIS Lung cancer has an overall 5 year survival rate of 10–12%.[2] At the time of diagnosis, 10–15% of people with lung cancer have localised disease. Of these, half will have died at 5 years despite potentially curative surgery. Over half of people have metastatic disease at the time of diagnosis. People with non-small cell cancer who undergo surgery have a 5 year survival of 60–80% for stage 1 disease and 25–50% for stage 2 disease.[2] In people with small cell cancer, those with limited stage disease who undergo combined chemotherapy and mediastinal irradiation have a median survival of 18–24 months, whereas those with extensive stage disease who are given palliative chemotherapy have a median survival of 10–12 months.[2] About 5–10% of people with small cell lung cancer present with central nervous system involvement, and half develop symptomatic brain metastases by 2 years. Of these, only half respond to palliative radiation, and their median survival is less than 3 months.[2]

Please refer to CD-ROM for full text and references.

Spontaneous pneumothorax

Search date April 2002

John Cunnington

What are the effects of treatments?

UNKNOWN EFFECTIVENESS

Chest tube drainage

We found no sufficiently large RCTs comparing chest tube drainage versus observation. Two small RCTs found that resolution is faster with chest tube drainage than with needle aspiration, but found no difference in recurrence rate. One of the RCTs found that chest tube drainage versus needle aspiration significantly increased pain, and increased the time spent in hospital by an average of 2 days.

Chest tube drainage plus suction

One small RCT found no significant difference in the rate of resolution whether chest tube drainage bottles were connected to suction or not, but the trial was too small to exclude a clinically important difference.

Needle aspiration

One small RCT found no good evidence of an improved rate of resolution with needle aspiration versus observation alone. Two small RCTs found that resolution is slower with needle aspiration than with chest tube drainage, but found no difference in recurrence rate. One of the RCTs found that people treated with needle aspiration versus chest tube drainage experienced significantly less pain and spent an average of two fewer days in hospital.

One way valves on chest tubes versus bottles with underwater seal

One small RCT found no significant difference in the rate of resolution with one way valves versus drainage bottles with an underwater seal, but the trial was too small to exclude a clinically important difference. People treated with one way valves required less analgesia and spent less time in hospital.

Small versus standard sized chest tubes

We found no RCTs comparing small versus standard sized chest tubes.

What are the effects of interventions to prevent recurrence?

TRADE OFF BETWEEN BENEFITS AND HARMS

Chemical pleurodesis

Two RCTs have found that chest tube drainage plus chemical pleurodesis versus chest tube drainage alone significantly reduces the rate of recurrence of spontaneous pneumothorax, but one of the RCTs found that treatment can be painful. The RCTs found no significant difference in length of hospital stay with pleurodesis versus chest tube drainage alone. One non-randomised prospective study found no significant difference in recurrence rate with chemical versus surgical pleurodesis. We found no RCTs or high quality cohort studies about the optimal timing of chemical pleurodesis.

UNKNOWN EFFECTIVENESS

Optimal timing of pleurodesis (after first, second, or third spontaneous pneumothorax)

We found no RCTs or high quality cohort studies assessing whether pleurodesis should take place after the first, second, or subsequent episodes of spontaneous pneumothorax.

Surgical pleurodesis

We found no RCTs comparing surgical pleurodesis versus chest tube drainage alone or versus chemical pleurodesis. One small RCT found that video-assisted thoracoscopic surgery versus thoracotomy significantly reduced hospital stay. It found no significant difference in the rate of recurrence after 3 years, but the limited evidence cannot exclude a clinically important difference.

DEFINITION A pneumothorax is air in the pleural space. A spontaneous pneumothorax occurs when there is no provoking factor, such as trauma, surgery, or diagnostic intervention. It implies a leak of air from the lung parenchyma through the visceral pleura into the pleural space.

INCIDENCE/PREVALENCE In a survey in Minnesota, USA, the incidence of spontaneous pneumothorax was 7/100 000 men and 1/100 000 for women.[1] Smoking increases the likelihood of spontaneous pneumothorax by 22 times for men and eight times for women. A dose–response relationship has been observed.[2]

AETIOLOGY/RISK FACTORS Spontaneous pneumothorax can be primary (typically in young fit people and thought to be because of a congenital abnormality of the pleura) or secondary (caused by underlying lung disease, typically occurring in older people with emphysema or pulmonary fibrosis).

PROGNOSIS Death from spontaneous pneumothorax is rare and in some cases a consequence of tension pneumothorax. Morbidity with pain and shortness of breath is common. Published recurrence rates vary; one cohort study in Denmark found that, after a first episode of primary spontaneous pneumothorax, 23% of people suffered a recurrence within 5 years, most within a year.[3] Recurrence rates had been thought to increase substantially after the first recurrence, but one case control study of military personnel found that 28% of men with a first spontaneous pneumothorax had a recurrence; 23% of the 28% had a second recurrence; and only 14% of that 23% had a third recurrence, giving a total recurrence rate of 35%.[4]

Please refer to CD-ROM for full text and references.

Upper respiratory tract infection

Search date June 2002

Chris Del Mar and Paul Glasziou

What are the effects of treatments?

BENEFICIAL

Analgesia/anti-inflammatories for symptom relief

One systematic review has found that analgesics or anti-inflammatory drugs versus placebo significantly reduce sore throat at 1–5 days. One RCT in people with acute sinusitis taking antibiotics found that steroid spray versus placebo significantly improved symptoms over 21 days.

Antibiotics for preventing (rare) complications of β haemolytic streptococcal pharyngitis

One systematic review has found that antibiotics versus no antibiotics can prevent non-suppurative complications of β haemolytic streptococcal pharyngitis, but in industrialised countries such complications are rare.

LIKELY TO BE BENEFICIAL

Antibiotics for reducing time to recovery in people with proven infection with *Haemophilus influenzae*, *Moraxella catarrhalis*, or *Streptococcus pneumoniae*

In a minority of people, the upper respiratory tract infection is caused by *H influenzae*, *M catarrhalis*, or *S pneumoniae*. One RCT found that in these people, antibiotics versus placebo significantly increased recovery at 5 days. However, we have no methods currently of easily identifying this subgroup within the majority of people with negative nasopharyngeal cultures.

Antihistamines for runny nose and sneezing

One systematic review has found that antihistamines versus placebo significantly reduce runny nose and sneezing after 2 days, but the clinical benefit is small.

β Agonists for reducing duration of cough in adults with bronchial hyperresponsiveness, wheezes, or airflow limitation

One systematic review found that β agonists versus placebo or erithromycin may reduce cough at 7 days in adults, but subgroup analysis suggests that this benefit may be confined to adults with bronchial hyperresponsiveness, wheezes, or airflow limitation. The review found that β agonists versus placebo significantly increased the proportion of adults with shaking, tremor, and nervousness. The review identified two small RCTs in children that found no significant difference with β agonists versus placebo in cough at 7 days. However, the RCTs may have been too small to exclude a clinically important difference.

Decongestants for short term relief of congestive symptoms

One systematic review found that a single dose of decongestant versus placebo significantly reduced nasal congestion over 3–10 hours.

Vitamin C

One systematic review found that vitamin C versus placebo slightly but significantly reduced the duration of cold symptoms, but the benefit was small and may be explained by publication bias.

Clin Evid Concise 2003;9:320–322.

TRADE OFF BETWEEN BENEFITS AND HARMS

Antibiotics for reducing time to recovery in people with acute bronchitis, sore throat, and sinusitis

Systematic reviews have found that antibiotics versus placebo slightly but significantly improve symptoms. Adverse effects (nausea, vomiting, headache, rash, vaginitis) were more common with antibiotics compared with placebo.

UNKNOWN EFFECTIVENESS

Echinacea for prevention

One systematic review found that echinachea versus no treatment significantly reduced the number of people who had one infection episode, but found insufficient evidence about the effects of echinachea versus placebo.

Echinacea for treatment

Systematic reviews found that some preparations of echinacea versus placebo may improve symptoms, but we found insufficient evidence about the effects of any specific product.

Steam inhalation

One systematic review found insufficient evidence about the effects of steam inhalation.

Zinc (intranasal gel or lozenges)

Two RCTs found that zinc intranasal gel versus placebo reduced the mean duration of cold symptoms, but the difference was significant in only one of the RCTs. Two systematic reviews found limited evidence that zinc gluconate or acetate lozenges versus placebo may reduce duration of symptoms at 7 days.

LIKELY TO BE INEFFECTIVE OR HARMFUL

Antibiotics in people with colds

Systematic reviews found no significant difference with antibiotics versus placebo in cure or general improvement at 6–14 days.

Decongestants for long term relief of congestive symptoms

One systematic review found no good evidence about the effects of repeated decongestants over several days. One case control study found weak evidence that phenylpropanolamine may increase the risk of haemorrhagic stroke.

DEFINITION Upper respiratory tract infection involves inflammation of the respiratory mucosa from the nose to the lower respiratory tree, but not including the alveoli. In addition to malaise, it causes localised symptoms that constitute several overlapping syndromes: sore throat (pharyngitis), rhinorrhoea (common cold), facial fullness and pain (sinusitis), and cough (bronchitis).

INCIDENCE/ PREVALENCE Upper respiratory tract infections, nasal congestion, throat complaints, and cough are responsible for 11% of general practice consultations in Australia.[1] Each year, children suffer about five such infections and adults two to three infections.[1]

AETIOLOGY/ RISK FACTORS Infective agents include over 200 viruses (with 100 rhinoviruses) and several bacteria. Transmission is mostly through hand to hand contact with subsequent passage to the nostrils or eyes rather than, as commonly perceived, through droplets in the air.[2]

Upper respiratory tract infection

PROGNOSIS Upper respiratory tract infections are usually self limiting. Although they cause little mortality or serious morbidity, upper respiratory tract infections are responsible for considerable discomfort, lost work, and medical costs. Clinical patterns vary and overlap between infective agents. In addition to nasal symptoms, half of sufferers experience sore throat and 40% experience cough. Symptoms peak within 1–3 days and generally clear by 1 week, although cough often persists.[2]

Please refer to CD-ROM for full text and references.

Bacterial vaginosis

Search date March 2002

M Joesoef and George Schmid

What are the effects of antianaerobic treatments?

BENEFICIAL

Antianaerobic treatment in symptomatic non-pregnant women

One systematic review has found no significant difference between oral and intravaginal antianaerobic drugs in cure rates after 5–10 days or at 4 weeks. Another systematic review has found that a 7 day course of twice daily oral metronidazole versus a single 2 g dose significantly increases cure rates at 3–4 weeks. Limited evidence from RCTs found no significant difference in cure rates with oral clindamycin versus oral metronidazole twice daily for 7 days, and no difference between once and twice daily dosing with intravaginal metronidazole gel. One RCT found no significant difference in cure rates at 35 days with intravaginal clindamycin ovules for 3 days versus intravaginal clindamycin cream for 7 days.

LIKELY TO BE BENEFICIAL

Antianaerobic treatment (except clindamycin) in pregnant women who have had a previous preterm birth

Limited evidence from a subgroup analysis in pregnant women with bacterial vaginosis who had a previous preterm birth found that oral antianaerobic treatment versus placebo significantly reduced the risk of premature delivery.

Oral antianaerobic treatment before surgical abortion

RCTs consistently found that oral antianaerobic treatment versus placebo in women with bacterial vaginosis about to undergo surgical abortion was associated with a lower risk of pelvic inflammatory disease, but the difference was only significant in the largest RCT.

UNKNOWN EFFECTIVENESS

Antianaerobic treatment before gynaecological procedures (other than abortion)

We found no evidence on the effects of antianaerobic treatment in women with bacterial vaginosis about to undergo gynaecological procedures other than abortion.

Antianaerobic treatment (except clindamycin) in low risk pregnancy

Two systematic reviews of antianaerobic treatment of bacterial vaginosis during pregnancy have found no significant difference in the risk of preterm delivery.

LIKELY TO BE INEFFECTIVE OR HARMFUL

Treating pregnant women with intravaginal clindamycin

Four RCTs found that intravaginal clindamycin cream versus placebo was associated with an increased risk of preterm delivery and low birth weight, but the increase was not significant.

Treating pregnant women without bacterial vaginosis

Subgroup analysis in two RCTs of pregnant women without bacterial vaginosis found that both intravaginal clindamycin cream and oral metronidazole plus erythromycin versus placebo were associated with an increased risk of preterm delivery before 34 weeks' gestation, although the difference was significant in only one of the RCTs.

Clin Evid Concise 2003;9:323–324.

What are the effects of interventions to prevent recurrence?

LIKELY TO BE INEFFECTIVE OR HARMFUL

Treating a woman's one steady male sexual partner

One systematic review has found that, in women with one steady male sexual partner, treating the partner with an oral antianaerobic agent does not reduce the woman's risk of recurrence.

DEFINITION Bacterial vaginosis is a microbial disease characterised by an alteration in the bacterial flora of the vagina from a predominance of *Lactobacillus* species to high concentrations of anaerobic bacteria. Diagnosis requires three out of four features: the presence of clue cells; a homogenous discharge adherent to the vaginal walls; pH of vaginal fluid greater than 4.5; and a "fishy" amine odour of the vaginal discharge before or after addition of 10% potassium hydroxide. The condition is asymptomatic in 50% of infected women. Women with symptoms have an excessive white to grey, or malodorous vaginal discharge, or both; the odour may be particularly noticeable during sexual intercourse.

INCIDENCE/ PREVALENCE Bacterial vaginosis is the most common infectious cause of vaginitis, being about twice as common as candidiasis.[1] Prevalences of 10–61% have been reported among unselected women from a range of settings.[2] Data on incidence are limited but one study found that, over a 2 year period, 50% of women using an intrauterine contraceptive device had at least one episode, as did 20% of women using oral contraceptives.[3] Bacterial vaginosis is particularly prevalent in lesbians.[4]

AETIOLOGY/ RISK FACTORS The cause is not understood fully. Risk factors include new or multiple sexual partners[1,3,5] and early age of sexual debut,[6] but no causative microorganism has been shown to be transmitted between partners. Use of an intrauterine contraceptive device[3] and douching[5] have also been reported as risk factors. Infection seems to be most common around the time of menstruation.[7]

PROGNOSIS The course of bacterial vaginosis varies and is poorly understood. Without treatment, symptoms may persist or resolve in both pregnant and non-pregnant women. Recurrence after treatment occurs in about a third of women. The condition is associated with complications of pregnancy: low birth weight; preterm birth (pooled OR from 10 cohort studies: 1.8, 95% CI 1.5 to 2.6);[8] preterm labour; premature rupture of membranes; late miscarriage; chorioamnionitis (48% *v* 22%, OR 2.6, 95% CI 1.0 to 6.6);[9] endometritis after normal delivery (8.2% *v* 1.5%, OR 5.6, 95% CI 1.8 to 17.2);[10] endometritis after caesarean section (55% *v* 17%, OR 5.8, 95% CI 3.0 to 10.9);[11] and surgery to the genital tract. Women who have had a previous premature delivery are especially at risk of complications in pregnancy, with a sevenfold increased risk of preterm birth (AR 24/428 [6%] in all women *v* 10/24 [42%] in women with a previous preterm birth).[12] Bacterial vaginosis can also enhance HIV acquisition and transmission.[13]

Please refer to CD-ROM for full text and references.

Genital chlamydial infection

Search date September 2002

Nicola Low and Frances Cowan

What are the effects of antibiotic treatment for men and non-pregnant women with uncomplicated genital chlamydial infection?

Short term microbiological cure is the outcome used in most RCTs, but this may not mean eradication of *Chlamydia trachomatis*. Long term cure rates have not been studied extensively because of high default rates and difficulty in distinguishing persistent infection from reinfection due to re-exposure.

BENEFICIAL

Doxycycline, teracycline, rosaramicin (multiple dose regimens)

Small RCTs with short term follow up and high withdrawal rates found that multiple dose regimens of tetracyclines (doxycycline, tetracycline) and macrolides (rosaramicin) achieve micrological cure in at least 95% of people with genital chlamydia.

LIKELY TO BE BENEFICIAL

Azithromycin (single dose)

One systematic review of short term RCTs hasfound no significant difference in microbiological cure of *Chlamydia trachomatis* between a single dose of azithromycin versus a 7 day course of doxycycline, although the RCTs may have lacked power to detect a clinically important difference. Rates of adverse effects were similar.

Erythromycin (multiple dose regimens)

Three small RCTs found that erythromycin achieved microbiological cure in 77–100% of people, with the highest cure rate with a 2 g versus a 1 g daily dose.

UNKNOWN EFFECTIVENESS

Ofloxacin, trovafloxacin, minocycline, lymecycline, clarithromycin, ampicillin, rifampicin (multiple dose regimens)

We found insufficient evidence on these regimens.

UNLIKELY TO BE BENEFICIAL

Ciprofloxacin (multiple dose)

Two RCTs found that ciprofloxacin cured 63–92% of people. Meta-analysis found that ciprofloxacin versus doxycycline significantly increased microbiological failure.

What are the effects of antibiotic treatment for pregnant women with uncomplicated genital chlamydial infection?

LIKELY TO BE BENEFICIAL

Azithromycin (single *v* multiple dose antibiotics)

One systematic review has found that a single dose of azithromycin versus a 7 day course of erythromycin significantly increases microbiological cure. Two subsequent unblinded RCTs found no significant difference in cure rate between single dose azithromycin versus multiple dose amoxicillin.

Erythromycin, amoxicillin (multiple dose regimens)

One systematic review of one small RCT has found erythromycin versus placebo significantly increased microbiological cure. The review found no significant difference between erythomycin and amoxicillin in microbiological cure, and high cure rates with both drugs.

UNKNOWN EFFECTIVENESS

Clindamycin (multiple dose)

One small RCT has found no significant difference in cure rates between clindamycin versus erythromycin.

DEFINITION Uncomplicated genital chlamydia is a sexually transmitted infection of the urethra in men and of the endocervix, urethra (or both) in women that has not ascended to the upper genital tract. Infection is asymptomatic in up to 80% of women, but may cause non-specific symptoms, including vaginal discharge and intermenstrual bleeding. Infection in men causes urethral discharge and urethral irritation or dysuria, but may also be asymptomatic in up to half of cases.[1] Complicated chlamydia infection includes spread to the upper genital tract (causing pelvic inflammatory disease [see pelvic inflammatory disease, p 336] in women and epididymo-orchitis in men) and extra genital sites, such as ocular infection.

INCIDENCE/ PREVALENCE Genital chlamydia is the most common bacterial sexually transmitted infection in developed countries. In the USA, over 642 000 cases of chlamydia were reported in the year 2000.[2] The prevalence of uncomplicated genital chlamydia in women attending general practice surgeries in the UK is reported to be 3–5%.[3] Prevalence is highest in young adults. Reported rates in 16–19 year old women are about 940/100 000 in the UK,[4] 1000/100 000 in Sweden,[1] and 2500/100 000 in the USA.[5]

AETIOLOGY/ RISK FACTORS Infection is caused by the bacterium *C trachomatis* serotypes D–K. It is transmitted primarily through sexual intercourse.

PROGNOSIS In women, untreated chlamydial infection that ascends to the upper genital tract causes pelvic inflammatory disease in an estimated 30–40% of women.[6] Tubal infertility has been found to occur in about 11% of women after a single episode of pelvic inflammatory disease, and the risk of ectopic pregnancy is increased six- to sevenfold.[7] Ascending infection in men causes epididymitis, but evidence that this causes male infertility is limited.[8] Maternal to infant transmission can lead to neonatal conjunctivitis and pneumonitis in 30–40% of cases.[1] Chlamydia may coexist with other genital infections and may facilitate transmission and acquisition of HIV infection.[1] Untreated chlamydial infection persists symptomatically in most women for at least 60 days and for a shorter period in men.[9] Spontaneous remission also occurs but data are insufficient to determine the rate of clearance.[9]

Please refer to CD-ROM for full text and references.

Genital herpes

Search date November 2002

Clinical Evidence freelance writers

What are the effects of treatments?

BENEFICIAL

Daily oral antiviral treatment in people with high rates of recurrence

RCTs have found that daily maintenance treatment with oral antiviral compared with placebo reduces the frequency of recurrences and improves psychosocial morbidity agents in people with frequent recurrence.

Oral antiviral treatment in first episodes

RCTs in people with a first episode of genital herpes have found that oral antiviral treatment versus placebo reduces the duration of symptoms, lesions, and viral shedding but found no significant difference in the time to recurrence or frequency of subsequent recurrences.

Oral antiviral treatment taken at the start of a recurrence

One systematic review and one subsequent RCT have found that oral antiviral treatment taken at the start of a recurrence reduces the duration of lesions, symptoms and viral shedding compared with placebo in people with recurrent genital herpes. RCTs found no significant differences among different antiviral agents.

UNKNOWN EFFECTIVENESS

Oral antiviral treatment in immunocompromise people with HIV infection

We found no RCTs evaluating antiviral treatment for genital herpes in people immunocompromised with HIV infection.

Psychotherapy to reduce recurrence

One systematic review found insufficient evidence on the effects of psychotherapy on genital herpes recurrence.

What are the effects of interventions to prevent transmission?

LIKELY TO BE BENEFICIAL

Male condom use to prevent sexual transmission to women*

Limited evidence from a prospective cohort study suggested that male condom use reduced the transmission of herpes simplex virus type 2 to women who had sexual partners with herpes simplex virus 2.

*Categorisation based on observational evidence.

UNKNOWN EFFECTIVENESS

Abdominal delivery in women with genital lesions at term

We found insufficient evidence of the effects of abdominal delivery on mother to baby transmission of genital herpes. The procedure carries the risk of increased maternal morbidity and mortality.

Antiviral treatment to prevent sexual transmission

We found no good evidence on the effects of antiviral treatments to prevent sexual transmission.

Daily oral antiviral treatment in late pregnancy (36 or more wks of gestation) in women with a history of genital herpes

We found insufficient direct evidence about effects on neonatal infection. One systematic review and one subsequent RCT found that aciclovir reduced the rate of genital lesions at term in women with first or recurrent episodes of genital herpes simplex virus during pregnancy.

Female condoms

We found no good evidence on the effects of female condoms to prevent transmission.

Male condoms to prevent sexual transmission to men

One prospective cohort study found no significant difference between male condom use versus no condom use in preventing transmission of herpes simplex virus type 2 to men who had sexual partners with genital herpes.

Serological screening and counselling in late pregnancy

The highest risk of mother to baby transmission is in women newly infected with genital herpes in late pregnancy. We found insufficient evidence of the effects of interventions to prevent infection in late pregnancy (such as serological screening and counselling).

UNLIKELY TO BE BENEFICIAL

Recombinant glycoprotein vaccine (gB2 and gD2)

One RCT found no significant difference between glycoprotein vaccine versus placebo in acquisition rates of herpes simplex virus 2. We found no good evidence on other forms of immunisation.

DEFINITION Genital herpes is an infection with herpes simplex virus type 1 or type 2, causing ulceration in the genital area. Herpes simplex virus infections can be defined on the basis of virological and serological findings. Types of infection include **first episode primary infection**, which is herpes simplex virus in a person without prior herpes simplex virus type 1 or type 2 antibodies; **first episode non-primary infection**, which is herpes simplex virus type 2 in a person with prior herpes simplex virus type 1 antibodies or vice versa; **first recognised recurrence**, which is herpes simplex virus type 2 (or type 1) in a person with prior herpes simplex virus type 2 (or type 1) antibodies; and **recurrent genital herpes**, which is caused by reactivation of latent herpes simplex virus.

INCIDENCE/ PREVALENCE Genital herpes infections are among the most common sexually transmitted diseases. Seroprevalence studies show that 22% of adults in the USA have herpes simplex virus type 2 antibodies.[1] A UK study found that 23% of adults attending sexual medicine clinics and 7.6% of blood donors in London had antibodies to herpes simplex virus type 2.[2] However, herpes simplex type 2 can cause other herpes infections such as ocular herpes.

AETIOLOGY/ RISK FACTORS Both herpes simplex virus type 1 and 2 can cause a first episode of genital infection, but herpes simplex virus type 2 is more likely to cause recurrent disease.[3] Most people with herpes simplex virus type 2 infection are not aware that they have genital herpes, as their symptoms are mild. However, these people can pass on the infection to sexual partners and newborns.[4,5]

PROGNOSIS Sequelae of herpes simplex virus infection include neonatal herpes simplex virus infection, opportunistic infections in immunocompromised people, recurrent genital ulceration, and psychosocial morbidity. Herpes simplex virus type 2 infection is associated with an increased risk of HIV transmission and acquisition.[6] The most common neurological complications are aseptic meningitis (reported in about 25% of women during primary infection) and urinary retention. The absolute risk of neonatal infection is high (41%, 95% CI 26% to 56%) in babies born to women who acquire infection near the time of labour[7,8] and low (< 3%) in women with established infection, even in those who have a recurrence at term. About 15% of neonatal infections result from postnatal transmission from oral lesions.

Please refer to CD-ROM for full text and references.

Genital warts

Search date January 2002

DJ Wiley

What are the effects of treatments?

BENEFICIAL

Cryotherapy (as effective as podophyllin, trichloroacetic acid, or electrosurgery)

We found no RCTs comparing cryotherapy versus placebo or no treatment. One RCT found limited evidence that cryotherapy versus podophyllin significantly increased clearance after 6 weeks' treatment, but follow up of the people with successful wart clearance found no significant difference in the proportion of people who had warts at 3–5 months. Two RCTs found no significant difference with cryotherapy versus trichloroacetic acid in clearance of warts after 6–10 weeks' treatment, and one of RCTs found no significant difference in recurrence of warts at 2 months after the end of treatment. One RCT found limited evidence that cryotherapy was significantly less effective for clearance than electrosurgery after 6 weeks' treatment, but follow up of the people with successful wart clearance found no significant difference in the proportion of people who had warts at 3–5 months. Another RCT found no significant difference in wart clearance at 3 months with cryotherapy versus electrosurgery.

Electrosurgery (more effective than intramuscular or subcutaneous interferon, as effective as cryotherapy)

We found no RCTs comparing electrosurgery versus no treatment. One RCT found limited evidence suggesting that electrosurgery may be more effective than intramuscular or subcutaneous interferon. One RCT found limited evidence that electrosurgery versus cryotherapy or podophyllin significantly improved clearance after 6 weeks' treatment, but follow up of the people with successful wart clearance found no significant difference in the proportion of people who had warts at 3–5 months. Another RCT found no significant difference in wart clearance at 3 months with electrosurgery versus cryotherapy.

Imiquimod

One systematic review has found that imiquimod cream versus placebo significantly increases wart clearance and reduces recurrence over 16 weeks in people with genital warts and without HIV. One RCT in people with HIV identified by the review found no significant difference in wart clearance over 16 weeks with imiquimod cream versus placebo.

Interferon, intralesional injection

RCTs have found that intralesional injection of interferon versus placebo significantly increases partial or total wart clearance

Interferon, topical

RCTs have found that topical interferon versus placebo significantly increases wart clearance at 4 weeks.

Laser surgery (as effective as surgical excision)

We found no RCTs comparing laser surgery versus placebo or no treatment. One RCT found no significant difference with laser versus surgical excision in wart clearance at 36 months.

Clin Evid Concise 2003;9:330–331.

Podophyllin (as effective as podophyllotoxin, cryotherapy, or electrosurgery)

We found no RCTs comparing podophyllin versus placebo. RCTs have found that podophyllin resin is as effective in clearing warts as podophyllotoxin, cryotherapy, and electrosurgery, but is significantly less effective than surgical excision.

Podophyllotoxin

RCTs have found that podophyllotoxin versus placebo significantly increases wart clearance within 16 weeks.

Surgical excision (as effective as laser surgery)

We found no RCTs comparing surgical excision versus placebo or no treatment. One RCT found no significant difference with surgical excision versus laser surgery in wart clearance.

UNKNOWN EFFECTIVENESS

Bi- and trichloroacetic acid

We found insufficient evidence to evaluate the efficacy of bi- and trichloroacetic acid versus placebo.

Interferon, topical as adjuvant treatment to laser surgery

RCTs found insufficient evidence on the effects of this intervention.

5-Fluorouracil cream; condoms in preventing human papillomavirus transmission; treatments to prevent human papillomavirus transmission

We found no RCTs on the effects of these interventions.

UNLIKELY TO BE BENEFICIAL

Systemic interferon

RCTs found no significant difference with systemic interferon versus placebo in wart clearance after 3 months and found that it was associated with a range of adverse effects.

DEFINITION External genital warts are benign epidermal growths on the external perianal and perigenital region. There are four morphological types: condylomatous, keratotic, papular, and flat warts.

INCIDENCE/ PREVALENCE In 1996, external and internal genital warts accounted for over 180 000 initial visits to private physicians' offices in the USA: about 60 000 fewer than were reported for 1995.[1] In the USA, 1% of sexually active men and women aged 18–49 years are estimated to have external genital warts.[2]

AETIOLOGY/ RISK FACTORS External genital warts are caused by the human papillomavirus (HPV). Although more than 70 types of HPV have been identified, most external genital warts in immunocompetent people are caused by HPV types 6 and 11.[3,4] HPV infections and, more specifically, external genital warts are sexually transmissible.

PROGNOSIS Clinical trials have found that recurrences are frequent and may necessitate repeated treatment. Without treatment, external genital warts may remain unchanged, may increase in size or number, or may completely resolve. They rarely, if ever, progress to cancer.[5] Juvenile laryngeal papillomatosis, a rare and sometimes life threatening condition, occurs in children of women with a history of genital warts. Its rarity makes it hard to design studies that can evaluate whether treatment in pregnant women alters the risk.[6,7]

Please refer to CD-ROM for full text and references.

Gonorrhoea

Search date May 2002

John Moran

What are the effects of treatments?

BENEFICIAL

Single dose regimens using selected fluoroquinolones, selected cephalosporins, or spectinomycin in uncomplicated infection in men and non-pregnant women*

One systematic review found limited evidence by combining cure rates across different arms of RCTs. It found that single dose regimens based on an antimicrobial agent other than a penicillin or a tetracycline achieved cure rates of 95% or higher in urogenital or rectal infection. Cure rates were lower (≤ 80%) for pharyngeal infection. Resistance is now widespread to penicillins, tetracyclines, and sulphonamides.

Single dose regimens using selected cephalosporins or spectinomycin in uncomplicated infection in pregnant women

RCTs comparing different antimicrobial agents have found that ceftriaxone and spectinomycin cure 89–97% of rectal, cervical, and pharyngeal infections.

LIKELY TO BE BENEFICIAL

Selected injectable fluoroquinolones or selected injectable cephalosporins in disseminated infection**

We found no RCTs published in the last 20 years assessing treatments for disseminated gonococcal infection, but there is strong consensus that multidose regimens using injectable cephalosporins or quinolones are the most effective treatment. We found no reports of treatment failures with these regimens.

UNKNOWN EFFECTIVENESS

Dual treatment for gonorrhoea and chlamydia infections in all people diagnosed with gonorrhoea

Dual treatment for gonorrhoea and chlamydia infections is based on theory and expert opinion rather than on evidence from RCTs. The balance between benefits and harms will vary with the prevalence of co-infection in each population.

*Based on comparisons of results across arms of different trials.
**Based only on non-RCT evidence and consensus.

DEFINITION Gonorrhoea is caused by infection with *Neisseria gonorrhoeae*. In men, uncomplicated urethritis is the most common manifestation, with dysuria and urethral discharge. Less typically, signs and symptoms are mild and indistinguishable from chlamydial urethritis. In women the most common manifestation is cervicitis, which produces symptoms (e.g. vaginal discharge, lower abdominal discomfort, and dyspareunia) in only half of the women. Co-infection with chlamydia is reported in 20–40% of people.[1]

INCIDENCE/ PREVALENCE Between 1975 and 1997, the incidence of reported gonorrhoea in the USA fell by 74%, reaching a level in 1996 of 122/100 000 people. Since 1997, between 122 and 132 cases have been reported per 100 000 people each year.[2] In the UK, diagnoses of gonorrhoea have increased since 1994, reaching 218/100 000 for 20–24 year old males and 184/100 000 for 16 to 19 year old females in 2001.[3] In poor communities, rates may be higher: the ▶

estimated incidence in people aged 15–59 years living in three inner London boroughs in 1994–1995 was 138/100 000 women and 292/100 000 men.[4] Rates are highest in younger people. In the USA in 2000, incidence was highest in women aged 15–19 years (716/100 000) and men aged 20–24 years (590/100 000).[2]

AETIOLOGY/ RISK FACTORS Most infections result from penile-vaginal, penile-rectal, or penile-pharyngeal contact. An important minority of infections are transmitted from mother to child during birth, which can cause ophthalmia neonatorum. Less common are ocular infections in older children and adults as a result of sexual exposure, poor hygiene, or the medicinal use of urine.

PROGNOSIS The natural history of untreated gonococcal infection is spontaneous resolution after weeks or months of unpleasant symptoms. During this time, there is a substantial likelihood of transmission to others and of complications developing in the infected individual.[5] Symptoms in most men are severe enough to cause them to seek treatment, but an estimated 1–3% of infected men remain asymptomatic. These men, and men who are infectious but not yet symptomatic, are largely responsible for the spread of the disease. In many women, the lack of readily discernible signs or symptoms of cervicitis means that infections go unrecognised and untreated. An unknown proportion of untreated infections causes local complications, including lymphangitis, periurethral abscess, bartholinitis, and urethral stricture; epididymitis in men; and in women involvement of the uterus, fallopian tubes, or ovaries causing pelvic inflammatory disease (see pelvic inflammatory disease, p 336). It is the association of gonorrhoea with pelvic inflammatory disease — a major cause of secondary infertility, ectopic pregnancy, and chronic pelvic pain — that makes gonorrhoea an important public health issue. Manifestations of disseminated infection are petechial or pustular skin lesions; asymmetrical arthropathies, tenosynovitis, or septic arthritis; and, rarely, meningitis or endocarditis.

Please refer to CD-ROM for full text and references.

Partner notification

Search date March 2002

Catherine Mathews, Nicol Coetzee, Merrick Zwarenstein, and Sally Guttmacher

What are the effects of different partner notification strategies in different groups of people and what are the effects of interventions to improve patient referral?

We found no good evidence on the effects of partner notification on relationships between patients and partners and, in particular, on the rate of violence, abuse, and abandonment of patient or partner.

We found no studies comparing the effects of an intervention across different groups, such as people with different diseases or combinations of diseases, or people from different settings.

LIKELY TO BE BENEFICIAL

Contract referral (as effective as provider referral in people with syphilis)

One systematic review of one RCT comparing different partner notification strategies in people with syphilis found no significant difference in the proportion of partners notified between provider referral Ⓖ and contract referral Ⓖ, when people receiving the contract referral option were given only 2 days to notify their partners.

Provider referral, contract referral, or offering a choice between provider and patient referral (*v* patient referral alone) in people with HIV, gonorrhoea, or chlamydia

One systematic review comparing different partner notification strategies found that in people with HIV, offering a choice between provider referral (where the identity of the index patient was not revealed) and patient referral Ⓖ was more effective than offering patient referral alone. It found that in people with gonorrhoea infections, contract referral versus patient referral significantly increased the number of partners presenting for treatment. In chlamydia infections, provider referral versus patient referral significantly increased the proportion of partners assessed per and of positive partners detected per patient. The systematic review found no good evidence on the effects of these strategies on relationships between patients and partners and, in particular, on the rate of violence, abuse, and abandonment of patient or partner.

UNKNOWN EFFECTIVENESS

Adding telephone reminders and contact cards to patient referral; patient referral with educational videos; patient referral by different types of healthcare professionals

We found insufficient evidence about the effects of these interventions in improving partner notification.

DEFINITION Partner notification is a process whereby the sexual partners of people with a diagnosis of sexually transmitted infection are informed of their exposure to infection. The main methods are patient referral, provider referral, contract referral, and outreach assistance Ⓖ.

Clin Evid Concise 2003;9:334–335.

INCIDENCE/ PREVALENCE A large proportion of people with sexually transmitted infections will have neither symptoms nor signs of infection. For example, 22–68% of men with gonorrhoea who were identified through partner notification were asymptomatic.[1] Partner notification is one of the two strategies to reach such individuals, the other strategy being screening. Managing infection in people with more than one current sexual partner is likely to have the greatest impact on the spread of sexually transmitted infections.[2]

PROGNOSIS Studies showing that partner notification results in a health benefit, either to the partner or to future partners of infected partners, are not available. Obtaining such evidence would be technically and ethically difficult. One RCT in asymptomatic women compared identifying, testing, and treating women at increased risk for cervical chlamydial infection versus usual care. It found these reduced incidence of pelvic inflammatory disease (RR 0.44, 95% CI 0.2 to 0.9).[3] This evidence suggests that partner notification, which also aims to identify and treat people who are largely unaware of infection, would provide a direct health benefit to partners who are infected.

Please refer to CD-ROM for full text and references.

Pelvic inflammatory disease

Search date April 2002

Jonathan Ross

What are the effects of treatments?

LIKELY TO BE BENEFICIAL

Antibiotics (symptoms improved and microbiological clearance in women with confirmed pelvic inflammatory disease)

One systematic review of observational studies and RCTs has found that several regimens of antibiotic treatment are effective in relieving the symptoms of pelvic inflammatory disease and achieving high rates of microbiological cure.

UNKNOWN EFFECTIVENESS

Different durations of antibiotic treatment

Systematic reviews found no good evidence on the optimal duration of treatment.

Empirical antibiotic treatment

We found no RCTs comparing empirical treatment with antibiotics (before receiving results of microbiological tests) versus delaying treatment until test results are available.

Oral versus parenteral antibiotics

Two RCTs found no significant difference between oral ofloxacin versus parenteral cefoxitin and doxycycline.

Routine antibiotic prophylaxis prior to intrauterine device insertion in people at high risk

We found no good evidence on the effects in people likely to be at high risk for pelvic inflammatory disease.

UNLIKELY TO BE BENEFICIAL

Routine antibiotic prophylaxis prior to intrauterine device insertion

One systematic review found no significant difference between routine prophylaxis with doxycycline versus placebo prior to intrauterine contraceptive device insertion in pelvic inflammatory disease. The absolute risk of pelvic inflammatory disease following intrauterine contraceptive device insertion was low. However, the systematic review may have lacked power to rule out a clinically important difference. We found no good evidence on the effects in people likely to be at high risk for pelvic inflammatory disease.

DEFINITION Pelvic inflammatory disease (PID) is inflammation and infection of the upper genital tract in women, typically involving the fallopian tubes, ovaries, and surrounding structures.

INCIDENCE/ PREVALENCE The exact incidence of PID is unknown because the disease cannot be diagnosed reliably from clinical symptoms and signs.[1–3] Direct visualisation of the fallopian tubes by laparoscopy is the best single diagnostic test, but it is invasive and not used routinely in clinical practice. PID is the most common gynaecological reason for admission to hospital in the USA, accounting for 49/10 000 recorded hospital discharges and a diagnosis of PID is made in 1/62 (1.6%) women aged 16–45 attending their primary care physician in

England and Wales.[4] However, because most PID diseases are asymptomatic, this figure underestimates the true prevalence.[1,5] A crude marker of PID in developing countries can be obtained from reported hospital admission rates, where it accounts for 17–40% of gynaecological admissions in sub-Saharan Africa, 15–37% in Southeast Asia, and 3–10% in India.[6]

AETIOLOGY/ RISK FACTORS Factors associated with PID mirror those for sexually transmitted infections: young age, reduced socioeconomic circumstances, African/Afro-Caribbean ethnicity, lower educational attainment, and recent new sexual partner.[2,7,8] Infection ascends from the cervix and initial epithelial damage caused by bacteria (especially *Chlamydia trachomatis* and *Neisseria gonorrhoeae*) allows the opportunistic entry of other organisms. Isolates from the upper genital tract are polymicrobial, including *Mycoplasma hominis* and anaerobes.[9] The spread of infection to the upper genital tract may be increased by vaginal douching and instrumentation of the cervix, but reduced by the barrier method and oral contraceptives compared with other forms of contraception.[10–13]

PROGNOSIS PID has high morbidity; about 20% of affected women become infertile, 20% develop chronic pelvic pain, and 10% of those who conceive have an ectopic pregnancy.[2] We found no placebo controlled trials of antibiotic treatment. Uncontrolled observations suggest that clinical symptoms and signs resolve in a significant number of untreated women.[14] Repeated episodes of pelvic inflammatory disease are associated with a four to six times increase in the risk of permanent tubal damage.[15] One case control study (76 cases and 367 controls) found that delaying treatment by even a few days is associated with impaired fertility (OR 2.6, 95% CI 1.2 to 5.9).[16]

Please refer to CD-ROM for full text and references.

Athlete's foot and fungally infected toe nails

Search date October 2001

Fay Crawford

What are the effects of treatments?

BENEFICIAL

Oral allylamines* for athlete's foot

One RCT identified by a systematic review found limited evidence that oral terbinafine versus placebo for 6 weeks significantly improved cure rates at 8 weeks. One RCT found that oral terbinafine versus oral itraconazole for 2 weeks significantly increased cure rates, but found no significant difference in cure rates with 2 weeks of oral terbinafine versus 4 weeks of oral itraconazole.

Oral azoles* for athlete's foot

One RCT identified by a systematic review found that oral itraconazole versus placebo for 1 week significantly increased cure rates at 8 weeks. The review found no significant difference in cure rates between individual azoles and oral allylamines, or between oral azoles and oral griseofulvin.

Topical allylamines* for athlete's foot

One systematic review and two subsequent RCTs have found that allylamines versus placebo significantly increase the proportion of people cured at 6–16 weeks. One systematic review and two additional RCTs have found that allylamines produce a faster response than azoles, but the cure rates are similar.

Topical azoles* for athlete's foot

One systematic review has found that azole creams versus placebo administered for 4–6 weeks significantly increase cure rates at 6–10 weeks. One systematic review and two additional RCTs have found that azoles produce a slower response than allylamines, but the cure rates are similar.

Topical tolnaftate* for athlete's foot

One systematic review has found that tolnaftate versus placebo for 4 weeks significantly reduces treatment failure after 5–8 weeks.

Topical undecenoic acid for athlete's foot

One systematic review has found that undecenoic acid versus placebo significantly reduces treatment failure after 4 weeks.

LIKELY TO BE BENEFICIAL

Topical acidified nitrite cream for athlete's foot

One systematic review of one RCT found limited evidence that topical nitrate plus salicylic acid versus salicylic acid alone for 4 weeks significantly improved cure rate.

Topical butenafine for fungal nail infections

RCTs found limited evidence that butenafine cream in combination with either urea or tea tree oil versus placebo significantly improved cure rates at 16–36 weeks.

Topical ciclopiroxolamine for athlete's foot

One systematic review of one RCT found that topical ciclopiroxolamine versus placebo for 4 weeks significantly reduced treatment failure at 6 weeks.

Topical ciclopiroxolamine for fungal nail infections

RCTs found that ciclopiroxolamine lacquer versus placebo significantly improved cure rates at 48 weeks.

Clin Evid Concise 2003;9:338–339.

Topical griseofulvin for athlete's foot

One systematic review of one RCT found that topical griseofulvin versus placebo significantly reduced treatment failure at 4 weeks.

*See table on the CD for a list of allylamines and azoles in common use.

DEFINITION Athlete's foot is a cutaneous fungal infection that causes the skin to itch, flake, and fissure. Nail involvement is characterised by ungual thickening and discolouration.

INCIDENCE/ PREVALENCE In the UK, athlete's foot is present in about 15% of the general population,[1] and 1.2 million people have fungally infected toe nails.[2]

AETIOLOGY/ RISK FACTORS Swimming pool users and industrial workers may have increased risk of fungal foot infection. However, one survey found fungal foot infection in only 9% of swimmers, with the highest incidence (20%) in men aged 16 years and over.[1]

PROGNOSIS Fungal infections of the foot are not life threatening in people with normal immunity, but in some people they cause persistent symptoms. Others are apparently oblivious of persistent infection. The infection can spread to other parts of the body and to other individuals.

Please refer to CD-ROM for full text and references.

Atopic eczema

Search date May 2002

Dominic Smethurst and Sarah Macfarlane

What are the effects of preventive interventions and treatments?

BENEFICIAL

Topical steroids

One systematic review has found that topical corticosteroids versus placebo improve atopic eczema after 1–4 weeks. Another systematic review comparing a variety of topical steroids versus each other found significant improvement in 22–100% of people after 1–6 weeks. One subsequent RCT in people with mild to moderate eczema found no significant difference in mean scratch free days over 18 weeks with 3 day treatment with betamethasone (a potent topical steroid) versus 7 day treatment with hydrocortisone (a mild topical steroid). Short term RCTs and one longer term cohort study found no serious systemic adverse effects or skin atrophy associated with topical steroids. Small volunteer studies have found that potent topical steroid preparations cause skin thinning after twice daily application for up to 6 weeks, although skin thickness returns to normal within 4 weeks of stopping treatment. One RCT found insufficient evidence of the effects of topical steroids in preventing relapse.

LIKELY TO BE BENEFICIAL

Control of house dust mite

RCTs found limited evidence suggesting that controlling house dust mite significantly reduced severity of symptoms at 6–12 months, but only if very low levels of mites were achieved. We found conflicting evidence about the effects on eczema severity of reducing dust mites in people with atopic eczema and positive mite radioallergosorbent test scores.

Dietary manipulation during lactation in mothers of predisposed infants

Limited evidence from one systematic review suggests that maternal dietary restriction during lactation may protect against the development of eczema at 12–18 months in infants with a family history of atopy.

Emollients

One systematic review has found that moisturising cream plus topical corticosteroid versus topical corticosteroid alone significantly improves clinical signs and symptoms of atopic eczema after 3 weeks.

UNKNOWN EFFECTIVENESS

Avoidance of biological washing detergents

One systematic review found no significant difference with washing detergents that contain enzymes versus washing detergents without enzymes in eczema severity at 1 month.

Avoidance of certain clothing textiles

RCTs found limited evidence that, in people with atopic eczema, the roughness of clothing textiles is a more important factor for skin irritation than the type of textile fibre (synthetic or natural). One RCT in infants with atopic eczema comparing cotton nappy/diaper versus cellulose core nappy/diaper versus cellulose core nappy/diaper containing absorbent gelling found no significant difference in eczema scores after 26 weeks.

Clin Evid Concise 2003;9:340–341.

◀ **Dietary manipulation**
One systematic review in children and adults with atopic eczema found inconclusive evidence about the effects of dietary manipulation, such as exclusion of egg and cows' milk.

Dietary manipulation during pregnancy in mothers of predisposed infants
One systematic review found no significant difference with maternal diet restriction during pregnancy versus no restriction in development of atopic eczema in the infant at 12–18 months.

Prolonged breast feeding in predisposed infants
One systematic review of prospective cohort studies suggests that exclusive breast feeding for at least 3 months may reduce the risk of eczema in infants with a family history of atopy.

Wet wrap dressing and bandaging
One systematic review identified no RCTs on the effects of wet wrap**G** or other forms of bandaging.

Avoidance of animal contact; avoidance of vaccination/immunisation; avoidance of all washing detergents
We found no RCTs about the effects of these preventive interventions.

UNLIKELY TO BE BENEFICIAL

Topical antimicrobial plus steroid combinations
One systematic review has found no significant difference with topical antimicrobial agents plus steroids versus topical steroids alone in improving the clinical signs and symptoms of atopic eczema.

DEFINITION Atopic eczema (atopic dermatitis) is an inflammatory skin disease characterised by an itchy erythematous poorly demarcated skin eruption with a predilection for skin creases.[1]

INCIDENCE/ PREVALENCE Atopic eczema affects 15–20% of school children in the UK and 2–3% of adults.[2] Prevalence has increased substantially over the past 30 years,[3] possibly because of environmental and lifestyle changes.

AETIOLOGY/ RISK FACTORS Aetiology is believed to be multifactorial. Recent interest has focused on airborne allergens (house dust mites, pollen, animal dander), outdoor pollution, climate, diet, and prenatal/early life factors such as infections.

PROGNOSIS Although there is currently no cure, several interventions can help to control symptoms. Atopic eczema clears in 60–70% of children by their early teens, although relapses may occur.

Please refer to CD-ROM for full text and references.

Cellulitis and erysipelas

Search date June 2002

Andrew Morris

What are the effects of treatments?

LIKELY TO BE BENEFICIAL

Antibiotics

We found no RCTs comparing antibiotics versus placebo. RCTs comparing different single antibiotic regimens found clinical cure in 50–100% of people at 4–30 days.

UNKNOWN EFFECTIVENESS

Different antibiotic regimens

RCTs comparing different antibiotic regimens were designed to test equivalence rather than to detect clinically significant differences in cure rates between antibiotics.

Oral versus intravenous antibiotics; short versus long courses of antibiotics

We found no RCTs comparing oral versus intravenous antibiotics, or different durations of treatment.

Treatment of predisposing factors to prevent recurrence

We found no RCTs or observational studies on the effects of treating predisposing factors for recurrence of cellulitis or erysipelas.

DEFINITION Cellulitis is a spreading bacterial infection of the dermis and subcutaneous tissues. It causes local signs of inflammation such as warmth, erythema, pain, lymphangitis, and frequently systemic upset with fever and raised white blood cell count. Erysipelas is a form of cellulitis and is characterised by pronounced superficial inflammation. The lower limbs are by far the most common sites, but any area can be affected. The term erysipelas is commonly used when the face is affected.

INCIDENCE/ PREVALENCE We found no specific data on the incidence of cellulitis, but cellulitis and abscess infections were responsible for 158 consultations per 10 000 person years at risk in the UK in 1991.[1] In 1985 in the UK, skin and subcutaneous tissue infections resulted in 29 820 hospital admissions and a mean occupancy of 664 hospital beds each day.[2]

AETIOLOGY/ RISK FACTORS The most common infective organisms for cellulitis and erysipelas in adults are *Streptococci* (particularly *S pyogenes*) and *Staphylococcus aureus*.[3] In children, *Haemophilus influenzae* is a frequent cause. Several risk factors for cellulitis and erysipelas have been identified in a case control study (167 cases and 294 controls): lymphoedema (OR 71.2, 95% CI 5.6 to 908.0), leg ulcer (OR 62.5, 95% CI 7.0 to 556.0), toe web intertrigo (OR 13.9, 95% CI 7.2 to 27.0), and traumatic wounds (OR 10.7, 95% CI 4.8 to 23.8).[4]

PROGNOSIS Cellulitis can spread through the bloodstream and lymphatic system. A retrospective case study of people admitted to hospital with cellulitis found that systemic symptoms such as fever and raised white blood cell count were present in up to 42% of cases at presentation.[5] Lymphatic involvement can lead to obstruction and damage the lymphatic system that predisposes to ▶

Clin Evid Concise 2003;9:342–343.

recurrent cellulitis. Recurrence can occur rapidly or after months or years. One study found that 29% of people with erysipelas had a recurrent episode within 3 years.[6] Local necrosis and abscess formation can also occur. It is not known whether the prognosis of erysipelas differs from that of cellulitis. We found no evidence about factors that predict recurrence, or a better or worse outcome. We found no good evidence on the prognosis of untreated cellulitis.

Please refer to CD-ROM for full text and references.

Chronic plaque psoriasis

Search date May 2002

Luigi Naldi and Bethold Rzany

What are the effects of treatments?

BENEFICIAL

Ingram regimen

One large RCT has found that the Ingram regimen**G** is of similar effectiveness to psoralen plus ultraviolet A in clearing moderate to severe psoriasis.

Psoralen plus ultraviolet A

One systematic review has found that clearing of psoriasis is more likely with higher versus lower doses of psoralen, and that the mean cumulative dose of ultraviolet A required for clearance is significantly reduced. Long term treatment risks include photoageing and skin cancer (mainly squamous cell carcinoma).

Vitamin D derivatives

Systematic reviews and additional long term uncontrolled studies have found that calcipotriol versus placebo improves plaque psoriasis and is at least as effective as topical steroids, coal tars, and dithranol. One review found that calcipotriol monotherapy caused more irritation than potent topical steroids.

LIKELY TO BE BENEFICIAL

Dithranol

Small RCTs have found that dithranol versus placebo improves chronic plaque psoriasis.

Topical retinoids (tazarotene)

RCTs have found that tazarotene versus placebo improves chronic plaque psoriasis in the short term. One RCT has found that tazarotene plus topical steroids versus calcipotriol improves short term outcomes.

Ultraviolet B

There is a consensus that ultraviolet B is effective, but one systematic review has found insufficient evidence on the effects of ultraviolet B versus other treatments, or on the effects of narrow band versus broad band ultraviolet B for either clearance or maintenance treatment.

TRADE OFF BETWEEN BENEFITS AND HARMS

Alefacept

One RCT found limited evidence that alefacept versus placebo may improve psoriasis. Adverse effects included dizziness, accidents, chills, and cough.

Ciclosporin

One systematic review has found optimal clearance rates with a ciclosporin dose of 5.0 mg/kg a day. Any advantage of doses greater than 5.0 mg/kg a day may be offset by an increase in dose related side effects, particularly increased renal toxicity.

Etanercept

One small RCT found limited evidence that etanercept versus placebo may improve psoriasis. Reported adverse effects include skin reactions, urticarial manifestations, and upper respiratory tract infections.

Infliximab

One RCT found limited evidence that infliximab versus placebo may improve psoriasis. Reported adverse effects include lupus-like syndrome and severe infections.

Oral retinoids (etretinate, acitretin, liarazole)

RCTs found limited evidence that oral retinoids alone may achieve complete clearance in people with plaque psoriasis. The number of people with complete clearance is increased by combination with psoralen ultraviolet A or ultraviolet B. We found insufficient evidence on the effects of liarozole. We found little reliable evidence on the effects of oral retinoids as maintenance treatment. Adverse effects lead to discontinuation of treatment in 10–20% of people. Teratogenicity renders oral retinoids less acceptable.

Topical steroids

RCTs have found that topical steroids improve psoriasis in the short term. Topical steroids may cause striae and atrophy, which increase with clinical potency and use of occlusive dressings. Continuous use may lead to adrenocortical suppression, and case reports suggest that severe flares of the disease may occur on withdrawal.

Tacrolimus

One RCT found limited evidence that tacrolimus versus placebo may improve psoriasis. Adverse effects are reported to be similar to those of ciclosporin.

UNKNOWN EFFECTIVENESS

Acupuncture; antistreptococcal treatments; balneotherapy; fish oil; heliotherapy; lifestyle changes; oral vitamin D; stress reduction; sunbeds

We found insufficient evidence on the effects of these interventions.

Emollients and keratolytics

We found no clear evidence on the effects of emollients and keratolytics.

Fumaric acid derivatives

One systematic review found limited evidence that oral fumaric acid esters provided short term improvement or complete clearing of psoriasis. Monoethylfumarate on its own has not been found to have a beneficial effect. The incidence of acute adverse effects (flushing and gastrointestinal symptoms) is high; 30–40% of people discontinue treatment because of adverse effects, non-compliance, or both. We found no evidence on the effects of fumaric acid derivatives as maintenance treatment.

Goeckerman treatment

We found no good evidence on the effects of the Goeckerman treatment**G**.

Methotrexate

Limited evidence from one small RCT in people with psoriatic arthritis suggests that methotrexate may improve skin lesions in psoriasis. Non-randomised evidence suggests that clearance can be maintained as long as treatment is continued. About half of people relapse within 6 months of stopping treatment. Methotrexate can induce acute myelosuppression. Long term methotrexate carries the risk of hepatic fibrosis and cirrhosis, which is related to the dose regimen employed.

Tars

Small RCTs have found conflicting results on the effects of tars in combination with ultraviolet B exposure.

Chronic plaque psoriasis

DEFINITION Chronic plaque psoriasis is a chronic inflammatory skin disease that is characterised by well demarcated erythematous scaly patches on the extensor surfaces of the body and scalp. The lesions may itch, sting, and occasionally bleed. Dystrophic nail changes are found in more than a third of people with chronic plaque psoriasis, and psoriatic arthropathy occurs in 1–3%. The condition waxes and wanes, with wide variations in course and severity among individuals. Other varieties of psoriasis include guttate, inverse, pustular, and erythrodermic psoriasis. This review deals with treatments for chronic plaque psoriasis.

INCIDENCE/ PREVALENCE Psoriasis affects 1–2% of the general population. It is believed to be less frequent in people from Africa and Asia, but we found no reliable epidemiological data.[1]

AETIOLOGY/ RISK FACTORS About a third of people with psoriasis have a family history of psoriasis, but physical trauma, acute infection, and some medications (e.g. lithium salts and β blockers) are believed to trigger the condition. A few observational studies have linked the onset or relapse of psoriasis with stressful life events and personal habits, including cigarette smoking and, less consistently, alcohol consumption. Others have found an association of psoriasis with body mass index**G** and an inverse association with intake of fruit and vegetables.

PROGNOSIS We found no long term prognostic studies. With the exceptions of erythrodermic and acute generalised pustular psoriasis (severe conditions that affect less than 1% of people with psoriasis and that require intensive hospital care), psoriasis is not known to affect mortality. Psoriasis may substantially affect quality of life.[2] At present there is no cure for psoriasis.

Please refer to CD-ROM for full text and references.

Head lice

Search date June 2002

Ian Burgess

What are the effects of treatments?

LIKELY TO BE BENEFICIAL

Insecticide based pharmaceutical products

One systematic review found that permethrin or malathion versus placebo significantly reduced the number of people with head lice at 1 week and at 2. Limited evidence from another systematic review suggests that permethrin versus lindane significantly reduces the number of people with head lice.

UNKNOWN EFFECTIVENESS

Mechanical removal of lice or viable eggs by combing

We found two RCTs comparing combing versus an insecticide treatment. The larger RCT found that wet combing with conditioner was significantly less effective than malathion in eradicating head lice 7 days after treatment. A smaller RCT found limited evidence that wet combing with conditioner was marginally more effective than phenothrin lotion plus combing in eradicating head lice after 14 days.

Essential oils and other chemicals used as repellents; herbal treatments

We found insufficient evidence on the effects of these interventions.

DEFINITION Head lice are obligate ectoparasites of socially active humans. They infest the scalp and attach their eggs to the hair shafts. Itching, resulting from multiple bites, is not diagnostic but may increase the index of suspicion. Infestation can be diagnosed only by finding living lice. Eggs glued to hairs, whether hatched (nits) or unhatched, are not proof of active infection, because eggs may retain a viable appearance for weeks after death.

INCIDENCE/ PREVALENCE We found no studies on incidence and no recent published prevalence results from any developed country. Anecdotal reports suggest that prevalence has increased in the past few years in most communities in the UK and USA.

AETIOLOGY/ RISK FACTORS Observational studies indicate that infections occur most frequently in school children, although there is no proof of a link with school attendance.[1,2] We found no evidence that lice prefer clean hair to dirty hair.

PROGNOSIS The infection is almost harmless. Sensitisation reactions to louse saliva and faeces may result in localised irritation and erythema. Secondary infection of scratches may occur. Lice have been identified as primary mechanical vectors of scalp pyoderma caused by streptococci and staphylococci usually found on the skin.[3]

Please refer to CD-ROM for full text and references.

Herpes labialis

Search date April 2002

Clinical Evidence freelance writers

What are the effects of preventive interventions?

LIKELY TO BE BENEFICIAL

Oral aciclovir

Limited evidence from RCTs suggests that prophylactic oral aciclovir versus placebo may reduce the frequency and severity of attacks, but the optimal timing and duration of treatment is uncertain.

Sunscreen

Two small crossover RCTs found that ultraviolet sunscreen versus placebo significantly reduced herpes recurrence.

UNKNOWN EFFECTIVENESS

Topical antiviral agents

We found no RCTs on the effects of topical antiviral agents used as prophylaxis.

What are the effects of treatments?

LIKELY TO BE BENEFICIAL

Oral aciclovir for first attack

One small RCT in children found that oral aciclovir verses placebo marginally but significantly reduced the mean duration of pain. One small RCT in children found that oral aciclovir versus placebo significantly reduced the median time to healing.

Oral aciclovir for recurrent attack

Two RCTs have found that oral aciclovir versus placebo (if taken early in the attack) marginally but significantly reduces the duration of symptoms and pain.

UNKNOWN EFFECTIVENESS

Topical anaesthetic agents

One small RCT found limited evidence that topical tetracaine versus placebo significantly reduced the mean time to scab loss.

Topical antiviral agents for first attack

We found no RCTs on the effects of topical antiviral agents in the first attack.

Topical antiviral agents for recurrent attacks

RCTs found conflicting evidence on the effects of topical antiviral agents.

Zinc oxide cream

One small RCT found limited evidence that zinc oxide cream versus placebo significantly reduced the time to resolution of skin lesions.

DEFINITION Herpes labialis is a mild self limiting infection with herpes simplex virus type 1. It causes pain and blistering on the lips and perioral area (cold sores); fever and constitutional symptoms are rare. Most people have no warning of an attack, but some experience a recognisable prodrome. ▶

Clin Evid Concise 2003;9:348–349.

Herpes labialis

INCIDENCE/ PREVALENCE Herpes labialis accounts for about 1% of primary care consultations in the UK each year; 20–40% of people have experienced cold sores at some time.[1]

AETIOLOGY/ RISK FACTORS Herpes labialis is caused by herpes simplex virus type-1. After the primary infection, which usually occurs in childhood, the virus is thought to remain latent in the trigeminal ganglion.[2] A variety of factors, including exposure to bright sunlight, fatigue, or psychological stress, can precipitate a recurrence.

PROGNOSIS In most people, herpes labialis is a mild, self limiting illness. Recurrences are usually shorter and less severe than the initial attack. Healing is usually complete in 7–10 days without scarring.[3] Rates of reactivation are unknown. Herpes labialis can cause serious illness in immunocompromised patients.

Please refer to CD-ROM for full text and references.

Malignant melanoma (non-metastatic)

Search date June 2002

David Crosby, Thomas Crosby, and Malcolm Mason

What are the effects of preventive interventions and treatments?

LIKELY TO BE BENEFICIAL

High dose adjuvant alfa interferon

One RCT has found that high dose alfa interferon versus no adjuvant treatment significantly extends the time to relapse at median follow up of 6.9 years, and may improve overall survival, but two RCTs found no significant difference in relapse rates or overall survival with high dose interferon versus no adjuvant treatment. Toxicity (myelosuppression, hepatotoxicity, and neurotoxicity) and withdrawal rates are high.

UNKNOWN EFFECTIVENESS

Low dose adjuvant alfa interferon

RCTs found inconsistent evidence on the effects of low dose alfa interferon versus no adjuvant treatment or relapse free and overall survival. Toxicity occurred in 10% of people.

Other adjuvant treatments (active specific immunotherapy, chemotherapy, coumarin, hormones, non-specific immunotherapy, retinoids)

RCTs found no evidence of improved survival with non-specific immunotherapy (e.g. bacille Calmette-Guérin or *Corynebacterium parvum*) or active specific immunotherapy, but may have been too small to exclude a clinically important benefit. RCTs found no difference in survival with single agent cytotoxic agents (especially dacarbazine), chemoimmunotherapy, and multi-agent cytotoxic treatments versus placebo, but may have been too small to exclude a clinically important benefit. Surveillance, hormones, coumarin, and retinoids have not yet been evaluated adequately in RCTs.

Sunscreens in prevention

We found no RCTs about the preventive effects of sunscreens. One systematic review of case control studies found inconclusive evidence about the effects of sunscreen for preventing malignant melanoma. However, the appropriate use of sunscreen seems a sensible measure to avoid excessive exposure to sunlight.

UNLIKELY TO BE BENEFICIAL

Prophylactic lymph node dissection

One systematic review found no significant difference in survival at 5 years with elective lymph node dissection versus delayed or no lymph node dissection in people with melanoma without clinically detectable lymph node metastases.

Wide primary excision (no better than narrower excision)

RCTs found no significant difference in local recurrence rates or overall survival with more radical local surgery (4–5 cm excision margins) versus less radical surgery (1–2 cm excision margins). One RCT found that wide versus narrow excision increased the need for skin grafting and the length of hospital stay.

DEFINITION Cutaneous malignant melanoma is a tumour derived from melanocytes in the basal layer of the epidermis. After undergoing malignant transformation, it becomes invasive by penetrating into and beyond the dermis.

Clin Evid Concise 2003;9:350–351.

Malignant melanoma (non-metastatic)

INCIDENCE/ PREVALENCE Incidence in developed countries has increased by 50% in the past 20 years. Incidence varies in different populations**T** and is about 10-fold higher in white than in non-white populations. Despite the rise in incidence, death rates have flattened and even fallen in some populations (e.g. in women and young men in Australia).[1,2] During the same period there has been a sixfold increase in the incidence of melanoma *in situ*, suggesting earlier detection.

AETIOLOGY/ RISK FACTORS The number of common, atypical, and dysplastic naevi on a person's body correlates closely with the risk of developing malignant melanoma. A genetic predisposition probably accounts for 5–10% of all cases. Although the risk of developing malignant melanoma is higher in fair skinned populations living close to the equator, the relation between sun exposure, sunscreen use, and skin type is not clear cut. Exposure to excessive sunlight and severe sunburn in childhood are associated with an increased risk of developing malignant melanoma in adult life. However, people do not necessarily develop tumours at sites of maximum exposure to the sun.

PROGNOSIS The prognosis of early malignant melanoma (stages I–III)**T** relates to the depth of invasion of the primary lesion, the presence of ulceration, and involvement of the regional lymph nodes, with the prognosis worsening with the number of nodes involved.[3] A person with a thin lesion (Breslow thickness**G** < 0.75 mm) and without lymph node involvement has a 3% risk of developing metastases and a 95% chance of surviving 5 years.[4] If regional lymph nodes are macroscopically involved there is a 20–50% chance of surviving 5 years. Most studies have shown a better prognosis in women and in people with lesions on the extremities compared with those with lesions on the trunk.

Please refer to CD-ROM for full text and references.

Scabies

Search date May 2002

Godfrey Walker and Paul Johnstone

What are the effects of treatments?

BENEFICIAL

Permethrin

One systematic review has found that permethrin versus crotamiton significantly increases clinical and parasitic cure after 28 days. The systematic review found conflicting results with permethrin versus lindane. One subsequent RCT found limited evidence that permethrin versus ivermectin significantly decreased failed clinical cure at 14 days.

LIKELY TO BE BENEFICIAL

Crotamiton

One systematic review has found a significantly lower proportion of people with clinical and parasitic cure with crotamiton versus permethrin after 28 days. One systematic review identified one RCT that found no significant difference with crotamiton versus lindane in clinical cure rates at 28 days.

Oral ivermectin

One systematic review identified one RCT that found that ivermectin versus placebo significantly increased clinical cure rates after 7 days. Another small RCT identified by the review found no significant difference with ivermectin versus benzyl benzoate in clinical cure rates at 30 days. One subsequent RCT found that ivermectin versus benzyl benzoate significantly increased clinical cure rates at 30 days. One systematic review identified one small RCT that found no significant difference with ivermectin versus lindane in cure rates at 15 days. One subsequent RCT found no significant difference with ivermectin versus lindane in failed clinical cure rates at 2 weeks, but found that ivermectin versus lindane significantly decreased failed clinical cure rates at 4 weeks. One RCT found limited evidence of a significantly higher proportion of people with failed clinical cure with ivermectin versus permethrin at 14 days. Experience of the use of oral ivermectin in onchocerciasis suggests that it is safe in younger adults, but no such experience exists for children, and there have been reports of increased risk of death in elderly people.

TRADE OFF BETWEEN BENEFITS AND HARMS

Lindane

One systematic review identified one RCT that found no significant difference with lindane versus crotamiton in clinical cure rates at 28 days. The systematic review found conflicting results with lindane versus permethrin after 28 days. Another small RCT identified by the review found no significant difference with lindane versus ivermectin in cure rates at 15 days. One subsequent RCT found no significant difference with lindane versus ivermectin in failed clinical cure rates at 2 weeks, but found a significantly higher proportion of people with failed clinical cure with lindane versus ivermectin at 4 weeks. We found reports of rare side effects such as convulsions and other severe adverse effects.

UNKNOWN EFFECTIVENESS

Benzyl benzoate

One systematic review identified one small RCT that found no significant difference with benzyl benzoate versus ivermectin in clinical cure rates at 30 days. One ▶

subsequent RCT found a significantly lower proportion of people with clinical cure with benzyl benzoate versus ivermectin at 30 days. One systematic review identified one RCT that found no significant difference with benzyl benzoate versus sulphur ointment in clinical cure at 8 or 14 days.

Malathion

One systematic review found no RCTs on the effects of malathion. Case series have reported cure rates in scabies of over 80%.

Sulphur compounds

One systematic review identified one RCT that found no significant difference with sulphur ointment versus benzyl benzoate in clinical cure at 8 or 14 days.

DEFINITION Scabies is an infestation of the skin by the mite *Sarcoptes scabiei*.[1] Typical sites of infestation are skin folds and flexor surfaces. In adults, the most common sites are between the fingers and on the wrists, although infection may manifest in elderly people as a diffuse truncal eruption. In infants and children, the face, scalp, palms, and soles are also often affected.

INCIDENCE/ PREVALENCE Scabies is a common public health problem with an estimated prevalence of 300 million cases worldwide, mostly affecting people in developing countries where prevalence can exceed 50%.[2] In industrialised countries, it is most common in institutionalised communities. Case studies suggest that epidemic cycles occur every 7–15 years and that these partly reflect the population's immune status.

AETIOLOGY/ RISK FACTORS Scabies is particularly common where there is social disruption, overcrowding with close body contact, and limited access to water.[3] Young children, immobilised elderly people, people with HIV/AIDS, and other medically and immunologically compromised people are predisposed to infestation and have particularly high mite counts.[4]

PROGNOSIS Scabies is not life threatening, but the severe, persistent itch and secondary infections may be debilitating. Occasionally, crusted scabies develops. This form of the disease is resistant to routine treatment and can be a source of continued reinfestation and spread to others.

Please refer to CD-ROM for full text and references.

Squamous cell carcinoma of the skin (non-metastatic)

Search date September 2002

Adèle Green and Robin Marks

What are the effects of preventive interventions?

LIKELY TO BE BENEFICIAL

Sunscreen in prevention (daily *v* discretionary use)

One RCT in adults in a subtropical Australian community found that daily versus discretionary use of sunscreen to the head, neck, arms, and hands significantly reduced the incidence of squamous cell carcinoma after 4.5 years.

Sunscreens to prevent development of new solar keratoses (*v* placebo)

One RCT in people with previous solar keratoses aged over 40 years and living in Victoria, Australia found that daily sunscreen versus placebo sunscreen significantly reduced the incidence of new solar keratoses after 7 months' use.

What are the effects of treatments?

UNKNOWN EFFECTIVENESS

Micrographically controlled surgery (unknown benefit compared with standard surgical excision)

We found no RCTs comparing the effects of micrographically controlled surgery**G** versus standard primary surgical excision on local recurrence rates.

Primary excision margin (unknown optimal margin of excision)

We found no RCTs relating size of primary excision margin to local recurrence rate.

Radiotherapy after surgery (unknown benefit compared with surgery alone)

We found no RCTs comparing the effects of radiotherapy after surgery versus surgery alone on local recurrence rates.

DEFINITION Cutaneous squamous cell carcinoma is a malignant tumour of keratinocytes arising in the epidermis, showing histological evidence of dermal invasion.

INCIDENCE/ PREVALENCE Incidence rates are often derived from surveys because few cancer registries routinely collect notifications of squamous cell carcinoma of the skin. Incidence rates on exposed skin vary markedly around the world according to skin colour and latitude, and range from negligible rates in black populations and white populations living at high latitudes to rates of about 1000/100 000 in white residents of tropical Australia.[1]

AETIOLOGY/ RISK FACTORS People with fair skin colour who sunburn easily without tanning, people with xeroderma pigmentosum**G**,[2–4] and those who are immunosuppressed[5] are susceptible to squamous cell carcinoma. The strongest environmental risk factor for squamous cell carcinoma is chronic sun exposure. Cohort and case control studies have found that clinical signs of chronic skin damage, especially solar keratoses, are also determinants of cutaneous squamous cell carcinoma.[3,4] For example, the risk of squamous cell carcinoma in people with the propensity to severe sunburn or with a history of multiple sunburns is three times greater than in people with no such propensity. In people with multiple solar keratoses (> 15), the risk of squamous cell carcinoma is 10–15 times greater than in people with no solar keratoses.[3,4]

Clin Evid Concise 2003;9:354–355.

Squamous cell carcinoma of the skin (non-metastatic)

PROGNOSIS Prognosis is related to the location and size of tumour, histological pattern, depth of invasion, perineural involvement, and immunosuppression.[6,7] A world-wide review of 95 case series, each comprising at least 20 people, found the overall metastasis rate for squamous cell carcinoma on the ear to be 11% and on the lip 14%, compared with an average for all sites of 5%.[7] A review of 71 case series found that lesions less than 2 cm in diameter compared with lesions greater than 2 cm have less than half the local recurrence rate (7% *v* 15%), and less than a third of the rate of metastasis (9% *v* 30%).[7]

Please refer to CD-ROM for full text and references.

Warts

Search date May 2002

Michael Bigby, Sam Gibbs, Ian Harvey, and Jane Sterling

What are the effects of treatments?

LIKELY TO BE BENEFICIAL

Topical treatments containing salicylic acid

One systematic review has found that simple topical treatments containing salicylic acid versus placebo significantly increase the number of people with complete wart clearance, successful treatment, or loss of one or more warts after 6–12 weeks.

Cryotherapy

One systematic review found limited evidence from two small RCTs that cryotherapy is no more effective than placebo in increasing the proportion of people with wart clearance after 2–4 months. But the review also identified two larger RCTs that found cryotherapy was as effective as salicylic acid in wart clearance at 3–6 months.

Contact immunotherapy (dinitrochlorobenzene)

One systematic review has found that contact immunotherapy**G** with dinitrochlorobenzene versus placebo significantly increases the number of people with wart clearance.

UNKNOWN EFFECTIVENESS

Carbon dioxide laser

One systematic review identified no RCTs about the effects of carbon dioxide laser.

Cimetidine

Three small RCTs found insufficient evidence about the effects of cimetidine versus placebo in the number of people with wart clearance after 12 weeks, and one RCT found insufficient evidence about the effects of cimetidine versus local treatments.

Distant healing

One RCT found insufficient evidence about the effects of distant healing on wart clearance.

Hypnotic suggestion

We found no RCTs on the effects of hypnotic suggestion in clearance of warts.

Inosine pranobex

One RCT found insufficient evidence about the effects of inosine pranobex on wart clearance.

Intralesional bleomycin

Five RCTs found conflicting evidence about the effects of intralesional bleomycin. Two RCTs found that intralesional bleomycin versus placebo significantly increased the number of warts cured after 6 weeks. One RCT found no significant difference with bleomycin versus placebo in the number of people with wart clearance after 30 days, and another RCT found that bleomycin cured fewer warts than placebo after 3 months. One RCT found no significant difference between different concentrations of bleomycin in the number of warts cured after 3 months.

Clin Evid Concise 2003;9:356–358.

Levamisole

Two RCTs and one controlled clinical trial found insufficient evidence about the effects of levamisole versus placebo on the clearance of warts. One RCT found that levamisole plus cimetidine versus cimetidine alone significantly increased the number of people with wart clearance.

Photodynamic treatment

RCTs found insufficient evidence about the effects of photodynamic treatment**G** on wart clearance.

Pulsed dye laser

One RCT found insufficient evidence about the effects of pulsed dye laser in number of warts cured.

Surgical procedures

One systematic review identified no RCTs about the effects of surgical procedures on wart clearance.

Systemic interferon α

We found no RCTs of sufficient quality about systemic interferon α.

UNLIKELY TO BE BENEFICIAL

Homeopathy

Two RCTs found no significant difference with homeopathy versus placebo in the number of people with wart clearance after 18 weeks.

DEFINITION Non-genital warts are an extremely common, benign, and usually self limiting skin disease. Infection of epidermal cells with the human papillomavirus results in cell proliferation and a thickened, warty papule on the skin. Any area of skin can be infected but the commonest sites involved are the hands and feet. Genital warts are not covered in this review (see topic p 330).

INCIDENCE/ PREVALENCE There are few reliable, population based data on the incidence and prevalence of common warts. Prevalence probably varies widely between different age groups, populations, and periods of time. Two large population based studies found prevalence rates of 0.84% in the USA[1] and 12.9% in Russia.[2] Prevalence rates are highest in children and young adults, and two studies in school populations have shown prevalence rates of 12% in 4–6 year olds in the UK[3] and 24% in 16–18 year olds in Australia.[4]

AETIOLOGY/ RISK FACTORS Warts are caused by human papillomavirus, of which there are over 70 different types. They are most common at sites of trauma such as the hands and feet, and probably result from inoculation of virus into minimally damaged areas of epithelium. Warts on the feet can be acquired from common bare foot areas. One observational study (146 adolescents) found that the prevalence of warts on the feet was 27% in those that used a communal shower room versus 1.3% in those that used the locker room.[5] Hand warts are also an occupational risk for butchers and meat handlers. One cross-sectional survey (1086 people) found that the prevalence of hand warts was 33% in abattoir workers, 34% in retail butchers, 20% in engineering fitters, and 15% in office workers.[6] Immunosuppression is another important risk factor. One observational study in immunosuppressed renal transplant recipients found that, at 5 years or longer after transplantation, 90% had warts.[7]

Warts

PROGNOSIS Non-genital warts in immunocompetent people are harmless and usually resolve spontaneously as a result of natural immunity within months or years. The rate of resolution is highly variable and probably depends on a number of factors including host immunity, age, human papillomavirus type, and site of infection. One cohort study (1000 institutionalised children) found that two thirds of warts resolved without treatment within a 2 year period.[8] One systematic review (search date 2000, 17 RCTs) comparing local treatments versus placebo found that about 30% of people taking placebo (range 0–73%) had no warts after about 10 weeks (range 4–24 wks).[9]

Please refer to CD-ROM for full text and references.

Wrinkles

Search date August 2002

Miny Samuel, Rebecca Brooke, and Christopher Griffiths

What are the effects of preventive interventions?

UNKNOWN EFFECTIVENESS

Sunscreens; vitamins (vitamin C and vitamin E)

We found no RCTs on the effects of these interventions in preventing wrinkles.

What are the effects of treatments?

BENEFICIAL

Tretinoin (for fine wrinkles after 6 months)

RCTs in people with mild to moderate photodamage have found that topical tretinoin versus vehicle cream applied for up to 48 weeks significantly improved fine wrinkles but found that the effect of tretinoin on coarse wrinkles differed between studies. Three RCTs in people with moderate to severe photodamageⒼ have found that topical tretinoin (0.01%–0.02%) versus vehicle cream applied for 6 months significantly improved fine and coarse wrinkles on the face. Common short term adverse effects with tretinoin included itching, burning, and erythema. Skin peeling was the most common persistent adverse effect, which is most frequent and severe at 12–16 weeks.

LIKELY TO BE BENEFICIAL

Tazarotene *New*

One RCT in people with moderate photodamage found that tazarotene cream improved fine wrinkling compared with placebo at 24 weeks. One RCT found no significant difference for tazarotene cream versus tretinoin in fine wrinkling at 24 weeks.

TRADE OFF BETWEEN BENEFITS AND HARMS

Isotretinoin

Two RCTs in people with mild to severe photodamage found that isotretinoin versus vehicle cream significantly improved fine and coarse wrinkles after 36 weeks. Severe facial irritation occurred in 5–10% of people using isotretinoin.

UNKNOWN EFFECTIVENESS

Carbon dioxide (CO_2) laser

We found no RCTs comparing CO_2 laser versus placebo or no treatment. Three small RCTs in women with perioral wrinkles found no significant difference with CO_2 laser versus dermabrasion in improvement in wrinkles at 4–6 months. One small RCT found limited evidence that CO_2 laser improved wrinkle score significantly less than chemical peel at 6 months. Two small RCTs found that CO_2 laser improved wrinkles more than erbium:YAG laserⒼ at 2 months and 6 months. Another RCT found no significant difference in wrinkle improvement with CO_2 laser versus erbium:YAG laser, but may have been too small to exclude a clinically important difference. One small RCT found no significant difference with CO_2 laser plus erbium: YAG laser versus CO_2 laser alone in improvement in upper lip wrinkles at 4 months.

Clin Evid Concise 2003;9:359–361.

Dermabrasion

We found no RCTs of dermabrasion versus placebo or no treatment. Three small RCTs in women with perioral wrinkles found no significant difference with dermabrasion versus CO_2 laser in improvement in wrinkles at 4–6 months. Adverse effects were commonly reported. Erythema was reported in all three RCTs, two of which found that erythema was significantly more common with laser versus dermabrasion.

Facelift

We found no RCTs on the effects of facelifts.

Oral natural cartilage polysaccharides

One RCT found limited evidence between an oral commercial preparation of cartilage polysaccharide versus placebo for reducing wrinkles at 3 months. Another RCT found that a different oral commercial preparation of cartilage polysaccharide versus placebo significantly reduced the number of women with moderate or severe wrinkles at 90 days. We found limited evidence that some commercial preparations may be more effective than others.

Retinyl esters

We found no systematic review or RCTs of retinyl esters that evaluated clinical outcomes.

Topical antioxidants (ascorbic acid)

One poor quality RCT found limited evidence that an ascorbic acid formulation versus a vehicle cream applied daily to the face for 3 months significantly improved fine and coarse wrinkles. Stinging and erythema were common but were not analysed by treatment.

Topical natural cartilage polysaccharides

One small RCT in people with moderate to severe facial wrinkles found limited evidence that a topical commercial preparation of natural cartilage polysaccharide versus placebo significantly reduced the number of fine and coarse wrinkles at 120 days.

DEFINITION Wrinkles, also known as rhytides, are visible creases or folds in the skin. Wrinkles less than 1 mm in width and depth are defined as fine wrinkles and those greater than 1 mm are coarse wrinkles. Most RCTs have studied wrinkles on the face, forearms, and hands.

INCIDENCE/ PREVALENCE We found no information on the incidence of wrinkles alone, only on the incidence of skin photodamage, which includes a spectrum of features such as wrinkles, hyperpigmentation, tactile roughness, and telangiectasia. The incidence of ultraviolet light associated skin disorders increases with age and develops over several decades. One Australian study (1539 people aged 20–55 years living in Queensland) found moderate to severe photoaging in 72% of men and 47% of women under 30 years of age.[1] The severity of photoaging was significantly greater with increasing age, and was independently associated with solar keratoses ($P < 0.01$) and skin cancer ($P < 0.05$). Wrinkling was more common in people with white skin, especially skin phototypes I and II. One study reported that the incidence of photodamage in European and North American populations with Fitzpatrick skin types I, II, and III Ⓖ is about 80–90%.[2] We found few reports of photodamage in black skin (phototypes V and VI).

AETIOLOGY/ RISK FACTORS Wrinkles may be caused by intrinsic factors (e.g. aging, hormonal status, and intercurrent diseases) and by extrinsic factors (e.g. exposure to ultraviolet radiation and cigarette smoke). These factors contribute to epidermal thinning, loss of elasticity, skin fragility, and creases and lines in the skin. The severity of photodamage varies with skin type, which includes skin colour and the capacity to tan.[3] One review of five observational studies found that facial wrinkles in men and women were more common in smokers than in non-smokers.[4] It also found that the risk of moderate to severe wrinkles in lifelong smokers was more than twice that in current smokers (RR 2.57, 95% CI 1.83 to 3.06). Oestrogen deficiency may contribute to wrinkles in postmenopausal women.[5]

PROGNOSIS Although wrinkles cannot be considered a medical illness requiring intervention, concerns about aging that affect quality of life are becoming increasingly common. Such concerns are likely to be influenced by geographical differences, culture, and personal values. In some cases, concerns about physical appearance can lead to difficulties with interpersonal interactions, occupational functioning, and self esteem.[6] In societies in which the aging population is growing and a high value is placed on the maintenance of a youthful appearance, there is a growing preference for interventions that ameliorate the visible signs of aging.

Please refer to CD-ROM for full text and references.

Insomnia

Search date November 2002

Clinical Evidence freelance writers

What are the effects of non-drug treatments in older people? New

LIKELY TO BE BENEFICIAL

Exercise programmes

One systematic review identified one small RCT. It found that sleep quality improved following a 16 week programme of regular, moderate intensity exercise four times weekly versus no treatment.

UNKNOWN EFFECTIVENESS

Cognitive behavioural therapy

One systematic review identified one small RCT, which found that individual or group cognitive behavioural therapy**G** improved sleep quality more than no treatment at 3 months, although mean sleep quality scores were consistent with continuing insomnia both with and without treatment.

Timed exposure to bright light

One systematic review found no RCTs about the effects of timed bright light exposure versus other treatments or no treatment.

DEFINITION Insomnia is defined by the US National Institutes of Health as experience of poor quality sleep, with difficulty in initiating or maintaining sleep, waking too early in the morning, or failing to feel refreshed. Chronic insomnia is defined as insomnia occurring for at least three nights per week for 1 month or more.[1] Primary insomnia is defined as chronic insomnia without specific underlying medical or psychiatric disorders such as sleep apnoea, depression, or dementia.

INCIDENCE/ PREVALENCE Across all adult age groups, up to 40% of people have insomnia.[2] However, prevalence increases with age, with estimates ranging from 31–38% in people aged 18–64 years to 45% in people aged 65–79 years.[3]

AETIOLOGY/ RISK FACTORS The aetiology of insomnia is uncertain. The risk of primary insomnia increases with age and may be related to age associated changes in circadian rhythms. Psychological factors and lifestyle changes may exacerbate perceived effects of age associated changes in sleep patterns, leading to reduced satisfaction with sleep.[4] Other risk factors in all age groups include hyperarousal, chronic stress, and daytime napping.[1,5]

PROGNOSIS We found few reliable data on long term morbidity and mortality in people with primary insomnia. Primary insomnia is a chronic and relapsing condition.[6] Likely consequences include reduced quality of life and increased risk of accidents due to daytime sleepiness. People with primary insomnia may be at greater risk of dependence on hypnotic medication, depression, dementia, and falls, and may be more likely to require residential care.[6,7]

Please refer to CD-ROM for full text and references.

Sleep apnoea

Search date November 2002

Michael Hensley

What are the effects of treatments?

BENEFICIAL

Nasal continuous positive airway pressure in moderate to severe obstructive sleep apnoea-hypopnoea syndrome (OSAHS)

Systematic reviews and subsequent RCTs have found that nasal continuous positive airway pressure**G**, versus placebo, oral appliances**G**, or no treatment reduces daytime sleepiness, improves vigilance and cognitive functioning, and reduces depression after 3–9 months in people with moderate to severe OSAHS.

LIKELY TO BE BENEFICIAL

Nasal continuous positive airway pressure in mild OSAHS

One systematic review of four RCTs in people with mild OSAHS found no significant difference with nasal continuous positive airway pressure versus conservative treatment or placebo tablets in daytime sleepiness, but found significant improvement in some measures of cognitive performance in people with mild OSAHS at about 4 weeks. One subsequent RCT in people with mild OSAHS found no significant difference with nasal continuous positive airway pressure plus conservative treatment versus conservative treatment alone in daytime sleepiness or functional or cognitive outcomes, but found significant improvement in sleep apnoea-hypopnoea related symptoms at 3 and 6 months.

Oral appliance in mild OSAHS

One RCT found that oral appliances that produce mandibular advancement significantly reduced apnoea**G** and hypopnoea**G**, but had no significant effect on daytime sleepiness or quality of life compared with uvulopalatopharyngoplasty in people with mild OSAHS.

Oral appliance in moderate to severe OSAHS

RCTs have found that oral appliances that produce anterior advancement of the mandible versus no treatment or versus control oral appliances significantly reduce daytime sleepiness and sleep disordered breathing**G** at 1–2 weeks.

UNKNOWN EFFECTIVENESS

Weight loss in mild OSAHS

One systematic review found no RCTs on the effects of weight loss in people with mild OSAHS.

Weight loss in moderate to severe OSAHS

One systematic review found no RCTs on the effects of weight loss in people with moderate to severe OSAHS.

DEFINITION OSAHS is abnormal breathing during sleep that causes recurrent arousals, sleep fragmentation, and nocturnal hypoxaemia. It is associated with daytime sleepiness, impaired vigilance and cognitive functioning, and reduced quality of life.[1,2] The diagnosis is made when a person with daytime symptoms has significant sleep disordered breathing revealed by polysomnography (study of sleep state, breathing, and oxygenation) or by more limited studies. Criteria for the diagnosis of significant sleep disordered breathing have not been rigorously assessed, but have been set by consensus and convention.[3,4] The criteria are based on the finding of sleep disordered breathing, reported as the number of abnormal breathing events in 1 hour of sleep (when full ▶

polysomnography is undertaken) or in 1 hour in bed for home based monitoring systems that do not include electroencephalography recordings. There are differences in the measurement techniques and criteria for diagnosis: hypopnoea may or may not include associated hypoxaemia or arousal, and the criteria vary for a significant obstructive event that is not apnoea or hypopnoea. In OSAHS, apnoeas and hypopnoeas are associated with absent or reduced airflow despite normal or increased inspiratory effort, but may also involve reduced inspiratory effort. However, many healthy people, especially the elderly, can have frequent apnoeas and hypopnoeas. Diagnostic criteria have variable sensitivity and specificity. For example, an apnoea/hypopnoea index(G) of 5–20 episodes per hour is often used to define borderline to mild OSAHS, 20–35 to define moderate OSAHS, and more than 35 to define severe OSAHS.[5] However, people with upper airway resistance syndrome(G) have an index below five episodes an hour[6] and many healthy elderly people have an index greater than 5 episodes an hour.[7] In an effort to obtain an international consensus, new criteria have been proposed but have not been widely adopted.[8] The most pragmatic test for clinically significant OSAHS is to show clinical improvement in daytime symptoms after treatment for sleep disordered breathing. In this topic, the criteria for OSAHS include apnoeas and hypopnoeas caused by upper airway obstruction. Central sleep apnoea and sleep associated hypoventilation syndromes are not covered here.

INCIDENCE/ PREVALENCE The Wisconsin Sleep Cohort Study of over 1000 people (mean age 47 years) in North America found a prevalence of apnoea/hypopnoea index greater than five episodes an hour in 24% of men and 9% of women, and of OSAHS with an index greater than five plus excessive sleepiness in 4% of men and 2% of women.[9] There are international differences in the occurrence of OSAHS, for which obesity is considered to be an important determinant.[10] Ethnic differences in prevalence have also been found after adjustment for other risk factors.[7,10] Little is known about the burden of illness in developing countries.

AETIOLOGY/ RISK FACTORS The site of the upper airway obstruction in the OSAHS is around the level of the tongue, soft palate, or epiglottis. Disorders that predispose to either narrowing of the upper airway or reduction in its stability (e.g. obesity, certain craniofacial abnormalities, vocal cord abnormalities, and enlarged tonsils) have been associated with an increased risk of OSAHS. It has been estimated that a 1 kg/m^2 increase in body mass index (3.2 kg for a person 1.8 m tall) leads to a 30% increase (95% CI 13% to 50%) in the relative risk of developing abnormal sleep disordered breathing (apnoea/hypopnoea index $\geq$ 5/h) over a period of 4 years.[10] Other strong associations include increasing age and sex (male to female ratio is 2 : 1). Weaker associations include menopause, family history, smoking, and night time nasal congestion.[10]

PROGNOSIS The long term prognosis of people with untreated severe OSAHS is poor with respect to quality of life, likelihood of motor vehicle accidents, hypertension, and possibly cardiovascular disease and premature mortality.[11] Unfortunately the prognosis of both treated and untreated OSAHS is unclear.[7] The limitations in the evidence include bias in the selection of participants, short duration of follow up, and variation in the measurement of confounders (e.g. smoking, alcohol use, and other cardiovascular risk factors). Treatment is widespread, making it difficult to find evidence on prognosis for untreated OSAHS. Observational studies support a causal association between OSAHS and systemic hypertension, which increases with the severity of OSAHS (OR 1.21 for mild OSAHS to 3.07 for severe OSAHS).[11] OSAHS increases the risk of motor vehicle accidents three- to sevenfold.[11,12] It is associated with increased risk of premature mortality, cardiovascular disease, and impaired neurocognitive functioning.[11]

Please refer to CD-ROM for full text and references.

Breast cancer (metastatic)

Search date April 2002

Stephen Johnston and Justin Stebbing

What are the effects of treatments?

BENEFICIAL

Chemotherapy

Anthracycline based regimens (CAF) containing doxorubicin as first line treatment

RCTs have found that combination chemotherapy regimens containing an anthracycline, such as doxorubicin (CAF**G**), versus other regimens as first line treatment**G** significantly increase response rates, time to progression**G**, and survival.

Classical combination chemotherapy (CMF)

One systematic review has found that classical combination chemotherapy**G** versus modified regimens as first line treatment significantly increases response rate and survival.

First line chemotherapy plus monoclonal antibody (in women with overexpressed HER2 neu oncogene)

One RCT found that, in women whose tumours overexpress HER2, standard chemotherapy**G** plus the monoclonal antibody trastuzumab versus standard chemotherapy alone as first line treatment significantly increased the time to disease progression, objective response**G**, and overall survival.

Hormone treatment

Selective aromatase inhibitors G as first line hormonal treatment G in postmenopausal women

RCTs have found that the aromatase inhibitor anastrozole as first line treatment in metastatic postmenopausal breast cancer is at least as effective as tamoxifen in reducing time to disease progression, and found that the aromatase inhibitor letrozole was superior to tamoxifen in reducing time to disease progression.

Selective aromatase inhibitors as second line hormonal treatment in postmenopausal women

RCTs in postmenopausal women who have relapsed during or after treatment with tamoxifen have found that the selective aromatase inhibitors anastrozole, letrozole, and exemestane versus progestins or aminoglutethimide significantly increase overall survival at 2–3 years, and are associated with fewer adverse effects.

Tamoxifen as first line treatment in oestrogen receptor positive disease

RCTs have found prolonged remission with tamoxifen in the first line treatment of women with oestrogen receptor positive metastatic breast cancer.

Radiotherapy

Radiotherapy plus appropriate analgesia

We found no RCTs comparing radiotherapy versus no treatment or versus bisphosphonates. We found limited evidence from non-randomised studies that persistent and localised bone pain can be treated successfully in over 80% of women with radiotherapy plus concomitant appropriate analgesia (from non-steroidal anti-inflammatory drugs to morphine and its derivatives). RCTs have found no evidence ▶

Clin Evid Concise 2003;9:365–367.

that short courses are less effective for pain relief than long courses of radiotherapy. One RCT found that different fractionation schedules can be used to treat neuropathic bone pain effectively.

Radiotherapy for spinal cord compression
We found no RCTs. Retrospective analyses found that early radiotherapy improved outcomes, but fewer than 10% of people walked again if severe deterioration of motor function occurred before radiotherapy.

Radiotherapy plus high dose steroids in spinal cord compression
One small RCT found that adding high dose steroids to radiotherapy improved the chance of walking after 6 months.

LIKELY TO BE BENEFICIAL

Bisphosphonates for bone metastasis
RCTs in women receiving standard chemotherapy for bone metastases secondary to metastatic breast cancer have found that bisphosphonates**G** versus placebo significantly reduce and delay skeletal complications. None of the RCTs found an impact on overall survival.

Combined gonadorelin analogues and tamoxifen as first line treatment in premenopausal women
One systematic review (in premenopausal women with oestrogen receptor positive metastatic breast cancer) has found that first line treatment with gonadorelin analogues**G** plus tamoxifen**G** versus gonadorelin analogues alone significantly improves response rates, overall survival, and progression free survival.

New cytotoxic drugs in anthracycline resistant disease G (such as taxanes G and semisynthetic vinca alkaloids) as second line treatment
RCTs suggest that second line treatment**G** with the docetaxel or vinorelbine versus standard relapse regimens may improve response rates, especially in women with anthracycline resistant disease**G**.

Radiotherapy to control cerebral and choroidal metastases
We found no RCTs. Retrospective studies suggest that whole brain radiation produces general improvement in neurological function in 40–70% of women with brain metastases secondary to breast cancer, and that radiotherapy benefits 70% of women with choroidal metastases.

TRADE OFF BETWEEN BENEFITS AND HARMS

Ovarian ablation as first line treatment in premenopausal women (*v* tamoxifen)
One systematic review and one subsequent RCT in premenopausal women found no significant difference in response rate, duration of response, or survival with ovarian ablation (surgery or irradiation) versus tamoxifen as first line treatment. Ovarian ablation is associated with substantial adverse effects such as hot flushes and "tumour flare".

Progestins as first line treatment (*v* tamoxifen, beneficial in women with bone pain or anorexia)
RCTs have found no significant difference in response rates, remission rates, or survival between progestins**G** versus tamoxifen as first line treatment, but found that progestins increased adverse effects including nausea, weight gain, and exacerbations of hypertension. One RCT found that medroxyprogesterone versus tamoxifen significantly improved bone pain. Observational evidence suggests that progestins may increase appetite, weight gain, and well being.

LIKELY TO BE INEFFECTIVE OR HARMFUL

High dose chemotherapy (v conventional chemotherapy) as first line treatment

One RCT (in women who had complete or partial response**G** to standard induction chemotherapy) found no significant difference in overall survival at 3 years with additional high dose versus standard dose chemotherapy as first line treatment.

Progestins (v aromatase inhibitors) as second line treatment

RCTs have found that in postmenopausal women with metastatic breast cancer who have relapsed on adjuvant tamoxifen or progressed during first line treatment with tamoxifen, the selective aromatase inhibitors**G** anastrozole, letrozole, and exemestane prolong survival compared with progestins or aminoglutethimide, with minimal adverse effects.

DEFINITION Metastatic or advanced breast cancer is the presence of disease at distant sites such as the bone, liver, or lung. It is not treatable by primary surgery and is currently considered incurable. However, young people with good performance status may survive for 15 to 20 years.[1] Symptoms may include pain from bone metastases, breathlessness from spread to the lung, and nausea or abdominal discomfort from liver involvement.

INCIDENCE/ PREVALENCE Breast cancer is the second most frequent cancer in the world (1.05 million people) and is by far the most common malignant disease in women (22% of all new cancer cases). Worldwide, the ratio of mortality to incidence is about 36%. It ranks fifth as a cause of death from cancer overall (although it is the leading cause of mortality in women — the 370 000 annual deaths represent 13.9% of cancer deaths in women). In the USA, metastatic breast cancer causes 46 000 deaths, and in the UK causes 15 000 deaths.[2] It is the most prevalent cancer in the world today and there are an estimated 3.9 million women alive who have had breast cancer diagnosed in the past 5 years (compared, for example, with lung cancer, where there are 1.4 million alive). The true prevalence of metastatic disease is high because some women live with the disease for many years. Since 1990, there has been an overall increase in incidence rates of about 1.5% annually.[3]

AETIOLOGY/ RISK FACTORS The risk of metastatic disease relates to known prognostic factors in the original primary tumour. These factors include oestrogen receptor negative disease, primary tumours 3 cm or more in diameter, and axillary node involvement — recurrence occurred within 10 years of adjuvant chemotherapy**G** for early breast cancer**G** in 60–70% of node positive women and 25–30% of node negative women in one large systematic review.[4]

PROGNOSIS Prognosis depends on age, extent of disease, and oestrogen receptor status. There is also evidence that overexpression of the product of the HER2/neu oncogene, which occurs in about a third of women with metastatic breast cancer, is associated with a worse prognosis.[5] A short disease free interval**G** (e.g. < 1 year) between surgery for early breast cancer and developing metastases suggests that the recurrent disease is likely to be resistant to the drug used for adjuvant treatment**G**.[6] In women who receive no treatment for metastatic disease, the median survival from diagnosis of metastases is 12 months.[7] The choice of first line treatment**G** (hormonal or chemotherapy) is based on a variety of clinical factors**T**.[8–11] In many countries there is evidence of a decrease in death rates in recent years, evident in the USA, Canada, and some European countries. This probably reflects improvements in treatment (and therefore improved survival) as well as earlier diagnosis.[2,12]

Please refer to CD-ROM for full text and references.

Breast cancer (non-metastatic)

Search date October 2002

J Michael Dixon, Kate Gregory, Stephen Johnston, and Alan Rodger

What are the effects of treatments for ductal carcinoma in situ?

LIKELY TO BE BENEFICIAL

Radiotherapy after breast conserving surgery (reduces recurrence)

RCTs found that radiotherapy**G** reduced the risk of local recurrence and invasive carcinoma, with no evidence of an effect on survival.

Tamoxifen plus radiotherapy after breast conserving surgery (reduces recurrence)

One RCT has found that adjuvant**G** tamoxifen**G** significantly reduces breast cancer events in women who have undergone wide excision and radiotherapy, but found no significant difference in overall survival at about 6 years.

What are the effects of treatments for operable breast cancer?

BENEFICIAL

Adjuvant chemotherapy

One systematic review has found that adjuvant chemotherapy versus no chemotherapy significantly reduces rates of recurrence and improves survival at 10 years. The benefit seems to be independent of nodal or menopausal status, although the absolute improvements are greater in women with node positive disease, and probably greater in younger women.

Adjuvant tamoxifen

One systematic review has found that adjuvant tamoxifen taken for up to 5 years reduces the risk of recurrence and death in women with oestrogen receptor positive tumours irrespective of age, menopausal status, nodal involvement, or the addition of chemotherapy. Tamoxifen slightly increases the risk of endometrial cancer, but we found no evidence of an overall adverse effect on non-breast cancer mortality.

Anthracycline regimens as adjuvant chemotherapy

One systematic review has found that adjuvant regimens containing an anthracycline**G** significantly reduce recurrence, and significantly improve survival compared with a standard multidrug chemotherapy regimen (CMF**G**) at 5 years.

Breast conserving surgery (similar survival to more extensive surgery)

Systematic reviews and long term results from included RCTs have found that, providing all local disease is excised, more extensive surgery does not increase survival up to 20 years. More extensive local resection in breast conserving surgery**G** gives worse cosmetic results.

Chemotherapy plus tamoxifen

One RCT found that adding chemotherapy (CMF) to tamoxifen significantly improves survival at 5 years.

Ovarian ablation in premenopausal women

One systematic review has found that in women less than 50 years of age, ovarian ablation**G** versus no ablation significantly improves survival for at least 15 years. ▶

Radiotherapy after breast conserving surgery (reduces local recurrence; no evidence of effect on survival)

One systematic review has found that adding radiotherapy to breast conserving surgery significantly reduces the risk of isolated local recurrence and loss of a breast, but does not increase survival at 10 years. Rates of survival and local recurrence are similar with radiotherapy plus either breast conserving surgery or mastectomy.

Radiotherapy after mastectomy in women at high risk of local recurrence

RCTs in high risk women receiving adjuvant chemotherapy after mastectomy have found that radiotherapy versus no radiotherapy significantly reduces local recurrence and increases survival at 10–15 years. Radiotherapy may be associated with late adverse effects, which are rare, including pneumonitis, pericarditis, arm oedema, brachial plexopathy, and radionecrotic rib fracture.

LIKELY TO BE BENEFICIAL

Neoadjuvant chemotherapy (reduces mastectomy rates *v* adjuvant chemotherapy; no evidence of effect on survival)

RCTs have found that neoadjuvantⒼ versus adjuvant chemotherapy reduces mastectomy rates, but found no significant difference in survival at 4–10 years.

Radiotherapy after mastectomy in node positive disease, large tumours, or where lymphovascular invasion is present

One systematic review has found that radiotherapy to the chest wall after mastectomy reduces the risk of local recurrence by about two thirds and the risk of death from breast cancer at 10 years, but found no evidence of effect on overall 10 year survival. One review of retrospective data found that greater axillary node involvement, larger tumour size, higher histological grade, presence of lymphovascular invasion, and involvement of tumour margins reduced the chance of successful treatment. Radiotherapy may be associated with late adverse effects, which are rare, including pneumonitis, pericarditis, arm oedema, brachial plexopathy, and radionecrotic rib fracture.

Total nodal radiotherapy in high risk disease

RCTs have found that, in women with high risk disease, total nodal irradiationⒼ versus no irradiation improves survival. An earlier systematic review found reduced locoregional recurrence, but no evidence of improved survival.

TRADE OFF BETWEEN BENEFITS AND HARMS

Axillary clearance (no evidence of survival benefit and increased morbidity compared with axillary sampling)

RCTs found no significant difference in survival at 5–10 years between axillary clearance versus axillary samplingⒼ, axillary radiotherapyⒼ, or sampling plus radiotherapyⒼ combined. One systematic review of mainly poor quality evidence found that the risk of arm lymphoedema was highest with axillary clearance plus radiotherapy, lower with axillary sampling plus radiotherapy, and lowest with sampling alone.

Axillary radiotherapy

One systematic review has found that axillary radiotherapy versus axilliary clearance significantly reduces isolated local recurrence, and has found no significant difference in mortality or overall recurrence at 10 years. One systematic review of mainly poor quality evidence found that radiotherapy plus axillary surgery was associated with arm lymphoedema.

Radiotherapy after mastectomy in women not at high risk of local recurrence

One systematic review has found that radiotherapy to the chest wall after mastectomy reduces the risk of local recurrence by about two thirds and the risk of death from breast cancer at 10 years, but found no evidence of an effect on overall 10 year survival. Radiotherapy may be associated with later adverse effects, which are rare, including pneumonitis, pericarditis, arm oedema, brachial plexopathy, and radionecrotic rib fracture.

UNKNOWN EFFECTIVENESS

Radiotherapy to the internal mammary chain

One RCT found no significant difference in overall survival or breast cancer specific survival at 2–3 years between radiotherapy versus no radiotherapy to the internal mammary chain. Treatment may increase radiation induced cardiac morbidity.

Radiotherapy to the ipsilateral supraclavicular fossa

We found insufficient evidence about the effects of irradiation of the ipsilateral supraclavicular fossa on survival. RCTs have found that radiotherapy reduces the risk of supraclavicular fossa nodal recurrence.

UNLIKELY TO BE BENEFICIAL

Enhanced dose regimens of adjuvant chemotherapy

RCTs found no significant improvement from enhanced dose regimens.

Prolonged chemotherapy (8–12 months *v* 4–6 months)

One systematic review found no additional benefit from prolonging adjuvant chemotherapy from 4–6 to 8–12 months.

Radical mastectomy (no greater survival than less extensive surgery)

Systematic reviews and long term follow up of one RCT have found no significant difference between radical, total, supraradical❻, or simple mastectomy in survival up to 25 years. More extensive surgery results in greater mutilation.

What are the effects of treatments for locally advanced breast cancer?

LIKELY TO BE BENEFICIAL

Radiotherapy

For locally advanced breast cancer❻ that is rendered operable, small RCTs found that radiotherapy or surgery as sole local treatments have similar effects on response rates, duration of response, and overall survival.

Radiotherapy after attempted curative surgery

One RCT found weak evidence that radiotherapy after attempted curative surgery versus no further local treatment may reduce local and/or regional recurrence.

Surgery

For locally advanced breast cancer that is rendered operable, small RCTs found that surgery or radiotherapy as sole local treatments have similar effects on response rates, duration of response, and overall survival.

Tamoxifen plus radiotherapy (*v* radiotherapy)

One RCT found that hormone treatment plus radiotherapy versus radiotherapy alone significantly improved locoregional recurrence at 6 years and improved median survival at 8 years.

UNLIKELY TO BE BENEFICIAL

Chemotherapy (cyclophosphamide/methotrexate/fluorouracil or anthracycline based regimens)

We found no evidence that the cytotoxic, multidrug chemotherapy regimen (CMF) improves survival, disease free survivalⒼ, or long term locoregional control.

DEFINITION **Ductal carcinoma *in situ*** is a non-invasiveⒼ tumour characterised by the presence of malignant cells in the breast ducts but with no evidence that they breach the basement membrane and invade into periductal connective tissues. **Invasive breast cancer** can be separated into three main groups: earlyⒼ or operable breast cancer, locally advanced disease, and metastatic breast cancer (see p 365). **Operable breast cancer** is apparently restricted to the breast and sometimes to local lymph nodes and can be surgically removed. Although these women do not have overt metastases at the time of stagingⒼ, they remain at risk of local recurrence and of metastatic spread. They can be divided into those women with tumours greater than 4 cm or multifocal cancers that can be treated by mastectomy, and those with tumours less than 4 cm that are unifocal that can be treated by breast conserving surgeryⒼ. **Locally advanced breast cancer** is defined according to the TNM staging system of the UICC TNMⓉ systemⒼ[1] as stage III B (includes T4 a–d; N2 disease, but absence of metastases). It is a disease presentation with evidence (clinical or histopathological) of skin and/or chest wall involvement and/or axillary nodes matted together by tumour extension. **Metastatic breast cancer** is presented in a separate topic (see p 365).

INCIDENCE/ PREVALENCE Breast cancer affects 1/10–1/11 women in the UK and causes about 21 000 deaths per year. Prevalence is about five times higher, with over 100 000 women living with breast cancer at any one time. Of the 15 000 new cases of breast cancer per annum in the UK, the majority will present with primary operable disease.[2]

AETIOLOGY/ RISK FACTORS The risk of breast cancer increases with age, doubling every 10 years up to the menopause. Risk factors include an early age at menarche, older age at menopause, older age at birth of first child, family history, atypical hyperplasia, excess alcohol intake, radiation exposure to developing breast tissue, oral contraceptive use, postmenopausal hormone replacement therapy, and obesity. Risk in different countries varies fivefold. The cause of breast cancer in most women is unknown. About 5% of breast cancers can be attributed to mutations in the genes *BRCA1* and *BRCA2*.[3]

PROGNOSIS **Primary carcinoma** of the breast is potentially curable. The risk of relapse depends on various clinico-pathological features, including axillary node involvement, oestrogen receptor status, and tumour size. Tumour size, axillary node status, histological grade, and oestrogen receptor status provide the most significant prognostic information. Seventy per cent of women with operable disease are alive 5 years after diagnosis and treatment (adjuvant drug treatment is given to most women after surgery). Risk of recurrence is highest during the first 5 years, but the risk remains even 15–20 years after surgery. Those with node positive disease have a 50–60% chance of recurrence within 5 years, compared with 30–35% for node negative disease. Recurrence within 10 years according to one large systematic review occurred in 60–70% of node positive women compared with 25–30% of node negative women.[4] The prognosis for a disease free survivalⒼ at 5 years is worse for stage III B (33%) than that for stage III A (71%). Five year overall survival is 44% and 84%, respectively.[5] Poor survival and high rates of local recurrence characterise locally advanced breast cancerⒼ.

Please refer to CD-ROM for full text and references.

Breast pain

Search date March 2002

Nigel Bundred

What are the effects of treatments?

LIKELY TO BE BENEFICIAL

Low fat, high carbohydrate diet

One RCT found limited evidence that advice to follow a low fat, high carbohydrate diet versus general dietary advice significantly reduced breast swelling and breast tenderness at 6 months.

TRADE OFF BETWEEN BENEFITS AND HARMS

Danazol

One RCT found that danazol versus placebo significantly reduced cyclical breast pain after 12 months, but significantly increased adverse effects (weight gain, deepening of the voice, menorrhagia, and muscle cramps). It found no significant difference in pain relief with danazol versus tamoxifen.

Gestrinone

One RCT found that gestrinone versus placebo significantly reduced breast pain after 3 months, but significantly increased adverse effects (greasy skin, hirsutism, acne, reduction in breast size, headache, and depression).

Tamoxifen

One RCT found that tamoxifen versus placebo significantly reduced breast pain after 3 months; another found that tamoxifen versus placebo significantly increased the number of women with greater than 50% reduction in mean pain score after 12. Tamoxifen increased adverse effects such as hot flushes, vaginal discharge, and gastrointestinal disturbances. Fewer adverse effects were found with the lower dose of 10 mg given between days 15 and 25 of the menstrual period.

UNKNOWN EFFECTIVENESS

Antibiotics; diuretics; evening primrose oil; gonadorelin analogues (luteinising hormone releasing hormone analogues); progestogens; pyridoxine; vitamin E

We found no RCTs on the effects of these interventions.

Lisuride maleate

One RCT found limited evidence that lisuride maleate versus placebo significantly reduced breast pain over 2 months.

Tibolone

One small RCT found limited evidence that tibolone versus hormone replacement therapy significantly reduced breast pain after 1 year.

UNLIKELY TO BE BENEFICIAL

Bromocriptine

Two RCTs found that bromocriptine versus placebo significantly reduced breast pain but one of these RCTs found that bromocriptine significantly increased adverse effects (including nausea, dizziness, postural hypotension, and constipation).

Hormone replacement therapy

One small RCT found limited evidence that women taking hormone replacement therapy had significantly more breast pain after 1 year than women taking tibolone.

Progesterones

We found limited evidence from two crossover RCTs that found no significant differences between progesterones versus placebo in breast pain.

DEFINITION Breast pain can be differentiated into cyclical mastalgia (worse before a menstrual period) or non-cyclical mastalgia (unrelated to the menstrual cycle).[1,2] Cyclical pain is often bilateral, usually most severe in the upper outer quadrants of the breast, and may refer to the medial aspect of the upper arm.[1–3] Non-cyclical pain may be caused by true breast pain or chest wall pain located over the costal cartilages.[1,2,4] Specific breast pathology and referred pain unrelated to the breasts are not included in this definition.

INCIDENCE/ PREVALENCE Up to 70% of women develop breast pain in their lifetime.[1,2] Of 1171 US women attending a gynaecology clinic, 69% suffered regular discomfort, which was judged as severe in 11% of women, and 36% had consulted a doctor about breast pain.[2]

AETIOLOGY/ RISK FACTORS Breast pain is more common in women aged 30–50 years.[1,2]

PROGNOSIS Cyclical breast pain resolves spontaneously within 3 months of onset in 20–30% of women.[5] The pain tends to relapse and remit, and up to 60% of women develop recurrent symptoms 2 years after treatment.[1] Non-cyclical pain responds poorly to treatment but may resolve spontaneously in about 50% of women.[1]

Please refer to CD-ROM for full text and references.

Candidiasis (vulvovaginal)

Search date July 2002
Jeanne Marrazzo

What are the effects of treatments for symptomatic vulvovaginal candidiasis in non-pregnant women?

BENEFICIAL

Intravaginal imidazoles

RCTs have found that intravaginal imidazoles (e.g. clotrimazole) versus placebo significantly reduce persistent symptoms of vulvovaginal candidiasis after 1 month. RCTs found no clear evidence that effects differ significantly among the various intravaginal imidazoles. RCTs found no clear evidence of any difference between shorter and longer durations of treatment (1–14 days).

Oral itraconazole

One RCT found that oral itraconazole versus placebo significantly reduced persistent symptoms at 1 week after treament. One systematic review has found no significant difference in persistant symptoms at 7 days or 28–35 days with oral itraconazole versus intravaginal imidazoles.

LIKELY TO BE BENEFICIAL

Intravaginal nystatin

One RCT found that intravaginal nystatin versus placebo significantly reduced the proportion of women with a poor symptomatic response after 14 days.

Oral fluconazole

We found no RCTs of oral fluconazole versus placebo or no treatment. A systematic review has found no significant difference with oral fluconazole versus intravaginal imidazoles in the symptoms of vulvovaginal candidiasis. RCTs have found that fluconazole versus intravaginal imidazoles is associated with increased frequency of mild nausea, headache, and abdominal pain.

TRADE OFF BETWEEN BENEFITS AND HARMS

Oral ketoconazole

We found no RCTs of oral ketoconazole versus placebo or versus no treatment. Four RCTs have found no significant difference with oral ketoconazole versus intravaginal imidazoles in the reduction of persistent symptoms, but found that ketoconazole significantly increased the frequency of minor adverse events (mainly nausea). Case reports have associated ketoconazole with a low risk of fulminant hepatitis (1/12 000 courses of treatment with oral ketoconazole).

UNKNOWN EFFECTIVENESS

Treating a male sexual partner

RCTs found no significant difference with treating versus not treating a woman's male sexual partner in the resolution of the woman's acute vulvovaginal candidiasis symptoms or in the rate of symptomatic relapse.

What are the effects of treatments in non-pregnant women with recurrent vulvovaginal candidiasis?

LIKELY TO BE BENEFICIAL

Oral itraconazole

One RCT found that oral itraconazole versus placebo significantly reduced the rate of recurrence over 6 months.

TRADE OFF BETWEEN BENEFITS AND HARMS

Prophylaxis with intermittent or continuous ketoconazole

One RCT found that oral ketoconazole (given either intermittently or continuously at a lower dose) versus placebo significantly reduced symptomatic recurrences over 6 months. Ketoconazole is associated with an increased frequency of gastrointestinal adverse effects, and case reports have associated ketoconazole with a low risk of serious fulminant hepatitis (1/12 000 courses of treatment with oral ketoconazole).

UNKNOWN EFFECTIVENESS

Regular prophylaxis with intravaginal imidazole

RCTs comparing regular prophylaxis with intravaginal imidazole versus placebo found inconsistent effects on the proportion of women with symptomatic relapse. One RCT found that regular prophylactic intravaginal imidazole versus treatment at the onset of symptoms reduced the frequency of episodes of symptomatic vaginitis, but the difference was not significant. The RCTs were too small to exclude a clinically important benefit.

Regular prophylaxis with oral fluconazole

We found no RCTs about the effects of fluconazole in preventing recurrence of vulvovaginal candidiasis.

DEFINITION Vulvovaginal candidiasis is symptomatic vaginitis (inflammation of the vagina), which often involves the vulva, caused by infection with a *Candida* yeast. Predominant symptoms are vulvar itching and abnormal vaginal discharge (which may be minimal, a "cheese like" material, or a watery secretion). Differentiation from other forms of vaginitis requires the presence of yeast on microscopy of vaginal fluid. The definition of recurrent vulvovaginal candidiasis varies among RCTs, but is commonly defined as four or more symptomatic episodes a year.[1] This summary excludes studies of asymptomatic women with vaginal colonisation by *Candida* species.

INCIDENCE/ PREVALENCE Vulvovaginal candidiasis is the second most common cause of vaginitis (after bacterial vaginosis). Estimates of its incidence are limited, and often derived from women attending hospital clinics. At least one episode of vulvovaginal candidiasis occurs during the lifetime of 50–75% of all women. About half of the women who have an episode develop recurrent vulvovaginal candidiasis.[2] Vulvovaginal candidiasis is diagnosed in 5–15% of women attending sexually transmitted disease and family planning clinics.[1]

AETIOLOGY/ RISK FACTORS *Candida albicans* accounts for 85–90% of vulvovaginal candidiasis infections. Development of symptomatic vulvovaginal candidiasis probably represents increased growth of yeast that previously colonised the vagina without causing symptoms. Risk factors for vulvovaginal candidiasis include pregnancy (RR 2–10), diabetes mellitus, and systemic antibiotics. The evidence that different types of contraceptives are risk factors is contradictory. The incidence of vulvovaginal candidiasis rises with initiation of sexual activity, but we found no direct evidence that vulvovaginal candidiasis is sexually transmitted.[3–5]

Candidiasis (vulvovaginal)

PROGNOSIS We found few descriptions of the natural history of untreated vulvovaginal candidiasis. Discomfort is the main complication and can include pain while passing urine or during sexual intercourse. Balanitis**G** in male partners of women with vulvovaginal candidiasis can occur, but it is rare.

Please refer to CD-ROM for full text and references.

Dysmenorrhoea

Search date June 2002

Cynthia Farquhar and Michelle Proctor

What are the effects of treatments?

BENEFICIAL

Non-steroidal anti-inflammatory drugs (other than aspirin)

Two systematic reviews found that naproxen, ibuprofen, mefenamic acid, and rofecoxib are all significantly more effective than placebo for pain relief. It remains unclear from direct comparisons which non-steroidal anti-inflammatory drugs are most effective and safe.

LIKELY TO BE BENEFICIAL

Aspirin, paracetamol, and compound analgesics

One systematic review has found that aspirin is significantly more effective for pain relief than placebo, but less effective than naproxen or ibuprofen. The review found no significant difference with paracetamol versus placebo, aspirin, or ibuprofen in pain relief. It found limited evidence that co-proxamolⒼ versus placebo significantly reduced pain, but compared to naproxen reduced pain significantly less and was associated with significantly more adverse effects. It also found that co-proxamol reduced dysmenorrhoea related symptoms significantly less than mefenamic acid.

Magnesium

Two RCTs found limited evidence that magnesium versus placebo significantly reduced pain after 5–6 months, but a third RCT found no significant difference.

Thiamine

One large RCT has found that thiamine versus placebo significantly reduces pain after 60 days.

Toki-shakuyaku-san (herbal remedy)

One systematic review found limited evidence that toki-shakuyaku-san versus placebo significantly reduced pain after 6 months and reduced the need for additional medication with diclofenac.

Topical heat *New*

One RCT found topical heat (about 39 °C) treatment to be as effective as ibuprofen and significantly more effective than placebo in reducing pain.

Transcutaneous electrical nerve stimulation

One systematic review found that high frequency transcutaneous electrical nerve stimulationⒼ is more effective than placebo transcutaneous electrical nerve stimulation for pain relief. There is insufficient evidence for other comparisons. A meta-analysis included in one systematic review found no significant difference in pain relief with low frequency transcutaneous electrical nerve stimulation, but two RCTs included in the review, but not in the meta-analysis, found that pain relief significantly improved with low placebo transcutaneous electrical nerve stimulation versus placebo transcutaneous electrical nerve stimulation or versus placebo tablets.

Vitamin E

One RCT found limited evidence that vitamin E versus placebo reduced pain. ▶

UNKNOWN EFFECTIVENESS

Acupuncture

One systematic review of one small RCT found limited evidence that acupuncture versus placebo acupuncture**G** or no treatment significantly reduced pain.

Behavioural interventions

Two RCTs found insufficient evidence about the effects of behavioural interventions**G**.

Combined oral contraceptives

One systematic review found insufficient evidence about the effects of combined oral contraceptives versus placebo for pain relief.

Dietary supplements (other than magnesium, thiamine, or vitamin E)

RCTs found insufficient evidence about the effects of fish oil or dietary change.

Herbal remedies (other than toki-shakuyaku-san)

We found no RCTs of other herbal remedies

Surgical interruption of pelvic nerve pathways

One small RCT found limited evidence suggesting that laparoscopic uterine nerve ablation**G** versus diagnostic laparoscopy significantly increased pain relief at 3 and 12 months. Another RCT comparing laparoscopic uterine nerve ablation versus laparoscopic presacral neurectomy**G** found no significant difference in pain relief at 3 months. It also found that laparoscopic presacral neurectomy versus laparoscopic uterine nerve ablation significantly reduced pain at 6 months and that laparoscopic uterine nerve ablation was significantly associated with increased risk of constipation.

UNLIKELY TO BE BENEFICIAL

Spinal manipulation

One systematic review has found inconclusive evidence on the effects of spinal manipulation versus placebo or no treatment for pain relief.

DEFINITION Dysmenorrhoea is painful menstrual cramps of uterine origin. It is commonly divided into primary dysmenorrhoea (pain without organic pathology) and secondary dysmenorrhoea (pelvic pain associated with an identifiable pathological condition, such as endometriosis or ovarian cysts). The initial onset of primary dysmenorrhoea is usually shortly after menarche (6–12 months) when ovulatory cycles are established. Pain duration is commonly 8–72 hours and is usually associated with the onset of menstrual flow. Secondary dysmenorrhoea may arise as a new symptom during a woman's fourth and fifth decade.[1]

INCIDENCE/ PREVALENCE Variations in the definition of dysmenorrhoea make it difficult to determine the precise prevalence. However, various types of study have found a consistently high prevalence in women of different ages and nationalities. A systematic review (search date 1996) of the prevalence of chronic pelvic pain, summarising both community and hospital surveys, estimated prevalence to be 45–95%.[2] Reports focus on adolescent girls and generally include only primary dysmenorrhoea, although this is not always specified**T**.[3–8]

AETIOLOGY/ RISK FACTORS A longitudinal study of a representative sample of women born in 1962 found that severity of dysmenorrhoea was significantly associated with duration of menstrual flow (average duration of menstrual flow was 5 days for women with no dysmenorrhoea and 5.8 days for women with severe dysmenorrhoea; $P < 0.001$; WMD –0.80, 95% CI –1.36 to –0.24); younger average menarcheal age (13.1 years in women without dysmenorrhoea *v* 12.6 years in women with severe dysmenorrhoea; $P < 0.01$; WMD 0.50, 95% CI 0.09 to 0.91); and cigarette smoking (41% of smokers and 26% of non-smokers experienced moderate or severe dysmenorrhoea).[9] There is also some evidence of a dose-response relationship between exposure to environmental tobacco smoke and increased incidence of dysmenorrhoea.[10]

PROGNOSIS Primary dysmenorrhoea is a chronic recurring condition that affects most young women. Studies of the natural history of this condition are sparse. One longitudinal study in Scandinavia found that primary dysmenorrhoea often improves in the third decade of a woman's reproductive life, and is also reduced after childbirth.[9]

Please refer to CD-ROM for full text and references.

Endometriosis

Search date March 2002

Cynthia Farquhar

What are the effects of treatments in women with pain attributed to endometriosis?

BENEFICIAL

Hormonal treatment at diagnosis (danazol, medroxyprogesterone, gonadorelin [gonadotrophin releasing hormone] analogues)

Small systematic reviews and small RCTs have found that hormonal treatments (except for dydrogesterone) versus placebo reduce pain attributed to endometriosis, and are of similar effectiveness.

LIKELY TO BE BENEFICIAL

Combined ablation of endometrial deposits and uterine nerve

One RCT found that ablation of deposits plus laparoscopic uterine nerve ablation reduced pain more than diagnostic laparoscopy at 6 months.

Cystectomy for ovarian endometrioma (better than drainage)

One RCT found that cystectomy versus drainage significantly improved pain caused by ovarian endometrioma at 2 years. Complication rates were similar.

Oral contraceptive pill

Two RCTs found no significant difference with combined oral contraceptives versus gonadorelin analogues in overall pain relief.

Postoperative hormonal treatment after conservative surgery

RCTs have found that postoperative hormonal treatment with danazol or medroxy-progesterone versus placebo for 6 months significantly reduces pain and delays the recurrence of pain at 12 and 24 months, but have found that treatment for 3 months does not seem to be effective. One RCT found no significant difference in recurrence of pain with combined oral contraceptives versus placebo at 6 months.

UNKNOWN EFFECTIVENESS

Dydrogesterone

Systematic reviews have found no significant difference in pain at 6 months with dydrogesterone and placebo given at two different doses in the luteal phase.

Laparoscopic ablation of endometrial deposits without ablation of the uterine nerve; laparoscopic uterine nerve ablation

We found insufficient evidence on the effects of these interventions. We found no RCTs comparing medical and surgical treatments.

Preoperative hormonal treatment

One RCT found no significant difference in ease of surgery with preoperative treatment with gonadorelin analogues for 3 months versus no treatment.

Postoperative hormonal treatment after oophorectomy

One RCT in women who previously had an oophorectomy found insufficient evidence on the effects of hormone replacement therapy versus no treatment in recurrence of endometriosis.

Clin Evid Concise 2003;9:380–381.

What are the effects of treatments in women with subfertility attributed to endometriosis?

LIKELY TO BE BENEFICIAL

Cystectomy for ovarian endometrioma (better than drainage)

One RCT found that cystectomy versus drainage significantly increased pregnancy in women with subfertility caused by ovarian endometrioma. Complication rates were similar.

Laparoscopic ablation/excision of endometrial deposits

One large RCT found that laparoscopic surgery versus diagnostic laparoscopy significantly increased cumulative pregnancy rates after 36 weeks, but a subsequent smaller RCT found no significant difference with laparoscopic surgery versus diagnostic laparoscopy in pregnancy rates at 12 months. We found no RCTs comparing medical and surgical treatments.

UNLIKELY TO BE BENEFICIAL

Hormonal treatment at diagnosis (danazol, medroxyprogesterone, gonadorelin [GnRH] analogues)

One systematic review and one subsequent RCT found no significant difference with hormonal treatments versus placebo in rates of pregnancy at 4–6 months.

Postoperative hormonal treatment (gonadorelin analogues and decapeptyl)

RCTs found no significant difference with gonadorelin analogues versus placebo after conservative surgery in rates of pregnancy or time to conception.

DEFINITION Endometriosis is characterised by ectopic endometrial tissue, which can cause dysmenorrhoea, dyspareunia, non-cyclical pelvic pain, and subfertility. Diagnosis is made by laparoscopy. Most endometrial deposits are found in the pelvis (ovaries, peritoneum, uterosacral ligaments, pouch of Douglas, and rectovaginal septum). Extrapelvic deposits, including those in the umbilicus and diaphragm, are rare. Severity of endometriosis Ⓖ is defined by the American Fertility Society: this review uses the terms mild (stage I and II), moderate (stage III), and severe (stage IV).[1] Endometriomas are cysts of endometriosis within the ovary.

INCIDENCE/ PREVALENCE In asymptomatic women, the prevalence of endometriosis ranges from 2–22%, depending on the diagnostic criteria used and the populations studied.[2–5] In women with dysmenorrhoea, the incidence of endometriosis ranges from 40–60%, and in women with subfertility from 20–30%.[3,6,7] The severity of symptoms and the probability of diagnosis increase with age.[8] Incidence peaks at about 40 years of age.[9] Symptoms and laparoscopic appearance do not always correlate.[10]

AETIOLOGY/ RISK FACTORS The cause of endometriosis is unknown. Risk factors include early menarche and late menopause. Embryonic cells may give rise to deposits in the umbilicus, whereas retrograde menstruation may deposit endometrial cells in the diaphragm.[11,12] Use of oral contraceptives reduces the risk of endometriosis, and this protective effect persists for up to 1 year after their discontinuation.[9]

PROGNOSIS We found two RCTs in which laparoscopy was repeated in the women treated with placebo.[13,14] Over 6–12 months, endometrial deposits resolved spontaneously in up to a third of women, deteriorated in nearly half, and were unchanged in the remainder.

Please refer to CD-ROM for full text and references.

Essential vulvodynia (vulval pain)

Search date May 2002

Clinical Evidence freelance writers

What are the effects of treatments?

UNKNOWN EFFECTIVENESS

Amitryptyline; pudendal nerve compression

We found no systematic review or RCTs on the effects of these interventions.

DEFINITION Essential vulvodynia is characterised by a diffuse, unremitting burning of the vulva, which may extend to the perineum, thigh, or buttock, and is often associated with urethral or rectal discomfort. Hyperaesthesia over a wide area is usually the only abnormal finding on physical examination. It is found primarily in postmenopausal women.

INCIDENCE/ PREVALENCE We found no data on the prevalence of essential vulvodynia.

AETIOLOGY/ RISK FACTORS The cause is unknown. The role of pudendal nerve compression is not clear; similar symptoms may be caused by pudendal nerve damage.[1–3]

PROGNOSIS Without treatment, the unremitting symptoms of essential vulvodynia may reduce the quality of life. Frequency of micturition, stress incontinence, and chronic constipation may rarely develop,[1–3] but we found no good data on prognosis without treatment.

Please refer to CD-ROM for full text and references.

Fibroids (uterine myomatosis, leiomyomas)

Search date August 2002

Anne Lethaby and Beverley Vollenhoven

What are the effects of medical treatment alone?

TRADE OFF BETWEEN BENEFITS AND HARMS

Gonadorelin analogues (gonadotropin releasing hormone analogues [GnRHa]) alone

RCTs have found that gonadorelin analogues reduce fibroid related symptoms compared with placebo, but are associated with important adverse effects. One RCT found that nafarelin versus placebo significantly increased amenorrhoea at 12 weeks. One systematic review found insufficient evidence to compare nafarelin versus buserelin. One RCT found that higher versus lower doses of nafarelin increased amenorrhoea at 16 weeks. Two RCTs found that nafarelin versus placebo significantly reduced bone density from baseline after 16 weeks' treatment, but that bone density returned to pretreatment levels 6 months after treatment was stopped. Two RCTs found that hot flushes were significantly more common with nafarelin versus placebo or buserelin.

Gonadorelin analogues (GnRHa) plus progestogen

One small RCT found that leuprorelin (leuprolide) acetate plus progesterone significantly reduced heavy bleeding compared with leuprorelin acetate alone. Two small RCTs found that gonadorelin analogue plus progesterone significantly reduced the proportion of women with hot flushes compared with gonadorelin analogue alone.

UNKNOWN EFFECTIVENESS

Gonadorelin analogue (GnRHa) plus tibolone

One small RCT found no significant difference with gonadorelin analogue alone versus gonadorelin analogue plus tibolone on uterine and fibroid size and fibroid related symptoms.

Gonadorelin analogues (GnRHa) plus combined oestrogen and progestogen

We found insufficient evidence from one small RCT to compare effects on fibroid related symptoms of gonadorelin analogue plus combined oestrogen and progestogen versus gonadorelin analogues plus progesterone alone.

Non-steroidal anti-inflammatory drugs

We found insufficient evidence from two small RCTs about the effects of non-steroidal anti-inflammatory drugs on heavy menstrual bleeding in women with uterine fibroids.

Gestrinone; levonorgestrel intrauterine system *New; **mifepristone***

We found no RCTs on the effects of these interventions.

What are the effects of preoperative medical interventions?

LIKELY TO BE BENEFICIAL

Gonadorelin analogues (GnRHa)

One systematic review and one additional RCT have found that gonadorelin analogues versus placebo or no treatment given at least 3 months before fibroid surgery increase haemoglobin and haematocrit and reduce uterine and pelvic ▶

symptoms and blood loss during surgery. Women having hysterectomy are more likely to have a vaginal rather than an abdominal procedure after gonadorelin treatment. However, women are more likely to experience adverse hypo-oestrogenic effects from preoperative treatment.

What are the effects of surgical interventions?

BENEFICIAL

Laparoscopic myomectomy (compared to abdominal myomectomy)

One RCT found that laparoscopic myomectomy**G** versus abdominal myomectomy resulted in less postoperative pain, and a shorter recovery time.

LIKELY TO BE BENEFICIAL

Abdominal hysterectomy*

We found no RCTs. There is consensus that abdominal hysterectomy is superior to no treatment in reducing fibroid related symptoms.

*Based on consensus.

UNKNOWN EFFECTIVENESS

Laparoscopic assisted vaginal hysterectomy

We found no RCTs comparing long term effects of laparoscopic assisted vaginal hysterectomy versus other treatments. One small RCT found limited evidence that women having laparoscopically assisted vaginal hysterectomy had shorter recovery and less postoperative pain compared with women having total abdominal hysterectomy**G**.

Thermal balloon endometrial ablation *New*

We found no RCTs comparing thermal balloon ablation**G** versus non-surgical treatment or versus hysterectomy. One RCT compared thermal balloon ablation versus rollerball endometrial ablation**G** in women with fibroids smaller than the average size of a 12 week pregnancy, all of whom had been pretreated with gonadorelin analogues. It found no significant difference between thermal balloon and rollerball ablation in hysterectomy rates, amenorrhoea rates, pictorial bleeding assessment chart score**G**, or haemoglobin at 12 months. It found that thermal balloon ablation reduced operation time and intraoperative complication rate compared with rollerball ablation. About a third of women reported being "not very satisfied" with either operation.

DEFINITION Fibroids (uterine leiomyomas) are benign tumours of the smooth muscle cells of the uterus. Women with fibroids can be asymptomatic or can present with menorrhagia (30%), dysmenorrhoea, pelvic pain, pressure symptoms, infertility, and recurrent pregnancy loss.[1] However, much of the data describing the relationship between the presence of fibroids and symptoms are based on uncontrolled studies that have assessed the effect of myomectomy on the presenting symptom.[2]

INCIDENCE/ PREVALENCE The reported incidence of fibroids varies from 5.4–77% depending on the method of diagnosis (the gold standard is histological evidence). A random sample of 335 Swedish women aged 25–40 years was reported to have an incidence of fibroids of 5.4% (95% CI 3.0% to 7.8%) based on transvaginal ultrasound examination. The prevalence of these tumours increased with age (age 25–32 years: 3.3%, 95% CI 0.7% to 6.0%; 33–40 years: 7.8%, 95% CI 3.6% to 12%).[3] Based on postmortem examination of women, 50% were found to have these tumours.[4] Gross serial sectioning at 2 mm intervals of 100 consecutive hysterectomy specimens revealed the presence of fibroids in

77%. These women were having hysterectomies for reasons other than fibroids.[5] The incidence of fibroids in black women is three times greater than that in white women, based on ultrasound or hysterectomy diagnosis.[6] Submucosal fibroids have been diagnosed in 6–34% of women having a hysteroscopy for abnormal bleeding, and in 2–7% of women having infertility investigations.[7]

AETIOLOGY/ RISK FACTORS The cause of uterine fibroids is unknown. It is known that each fibroid is of monoclonal origin and arises independently.[8,9] Factors thought to be involved include the sex steroid hormones oestrogen and progesterone as well as the insulin-like growth factors, epidermal growth factor and transforming growth factor. Risk factors for fibroid growth include nulliparity and obesity. There is a risk reduction to a fifth with five term pregnancies, compared with nulliparous women ($P < 0.001$).[10] Obesity increases the risk of fibroid development by 21% with each 10 kg weight gain ($P = 0.008$).[10] Factors associated with reduced incidence of fibroids include cigarette smoking and hormonal contraception. Women who smoke 10 cigarettes a day have an 18% lowered risk of fibroid development compared with non-smokers ($P = 0.036$).[10] The combined oral contraceptive pill reduces the risk of fibroids with increasing duration of use compared with never users (users for 4–6 years: OR 0.8, 95% CI 0.5 to 1.2; users for ≥ 7 years: OR 0.5, 95% CI 0.3 to 0.9).[11] Women who have used injections containing 150 mg depot medroxyprogesterone acetate also have a reduced incidence compared with women who have never used (OR 0.44, 95% CI 0.36 to 0.55).[12]

PROGNOSIS There are few data on the long term untreated prognosis of these tumours, particularly in women who are asymptomatic at diagnosis. One small case control study reported that in a group of 106 women treated with observation alone over 1 year there was no significant change in symptoms and quality of life over that time.[13]

Please refer to CD-ROM for full text and references.

Infertility and subfertility

Search date October 2002

Kirsten Duckitt

What are the effects of treatments in women with infertility caused by ovulation disorders?

LIKELY TO BE BENEFICIAL

Clomifene

One systematic review has found that clomifene significantly increases pregnancy rate compared with placebo in women who ovulate infrequently. Four other studies comparing clomifene versus tamoxifen have found no significant difference in ovulation or pregnancy rates. One RCT found that clomifene plus metformin significantly increased pregnancy rate compared with clomifene alone after 6 months' treatment.

UNKNOWN EFFECTIVENESS

Cyclofenil

One RCT found no significant difference in pregnancy rates with cyclofenil versus placebo.

Gonadotrophins

One systematic review found no significant difference between human menopausal gonadotrophins and urofollitropin (urofollitrophin, urinary follicle stimulating hormone) in pregnancy rates. Two RCTs found no significant difference in cumulative pregnancy or live birth rates with follitropin (recombinant follicle stimulating hormone) versus urofollitropin. The review found that urofollitropin versus human menopausal gonadotrophins significantly reduced the risk of ovarian hyperstimulation syndrome(G), although this was confined to women who were not treated with concomitant gonadotrophin releasing hormone analogues. Observational evidence suggests that gonadotrophins may be associated with an increased risk of non-invasive ovarian tumours and multiple pregnancies.

Laparoscopic ovarian drilling

One systematic review and one subsequent small RCT found no significant difference in pregnancy rate with laparoscopic ovarian drilling(G) versus gonadotrophins, but found that laparoscopic ovarian drilling significantly reduced rates of multiple pregnancies.

Pulsatile gonadotrophin releasing hormone

One systematic review found insufficient evidence on the effects of pulsatile gonadotrophin releasing hormone treatment.

What are the effects of treatments in women with tubal infertility?

LIKELY TO BE BENEFICIAL

Tubal flushing with oil soluble media *New*

One systematic review found that tubal flushing with oil soluble media versus no intervention increased pregnancy rate. The review found that tubal flushing with oil soluble media increased the live birth rate compared with flushing with water soluble media.

Clin Evid Concise 2003;9:386–389.

Tubal surgery (before in vitro fertilisation)
One systematic review in women undergoing in vitro fertilisation has found that tubal surgery significantly increases pregnancy and live birth rates compared with no treatment or medical treatment. Another review found no significant difference in pregnancy rates between different types of tubal surgery. One systematic review found no significant difference in pregnancy rates with tubal surgery plus additional treatments versus tubal surgery alone to prevent adhesion formation (steroids, dextran, noxytioline).

UNKNOWN EFFECTIVENESS

In vitro fertilisation
We found no RCTs of in vitro fertilisation versus no treatment. One RCT found that immediate versus delayed in vitro fertilisationⒼ significantly increased numbers of pregnancies and live births. Three RCTs found no significant difference in numbers of live births with in vitro fertilisation versus intracytoplasmic sperm injection. Observational evidence suggests that adverse effects associated with in vitro fertilisation include multiple pregnancies and ovarian hyperstimulation syndrome.

Selective salpingography plus tubal catheterisation
We found no RCTs on the effects of selective salpingography plus tubal catheterisation.

Tubal flushing with water soluble media *New*
One systematic review found no RCTs of tubal flushing with water soluble media versus no intervention. It found that tubal flushing with water soluble media decreased live birth rate compared with flushing with oil soluble media.

What are the effects of interventions in women with infertility associated with endometriosis?

LIKELY TO BE BENEFICIAL

Intrauterine insemination plus gonadotrophins
One RCT found that intrauterine insemination plus gonadotrophins significantly increased live birth rates compared with no treatment. A second RCT found no significant difference in birth rates between expectant management versus intrauterine insemination plus pituitary down regulation plus gonadotrophins. A third RCT found that intrauterine insemination plus gonadotrophins significantly increased pregnancy rates compared with intrauterine insemination alone after the first treatment cycle.

UNKNOWN EFFECTIVENESS

In vitro fertilisation
We found no RCTs in women with endometriosis related infertility.

Laparoscopic surgical treatment
Two RCTs found inconsistent evidence about effects on pregnancy and live birth rates of laparoscopic surgery compared with diagnostic laparoscopy.

LIKELY TO BE INEFFECTIVE OR HARMFUL

Drug-induced ovarian suppression
One systematic review found no significant difference in pregnancy rates between drugs that induce ovarian suppression versus placebo. The review found that

ovulation suppression agents cause adverse effects, including weight gain, hot flushes, and osteoporosis, and that danazol may cause dose related weight gain and androgenic effects.

What are the effects of interventions in couples with male factor infertility?

BENEFICIAL

Intrauterine insemination

Two systematic reviews have found that intrauterine insemination significantly increases pregnancy rate compared with intracervical insemination or natural intercourse.

UNKNOWN EFFECTIVENESS

Donor insemination

We found no good evidence on the effects of donor insemination.

Intracytoplasmic sperm injection plus in vitro fertilisation

One systematic review found insufficient evidence on the effects of intracytoplasmic sperm injection plus in vitro fertilisation versus in vitro fertilisation alone.

In vitro fertilisation versus gamete intrafallopian transfer

One RCT found insufficient evidence on the effects of in vitro fertilisation versus gamete intrafallopian transfer.

What are the effects of interventions in couples with unexplained infertility?

BENEFICIAL

Intrauterine insemination (plus ovarian stimulation treatment)

Two systematic reviews and one subsequent RCT in couples undergoing ovarian stimulation treatment have found that intrauterine insemination significantly increases pregnancy rates compared with timed intercourse or intracervical insemination. One systematic review found no significant difference with intrauterine insemination versus timed intercourse or intracervical insemination in pregnancy rates, but found that adding ovarian stimulation to any of the three interventions significantly increased pregnancy rate per cycle. One systematic review and one subsequent RCT have found that fallopian tube sperm perfusion significantly increased pregnancy rates compared with intrauterine insemination. One systematic review found no significant difference between intrauterine insemination with or without ovarian stimulation versus in vitro fertilisation for live birth rate.

LIKELY TO BE BENEFICIAL

Clomifene

One systematic review found limited evidence that clomifene versus placebo significantly increased rates of pregnancy per cycle.

Fallopian tube sperm perfusion (v intrauterine insemination)

One systematic review and one subsequent RCT have found that fallopian tube sperm perfusion(G) significantly increases pregnancy rates compared with intrauterine insemination.

UNKNOWN EFFECTIVENESS

Gamete intrafallopian transfer

We found no RCTs of gamete intrafallopian transfer versus no treatment. RCTs found conflicting effects on pregnancy rates of gamete intrafallopian transfer versus other treatments (intrauterine insemination, timed intercourse, and in vitro fertilisation).

In vitro fertilisation

One systematic review found no significant difference between in vitro fertilisation and expectant management for pregnancy rate. It found no significant difference between in vitro fertilisation versus gamete intrafallopian transfer or versus intraterine insemination with or without ovarian stimulation for live birth rate.

DEFINITION Normal fertility has been defined as achieving a pregnancy within 2 years by regular sexual intercourse.[1] However, many define infertility as the failure to conceive after 1 year of unprotected intercourse. Infertility can be primary, in couples who have never conceived, or secondary, in couples who have previously conceived. Infertile couples include those who are sterile (who will never achieve a natural pregnancy) and those who are subfertile (who could eventually achieve a pregnancy).

INCIDENCE/ PREVALENCE Although there is no evidence of a major change in the prevalence of infertility, many more couples are seeking help than previously. Currently, about 1/7 couples in industrialised countries will seek medical advice for infertility.[2] Rates of primary infertility vary widely between countries, ranging from 10% in Africa to about 6% in North America and Europe.[1] Reported rates of secondary infertility are less reliable.

AETIOLOGY/ RISK FACTORS In the UK, nearly a third of infertility cases are unexplained. The rest are caused by ovulatory failure (27%), low sperm count or quality (19%), tubal damage (14%), endometriosis (5%), and other causes (5%).[3]

PROGNOSIS In developed countries, 80–90% of couples attempting to conceive are successful after 1 year and 95% after 2 years.[3] The chances of becoming pregnant vary with the cause and duration of infertility, the woman's age, the couple's previous pregnancy history, and the availability of different treatment options.[4,5] For the first 2–3 years of unexplained infertility, cumulative conception rates remain high (27–46%) but decrease with increasing age of the woman and duration of infertility. The background rates of spontaneous pregnancy in infertile couples can be calculated from longitudinal studies of infertile couples who have been observed without treatment.[4]

Please refer to CD-ROM for full text and references.

Menopausal symptoms

Search date March 2002

Edward Morris and Janice Rymer

What are the effects of medical treatments?

BENEFICIAL

Oestrogens

One systematic review and two subsequent RCTs have found that oestrogen versus placebo significantly improves vasomotor symptoms. Two systematic reviews and three subsequent RCTs have found that oestrogen prevents urinary tract infection and improves urogenital symptoms. One systematic review found that oestrogen reduced depressed mood. Four RCTs have found that oestrogen improves quality of life in the short term. Important adverse effects include venous thromboembolic disease, breast cancer, and endometrial cancer.

Progestogens

One systematic review and six additional RCTs found that progestogens reduce vasomotor symptoms. We found no good quality evidence on other outcomes, including quality of life.

Tibolone

One RCT has found that tibolone versus placebo significantly reduces vasomotor symptoms. A second RCT found that tibolone was not less effective than oestrogen/progestogen replacement therapy in reducing vasomotor symptoms. A third RCT found no significant differences in vasomotor symptoms between tibolone and oestrogen/progestogen replacement therapy. One RCT found no significant differences in vaginal dryness between tibolone and continuous hormone replacement therapy after 48 weeks, but found a significant improvement in sexual satisfaction with tibolone versus oestradiol plus noresthisterone. One RCT found that tibolone versus placebo improved sexual fantasies and arousability over 3 months. One RCT found that tibolone versus conjugated oestrogen significantly improved sexual desire and coital frequency.

LIKELY TO BE BENEFICIAL

Phyto-oestrogens

One RCT found that soy protein versus no phyto-oestrogens reduces the severity but not the frequency of vasomotor symptoms at 6 weeks. One RCT found no significant differences in vasomotor symptoms between isoflavone and placebo after 12 weeks, and another RCT found that isoflavone versus placebo reduced the severity of vasomotor symptoms over 12 weeks. One RCT found that soy flour versus placebo significantly reduced mean number of weekly hot flushes after 12 weeks, but another RCT found no significant difference between soy protein and placebo in vasomotor symptoms. One RCT found no significant difference in vasomotor symptoms between soy flour versus wheat flour over 12 weeks. One RCT (94 women) found no significant difference between soy protein and placebo at 3 months for psychological, musculoskeletal, and genitourinary symptoms.

UNKNOWN EFFECTIVENESS

Antidepressants

We found no RCTs on the effects of antidepressants on menopausal symptoms. ▶

Clonidine

One RCT found that transdermal clonidine versus placebo for 8 weeks reduced the number of women reporting hot flushes, and increased the number of women reporting reductions in intensity of hot flushes.

Testosterone

One RCT comparing methyltestosterone plus oestrogen versus oestrogen alone found that the addition of methyltestosterone significantly reduced hot flushes and a second RCT found no significant differences after 6 months. One crossover RCT found limited evidence that testosterone improved sexual enjoyment and libido and another RCT found no significant differences at 6 months. We found no RCTs evaluating effects on other commonly experienced menopausal symptoms with testosterone alone.

DEFINITION Menopause is defined as the end of the last menstrual period. A woman is deemed to be postmenopausal 1 year after her last period. For practical purposes most women are diagnosed as menopausal after 1 year of amenorrhoea. Menopausal symptoms often begin in the perimenopausal years.

INCIDENCE/PREVALENCE In the UK, the mean age for the start of the menopause is 50 years and 9 months. The median onset of the perimenopause is between 45.5–47.5 years. One Scottish survey (6096 women aged 45–54 years) found that 84% of women had experienced at least one of the classic menopausal symptoms, with 45% finding one or more symptoms a problem.[1]

AETIOLOGY/RISK FACTORS Urogenital symptoms of menopause are caused by decreased oestrogen concentrations, but the cause of vasomotor symptoms and psychological effects is complex and remains unclear.

PROGNOSIS Menopause is a physiological event. Its timing may be determined genetically. Although endocrine changes are permanent, menopausal symptoms such as hot flushes, which are experienced by about 70% of women, usually resolve with time.[2] However, some symptoms may remain the same or worsen, for example genital atrophy.

Please refer to CD-ROM for full text and references.

Menorrhagia

Search date June 2002

Kirsten Duckitt

What are the effects of treatments?

BENEFICIAL

Endometrial thinning before hysteroscopic surgery

One systematic review has found that gonadotrophin releasing hormone analogues versus placebo or versus no treatment significantly reduce the duration of surgery, operative difficulty, and the risk of continuing to have moderate or heavy periods, and significantly increase the rate of postoperative amenorrhoea after 6–12 months. The review has found that gonadotrophin releasing hormone analogues versus danazol significantly increase the rate of postoperative amenorrhoea and significantly reduce the duration of surgery, but found no significant difference in operative difficulty. One small RCT found no significant difference between perioperative depot medroxyprogesterone acetate versus no perioperative hormonal treatment in amenorrhoea after 4 years' follow up.

Hysterectomy (*v* endometrial destruction) after medical failure

Systematic reviews have found that hysterectomy versus endometrial destruction significantly reduces menstrual blood loss, significantly increases patient satisfaction at 1 year, and significantly reduces the number of women requiring further operations within 1–4 years. RCTs have found no differences between different types of hysterectomy. One large cohort study reported major or minor complications in about a third of women undergoing hysterectomy.

Non-steroidal anti-inflammatory drugs

One systematic review has found that non-steroidal anti-inflammatory drugs versus placebo significantly reduce mean menstrual blood loss. One systematic review found no significant difference in menstrual blood loss with mefenamic acid versus naproxen, or with non-steroidal anti-inflammatory drugs versus oral progestogens, oral contraceptives, or progesterone releasing intrauterine devices.

Tranexamic acid

Systematic reviews have found that tranexamic acid versus placebo significantly reduces menstrual blood loss. One systematic review and several additional RCTs have found that tranexamic acid versus other drugs (oral progestogens, mefenamic acid, etamsylate, flurbiprofen, and diclofenac) also significantly reduces menstrual blood loss. Adverse effects of tranexamic acid include leg cramps and nausea in around a third of women. One long term observational study found no evidence to confirm the possibility of an increased risk of thromboembolism with tranexamic acid.

LIKELY TO BE BENEFICIAL

Hysteroscopic versus non-hysteroscopic endometrial destruction after medical failure

One systematic review found that hysteroscopic methods versus non-hysteroscopic methods of endometrial destruction significantly increased amenorrhoea at 12 months, although it found no significant differences with different types of hysteroscopic procedure versus each other in amenorrhoea or satisfaction rates.

Clin Evid Concise 2003;9:392–394.

TRADE OFF BETWEEN BENEFITS AND HARMS

Danazol

One systematic review found that danazol versus placebo, luteal phase oral progestogens, mefenamic acid, naproxen, or oral contraceptives reduced blood loss but that danazol versus either NSAIDs or oral progestogens significantly increased adverse effects. A second review found that danazol versus placebo significantly reduced menstrual blood loss after 2–3 months.

UNKNOWN EFFECTIVENESS

Combined oral contraceptives

One systematic review found insufficient evidence on the effects of oral contraceptives in the treatment of menorrhagia.

Endometrial resection versus medical treatment

One systematic review and one additional RCT compared transcervical endometrial resection versus medical treatment and found conflicting results. RCTs have found complications in 0–15% of women undergoing endometrial destruction.

Etamsylate

One RCT found limited evidence that etamsylate versus tranexamic acid or versus mefenamic acid significantly increased menstrual blood loss.

Intrauterine progestogens

We found no RCTs comparing intrauterine progestogens versus placebo. Two systematic reviews and two subsequent RCTs found conflicting evidence about menstrual blood loss, satisfaction rates, and quality of life scores with levonorgestrel releasing intrauterine devices versus other treatments (endometrial resection, norethisterone, medical treatment, non-steroidal anti-inflammatory drugs, and hysterectomy).

Dilatation and curettage after medical failure; gonadorelin (GnRH; gonadotrophin releasing hormone) analogues; myomectomy after medical failure

We found no RCTs on the effects of these interventions.

UNLIKELY TO BE BENEFICIAL

Oral progestogens (longer cycle)

We found no RCTs comparing oral progestogens versus placebo. One RCT found no significant difference in menstrual blood loss with 21 days per cycle of oral progestogen (oral noresthisterone) versus a levonorgestrel releasing intrauterine device.

LIKELY TO BE INEFFECTIVE OR HARMFUL

Oral progestogens in luteal phase only

We found no RCTs comparing oral progestogens versus placebo. One systematic review has found that luteal phase oral progestogens versus danazol, tranexamic acid, or a progesterone releasing intrauterine device significantly increase mean menstrual blood loss.

DEFINITION Menorrhagia is defined as heavy but regular menstrual bleeding. Idiopathic ovulatory menorrhagia is regular heavy bleeding in the absence of recognisable pelvic pathology or a general bleeding disorder. Objective menorrhagia is taken to be a total menstrual blood loss of 80 mL or more each menstruation.[1] Subjectively, menorrhagia may be defined as a complaint of regular excessive menstrual blood loss occurring over several consecutive cycles in a woman of reproductive years.

Menorrhagia

INCIDENCE/ PREVALENCE In the UK, 5% of women (aged 30–49 years) consult their general practitioner each year with menorrhagia.[2] In New Zealand, 2–4% of primary care consultations by premenopausal women are for menstrual problems.[3]

AETIOLOGY/ RISK FACTORS Idiopathic ovulatory menorrhagia is thought to be caused by disordered prostaglandin production within the endometrium.[4] Prostaglandins may also be implicated in menorrhagia associated with uterine fibroids, adenomyosis, or the presence of an intrauterine device. Fibroids have been reported in 10% of women with menorrhagia (80–100 mL/cycle) and 40% of those with severe menorrhagia (≥ 200 mL/cycle).[5]

PROGNOSIS Menorrhagia limits normal activities and causes iron deficiency anaemia in two thirds of women proved to have objective menorrhagia.[1,6,7] One in five women in the UK and one in three women in the USA will have a hysterectomy before the age of 60 years; menorrhagia is the main presenting problem in at least 50% of these women.[8–10] About 50% of the women who have a hysterectomy for menorrhagia have a normal uterus removed.[11]

Please refer to CD-ROM for full text and references.

Ovarian cancer

Search date February 2002

Hani Gabra, Charles Redman, and Jennifer Byrom

What are the effects of treatments for ovarian cancer that is advanced at first presentation?

BENEFICIAL

Adding platinum to chemotherapy regimens

One systematic review has found that adding platinum to any non-platinum regimen significantly improves survival, particularly if platinum is added to a combination regimen.

LIKELY TO BE BENEFICIAL

Adding paclitaxel to platinum regimens

One systematic review and one additional RCT have found that adding paclitaxel to platinum based chemotherapy versus platinum based chemotherapy alone significantly improves progression free survival and overall survival after primary surgery for advanced ovarian cancer.

Combination platinum regimens versus combination non-platinum regimens

Seven RCTs have compared combination platinum regimens versus many different non-platinum combination regimens. Most RCTs have found that platinum regimens improve outcomes, although benefits and harms depend on the regimens being compared. None have found that platinum significantly decreased progression free survival or overall survival.

TRADE OFF BETWEEN BENEFITS AND HARMS

Combination platinum regimens versus single agent platinum regimens

One systematic review and three additional RCTs found no evidence that combination platinum based regimens improved progression free survival or overall survival compared with single agent platinum regimens.

UNKNOWN EFFECTIVENESS

Carboplatin plus paclitaxel versus carboplatin plus docetaxel

We found no RCTs of sufficient quality comparing the effects of carboplatin plus paclitaxel versus carboplatin plus docetaxel.

Paclitaxel plus cisplatin versus paclitaxel plus carboplatin

One RCT found no significant difference in progression free survival or overall survival between paclitaxel plus cisplatin versus paclitaxel plus carboplatin, although it may have lacked power to exclude a clinically important difference.

Routine interval debulking after primary surgery plus chemotherapy

One RCT found that interval debulking**G** after primary surgery plus chemotherapy versus continued chemotherapy without debaulking significantly improved overall survival over about 3.5 years. A second RCT found that interval debaulking had no significant effect on survival, but it was was probably underpowered to detect a clinically important effect.

Primary surgery versus no surgery; Primary surgery plus chemotherapy versus chemotherapy alone

We found no RCTs about the effects of these interventions.

Clin Evid Concise 2003;9:395–396.

UNLIKELY TO BE BENEFICIAL

Routine second look surgery

Two RCTs have no evidence that routine second look surgery**G** improves overall survival compared with watchful waiting in women undergoing chemotherapy after primary surgery for advanced ovarian cancer.

DEFINITION Ovarian tumours are classified according to the assumed cell type of origin (surface epithelium, stroma, or germ cells). Most malignant ovarian tumours (85–95%) are derived from the epithelium of the ovarian surface, and are thus termed epithelial.[1] These can be further grouped into histological types (serous, mucinous, endometroid, and clear cell). Epithelial ovarian cancer is staged using the FIGO classification**T**. This review concerns only advanced epithelial ovarian cancer, which is regarded as FIGO stages II–IV.

INCIDENCE/ PREVALENCE The worldwide annual incidence of ovarian cancer exceeds 140 000.[2] Rates vary between countries. Differences in reproductive patterns, including age of menarche and menopause, gravidity, breast feeding, and use of the oral contraceptive pill may contribute to this variation. Rates are highest in Scandinavia, Northern America and the UK and lowest for Africa, India, China, and Japan.[3] In the UK, ovarian cancer is the fourth most common malignancy in women and is the leading cause of death from gynaecological cancers, with a lifetime risk of about 2%.[4] In the UK, the incidence was 5174 in 1988[5] and 6880 in 1998.[6] The incidence of ovarian cancer seems to be stabilising in some other countries, and in more affluent countries (Finland, Denmark, New Zealand, and the USA) rates are declining.

AETIOLOGY/ RISK FACTORS Risk factors include increasing age, family history of ovarian cancer, low fertility, use of fertility drugs, and low parity.[7–11] Case control studies found that using the combined oral contraceptive pill for more than 5 years was associated with a 40% reduction in the risk of ovarian cancer.[3,7,12,13]

PROGNOSIS Over 80% of women present with advanced disease, and the overall 5 year survival rates are poor (< 30%).[14] For advanced disease the major independent prognostic factors seem to be stage, and residual tumour mass after surgery.

Please refer to CD-ROM for full text and references.

Premalignant vulval disorders

Search date May 2002

Clinical Evidence freelance writers

What are the effects of treatments for lichen sclerosus?

LIKELY TO BE BENEFICIAL

Topical clobetasol propionate (0.05%)

One small RCT found that topical clobetasol propionate controlled symptoms more effectively than topical testosterone propionate or petroleum jelly after 3 months' treatment. Good quality prospective observational studies reported minimal adverse effects when clobetasol propionate was used as required for maintenance treatment.

TRADE OFF BETWEEN BENEFITS AND HARMS

Oral retinoids (acitretin)

One small RCT found acitretin significantly reduced itching and extent of compared with placebo after 20–22 weeks, but was associated with severe skin peeling and hair.

UNKNOWN EFFECTIVENESS

Surgery (vulvectomy⊕, cryosurgery, laser)

We found insufficient evidence on the effects of surgery in women with lichen sclerosis.

LIKELY TO BE INEFFECTIVE OR HARMFUL

Topical testosterone

Two small RCTs found no evidence that testosterone propionate improved symptoms more than petroleum jelly, either as initial treatment for 12 months or after 16 weeks' treatment in women previously treated with clobetasol propionate. Testosterone propionate is associated with virilisation.

What are the effects of treatments for vulval intraepithelial neoplasia?

UNKNOWN EFFECTIVENESS

Surgical treatments, topical α interferon

We found insufficient evidence on the effects of surgical or topical treatments in women with vulval intraepithelial neoplasia.

DEFINITION There are two recognised premalignant conditions of the vulva. **Lichen sclerosus** is characterised by epithelial thinning, inflammation, and distinctive histological changes in the dermis. It affects all age groups but is typically found in the anogenital region in postmenopausal women. The most common presentation is severe intractable itching (pruritus vulvae) and vaginal soreness with dyspareunia. **Vulval intraepithelial neoplasia (VIN)** is dysplasia of the vulval epithelium, categorised as mild (VIN I), moderate (VIN II), or severe (VIN III). The vulval lesions are often multifocal and are usually associated with itching and pain.

INCIDENCE/ PREVALENCE We found no data on the prevalence of lichen sclerosus. The true incidence of vulval intraepithelial neoplasia is unknown, but it is being diagnosed with increased frequency in the UK and the USA. This may be because of increased recognition of the disease or a true increase in incidence.[1–3]

▶

Clin Evid Concise 2003;9:397–398.

Premalignant vulval disorders

AETIOLOGY/ RISK FACTORS The cause is unknown. Vulval intraepithelial neoplasia is associated with human papilloma virus 16.[1]

PROGNOSIS There is currently no cure for lichen sclerosus. The risk of progression to vulval carcinoma ranges from 0–9%.[4] People with concomitant squamous cell hyperplasia are at increased risk of malignancy.[5] Malignant transformation has been reported in 2–4% of women with VIN III but the incidence appears to be lower in women with VIN I and II.[2,6] About 30% of vulval carcinomas are associated with vulval intraepithelial neoplasia.[1]

Please refer to CD-ROM for full text and references.

Premenstrual syndrome

Search date October 2002

Katrina Wyatt

What are the effects of treatments?

BENEFICIAL

Diuretics

RCTs have found that spironolactone improves symptoms of premenstrual syndrome including breast tenderness and bloating, compared to placebo. Two RCTs have found that metolazone or ammonium chloride versus placebo reduce premenstrual swelling and weight gain.

Non-steroidal anti-inflammatory drugs

RCTs found that prostaglandin inhibitors significantly improved a range of premenstrual symptoms but did not reduce premenstrual breast pain, compared to placebo.

Selective serotonin reuptake inhibitors

One systematic review and subsequent RCTs have found that selective serotonin reuptake inhibitors significantly improve premenstrual symptoms, but cause frequent adverse events compared to placebo.

LIKELY TO BE BENEFICIAL

Cognitive behavioural therapy

RCTs found that cognitive behavioural therapy significantly reduced premenstrual symptoms compared to control treatments, but the evidence is insufficient to define the size of an effect.

Exercise

One RCT has found that aerobic exercise significantly improves premenstrual symptoms compared to placebo. Another RCT has found that high intensity aerobic exercise improves symptoms significantly more than low intensity.

Oestrogens

Limited evidence from small RCTs suggests that oestradiol improves symptoms compared to placebo, but the magnitude of any effect remains unclear.

Oral contraceptives

RCTs found limited evidence that oral contraceptives improved premenstrual symptoms compared to placebo.

TRADE OFF BETWEEN BENEFITS AND HARMS

Bromocriptine (breast symptoms only)

RCTs have found limited evidence that bromocriptine relieves breast tenderness compared to placebo, although adverse effects are common.

Danazol

RCTs have found that danazol significantly reduces premenstrual symptoms compared to placebo, but has important adverse effects associated with masculinisation when used continuously in the long term.

Gonadorelin analogues

RCTs have found that gonadorelin analogues (GnRH in previous nomenclatrues) significantly reduce premenstrual symptoms compared to placebo. RCTs have found that gonadorelin plus oestrogen plus progestogen (addback treatment) improves symptom scores less than that gonadorelin analogue alone but more ▶

than placebo. One small RCT found a similar reduction in symptom scores with gonadorelin analogue plus tibolone compared to gonadorelin analogue plus placebo. Treatment with gonadorelin analogues for more than 6 months carries a significant risk of osteoporosis, limiting their usefulness for long term treatment.

Non-selective serotonin reuptake inhibitor antidepressants/anxiolytics

RCTs have found that non-selective serotonin reuptake inhibitor antidepressants and anxiolytic drugs significantly improve at least one symptom of premenstrual syndrome compared to placebo, but a proportion of women stop treatment because of adverse effects. We found insufficient evidence from small RCTs about effects of β blockers and lithium.

UNKNOWN EFFECTIVENESS

Hysterectomy with or without bilateral oophorectomy

We found no RCTs. Observational studies have found that hysterectomy plus bilateral oophorectomy is curative. Hysterectomy alone may reduce symptoms, but evidence is limited because of the difficulty in providing controls. The risks are those of major surgery. Infertility is an irreversible consequence of bilateral oophorectomy.

Progestogens

We found insufficient evidence from one small RCT about the effects of progestogens compared to placebo.

Pyridoxine

One systematic review of poor quality RCTs found insufficient evidence about the effects of pyridoxine (vitamin B_6). In the review, an analysis of weak RCTs suggested that pyridoxine significantly reduced symptoms compared to placebo. Additional RCTs with weak methods found conflicting evidence on the effects of pyridoxine.

Tibolone

One small RCT found limited evidence that tibolone improved premenstrual symptom score compared to placebo (multivitamins).

Chiropractic treatment; dietary supplements; endometrial ablation; evening primrose oil; laparoscopic bilateral oophorectomy; reflexology; relaxation treatment

We found insufficient evidence about the effects of these interventions.

LIKELY TO BE INEFFECTIVE OR HARMFUL

Progesterone

One systematic review of progesterone has found a small but significant improvement in overall premenstrual symptoms and no increase in the frequency of withdrawals caused by adverse effects, compared to placebo. However, the improvement is unlikely to be clinically important. It remains unclear whether the route or timing of administration of progesterone is important.

DEFINITION A woman has premenstrual syndrome if she complains of recurrent psychological or somatic symptoms (or both) occurring specifically during the luteal phase of the menstrual cycle and resolving by the end of menstruation Ⓣ.[1]

INCIDENCE/ PREVALENCE Premenstrual symptoms occur in 95% of all women of reproductive age; severe, debilitating symptoms (premenstrual syndrome) Ⓖ occur in about 5% of those women.[1]

AETIOLOGY/ RISK FACTORS The aetiology is unknown, but hormonal and other (possibly neuroendocrine) factors probably contribute.[2,3] There may be enhanced sensitivity to progesterone, possibly caused by a deficiency of serotonin.[2]

PROGNOSIS Except after oophorectomy, symptoms usually recur when treatment is stopped.

Please refer to CD-ROM for full text and references.

Pyelonephritis in non-pregnant women

Search date March 2002

Bruce Cooper

What are the effects of treatments?

LIKELY TO BE BENEFICIAL

Intravenous antibiotics (ampicillin, co-trimoxazole) in women admitted to hospital with uncomplicated infection

We found no RCTs comparing intravenous antibiotics versus no antibiotics, however, it is unlikely that such an RCT would now be performed. One RCT in women admitted to hospital with uncomplicated pyelonephritis found no significant difference with intravenous ampicillin plus intravenous gentamicin versus intravenous co-trimoxazole plus intravenous gentamicin in clinical response or recurrence of bacteria in the urine. One RCT in women admitted with uncomplicated pylonephritis found no significant difference with a single dose of intravenous tobramycin plus oral ciprofloxacin versus oral ciprofloxacin plus placebo in rates of clinical success with treatment. We found no well designed trials comparing newer intravenous antibiotics versus older regimens.

Oral antibiotics (co-trimoxazole, co-amoxiclav, or a fluoroquinolone) for women with uncomplicated infection

We found no RCTs comparing oral antibiotics versus no antibiotics; however, it is unlikely that such an RCT would now be performed. One systematic review and one subsequent RCT in women with uncomplicated pyelonephritis have found no consistent differences between oral co-trimoxazole, co-amoxiclav, or a fluoroquinolone (ciprofloxacin, norfloxacin, levofloxacin, or lomefloxacin) in bacteriological or clinical cure rates.

UNKNOWN EFFECTIVENESS

Inpatient versus outpatient management

We found no RCTs comparing inpatient versus outpatient management of women with acute uncomplicated pyelonephritis.

DEFINITION Acute pyelonephritis, or upper urinary tract infection, is an infection of the kidney characterised by pain when passing urine, fever, flank pain, nausea and vomiting. White blood cells are almost always present in the urine and occasionally white blood cell casts are also seen on urine microscopy. Uncomplicated infection occurs in an otherwise healthy person without any other underlying disease. Complicated infection occurs in people with structural or functional urinary tract abnormalities or additional diseases. People with acute pyelonephritis may also be divided into those able to take oral antibiotics and without signs of sepsis who may be managed at home, and those requiring treatment delivered by injection whilst in hospital.

INCIDENCE/ PREVALENCE In the USA, there are 250 000 cases of acute pyelonephritis a year.[1] Worldwide prevalence and incidence are unknown.

Pyelonephritis in non-pregnant women

AETIOLOGY/ RISK FACTORS Pyelonephritis is most commonly caused when bacteria in the bladder ascend the ureters and invade the kidneys. In some cases, this may result in bacteria entering and multiplying in the bloodstream.

PROGNOSIS Complications include sepsis, infection that spreads to other organs, renal impairment, and renal abscess formation. Conditions such as underlying renal disease, diabetes mellitus, and immunosuppression may worsen prognosis, with a potential increase in risk of sepsis and death, but we found no good long term evidence about such people.

Please refer to CD-ROM for full text and references.

Recurrent cystitis in non-pregnant women

Search date August 2002

Clinical Evidence freelance writers

What are the effects of interventions to prevent further recurrence of cystitis?

BENEFICIAL

Continuous antibiotic prophylaxis (trimethoprim, co-trimoxazole, nitrofurantoin, cefaclor, or a quinolone)

RCTs have found that continuous antibiotic prophylaxis lasting 6–12 months with trimethoprim, co-trimoxazole, nitrofurantoin, cefaclor, or a quinolone significantly reduces rates of recurrent cystitis compared with placebo**T**. However, the RCTs found no consistent difference in recurrence rate among different regimens. One RCT comparing continuous daily antibiotic prophylaxis versus postcoital antibiotic prophylaxis found no significant difference in rates of positive urine culture after 1 year.

Postcoital antibiotic prophylaxis (co-trimoxazole, nitrofurantoin, or a quinolone)

Four RCTs have found that co-trimoxazole, nitrofurantoin, or a quinolone up to 2 hours after sexual intercourse significantly reduces the rates of cystitis compared with placebo**T**. One RCT comparing continuous daily antibiotic prophylaxis versus postcoital antibiotic prophylaxis found no significant difference in rates of positive urine culture after 1 year.

UNKNOWN EFFECTIVENESS

Cranberry juice and cranberry products

One systematic review found insufficient evidence on the effects of cranberry juice and other cranberry products on recurrent cystitis.

Prophylaxis with methenamine hippurate

We found no reliable RCTs on the effects of methenamine hippurate (hexamine hippurate).

Single dose self administered co-trimoxazole

One small RCT found that continuous co-trimoxazole prophylaxis versus single dose self administered co-trimoxazole started at the onset of cystitis symptoms significantly reduced the number of episodes of cystitis within 1 year. However, evidence was too limited to draw firm conclusions.

DEFINITION Cystitis is an infection of the lower urinary tract, which causes pain when passing urine, and causes frequency, urgency, haematuria, or suprapubic pain not associated with passing urine. White blood cells and bacteria are almost always present in the urine. The presence of fever, flank pain, nausea, or vomiting suggests pyelonephritis (upper urinary tract infection) (see pyelonephritis in non-pregnant women, p 402). Recurrent cystitis may be either a reinfection (after successful eradication of infection) or a relapse after inadequate treatment.

INCIDENCE/ PREVALENCE The incidence of cystitis among premenopausal sexually active women is 0.5–0.7 infections per person year,[1] and 20–40% of women will experience cystitis during their lifetime. Of those, 20% will develop recurrence, almost always (90% of cases) because of reinfection rather than relapse. Rates of infection fall during the winter months.[2]

Clin Evid Concise 2003;9:404–405.

Recurrent cystitis in non-pregnant women

AETIOLOGY/ RISK FACTORS Cystitis is caused by uropathogenic bacteria in the faecal flora that colonise the vaginal and periurethral openings, and ascend the urethra into the bladder. Prior infection, sexual intercourse, and exposure to vaginal spermicide are risk factors for developing cystitis.[3,4]

PROGNOSIS We found little evidence on the long term effects of untreated cystitis. One study found that progression to pyelonephritis was infrequent, and that most cases of cystitis regressed spontaneously, although symptoms sometimes persisted for several months.[5] Women with a baseline rate of more than two infections a year, over many years, are likely to have ongoing recurrent infections.[6]

Please refer to CD-ROM for full text and references.

Bites (mammalian)

Search date July 2002

Iara Marques de Medeiros and Humberto Saconato

What are the effects of interventions to prevent and treat mammalian bites?

LIKELY TO BE BENEFICIAL

Antibiotics for treatment of infected mammalian bites*

We found no RCTs of antibiotics versus placebo for infected mammalian bites. However, there is consensus that antibiotics are likely to be beneficial

Antibiotic prophylaxis

Limited evidence from one systematic review found no significant difference with antibiotics versus control in the infection rate in people bitten by a dog, cat, or human in the preceding 24 hours. Meta-analysis according to the site of the wound found that antibiotics significantly reduced infections of the hand. One small RCT in the review found that in people with human bites, antibiotics versus control significantly reduced the rate of infection.

Debridement, irrigation, and decontamination*

We found no reliable studies assessing debridement, irrigation, decontamination measures, or serum infiltration in the wound. However, there is consensus that such measures are likely to be beneficial.

Education to prevent bites

We found no RCTs of the effect of education programmes on the incidence of mammalian bites. One RCT found that an educational programme versus no education in school children significantly increased precautionary behaviour around dogs.

*No RCT evidence, but there is consensus that treatment is likely to be beneficial.

UNKNOWN EFFECTIVENESS

Comparative effectiveness of different antibiotics for treatment of infected mammalian bites

One RCT in people with infected and uninfected animal and human bites comparing penicillin with or without dicloxacillin versus amoxicillin/clavulanic acid found no significant difference in failure rate (which was undefined).

Education to prevent bites in specific occupational groups

We found no RCTs of education to prevent bites in specific occupational groups.

Primary wound closure

One poor quality RCT comparing primary wound closure versus no closure in people with dog bites found no significant difference in the incidence of infection, but the RCT was too small to exclude clinically important effects.

Tetanus toxoid after mammalian bites

We found no evidence on the effects of tetanus toxoid in preventing tetanus after human or animal bites.

DEFINITION Bite wounds are mainly caused by humans, dogs, or cats. They include superficial abrasions(G) (30–43%), lacerations(G) (31–45%), and puncture(G) wounds (13–34%).[1]

Clin Evid Concise 2003;9:406–407.

INCIDENCE/ PREVALENCE In areas where rabies is poorly controlled among domestic animals, dogs account for 90% of reported mammalian bites compared with less than 5% in areas where rabies is well controlled. In the USA, an estimated 3.5–4.7 million dog bites occur each year.[2] About one in five people bitten by a dog seek medical attention, and 1% of those require admission to hospital.[3,4] Between a third and half of all mammalian bites occur in children.[5]

AETIOLOGY/ RISK FACTORS In over 70% of cases, people are bitten by their own pets or by an animal known to them. Males are more likely to be bitten than females, and are more likely to be bitten by dogs, whereas females are more likely to be bitten by cats.[2] One study found that children under 5 years old were significantly more likely than older children to provoke animals before being bitten.[6] One study of infected dog and cat bites found that the most commonly isolated bacteria was *Pasteurella*, followed by *Streptococci*, *Staphylococci*, *Moraxella*, *Corynebacterium*, and *Neisseria*.[7] Mixed aerobic and anaerobic infection was more common than anaerobic infection alone.

PROGNOSIS In the USA, dog bites cause about 20 deaths a year.[8] In children, dog bites frequently involve the face, potentially resulting in severe lacerations and scarring.[9] Rabies, a life threatening viral encephalitis, may be contracted as a consequence of being bitten or scratched by a rabid animal. More than 99% of human rabies is in developing countries where canine rabies is endemic.[10]

Please refer to CD-ROM for full text and references.

Pressure sores

Search date February 2002

Nicky Cullum, E Andrea Nelson, and Jane Nixon

What are the effects of preventive interventions?

BENEFICIAL

Foam alternatives (*v* standard foam mattresses)

A meta-analysis of five RCTs has found that foam alternatives versus standard hospital foam mattresses significantly reduce the incidence of pressure sores after 10–14 days in people at high risk.

Pressure relieving overlays on operating tables

One systematic review has found that the use of pressure relieving overlays on operating tables significantly reduces the incidence of pressure sores.

LIKELY TO BE BENEFICIAL

Low air loss beds in intensive care (*v* standard beds)

One RCT found that low air loss beds**G** versus standard beds significantly reduced the risk of new pressure sores over the duration of the trial (not specified).

Medical sheepskin overlays

One RCT in people aged 60 years or over undergoing orthopaedic surgery has found that medical sheepskins versus standard treatment significantly reduces the incidence of pressure sores after an unstated period.

UNKNOWN EFFECTIVENESS

Alternating pressure surfaces G; different seat cushions; electric profiling beds; low air loss hydrotherapy beds; low tech constant low pressure supports G; repositioning (regular "turning"); topical lotions and dressings

We found insufficient evidence about the effects of these interventions in preventing pressure sores.

LIKELY TO BE INEFFECTIVE OR HARMFUL

Air filled vinyl boots with foot cradle

One small RCT found that air filled vinyl boots with foot cradles versus hospital pillows were associated with a significantly faster rate of development of pressure sores.

What are the effects of treatments?

LIKELY TO BE BENEFICIAL

Air fluidised supports (*v* standard care)

Two RCTs in people in hospital found that air fluidised supports**G** versus standard care healed more established sores. One RCT in people cared for at home found no significant difference with air fluidised supports versus standard care in healing; this trial had a high withdrawal rate.

Clin Evid Concise 2003;9:408–409.

UNKNOWN EFFECTIVENESS

Alternating pressure surfaces; debridement; electrotherapy; hydrocolloid dressings (*v* gauze soaked in saline or hypochlorite); low air loss beds; low level laser therapy; low tech constant low pressure supports; nutritional supplements; other dressings; seat cushions; surgery; topical negative pressure⊖; topical phenytoin; therapeutic ultrasound

We found insufficient evidence on the effects of these interventions in healing pressure sores.

DEFINITION Pressure sores (also known as pressure ulcers, bed sores, and decubitus ulcers) may present as persistently hyperaemic, blistered, broken, or necrotic skin, and may extend to underlying structures, including muscle and bone. Whether blanching and non-blanching erythema constitute pressure sores remains controversial.

INCIDENCE/ PREVALENCE The most comprehensive data on prevalence and incidence come from hospital populations. Studies have found prevalences of 6–10% in National Health Service hospitals in the UK,[1] and 8% in a teaching hospital in the USA.[2]

AETIOLOGY/ RISK FACTORS Pressure sores are caused by unrelieved pressure, shear, or friction, and are most common below the waist and at bony prominences such as the sacrum, heels, and hips. They occur in all healthcare settings. Increased age, reduced mobility, and impaired nutrition emerge consistently as risk factors.[3] However, the relative importance of these and other factors is uncertain.

PROGNOSIS The presence of pressure sores has been associated with a two- to fourfold increased risk of death in elderly people and people in intensive care.[4,5] However, pressure sores are a marker for underlying disease severity and other comorbidities rather than an independent predictor of mortality.[4] Pressure sores vary considerably in size and severity.

Please refer to CD-ROM for full text and references.

Venous leg ulcers

Search date February 2002

E Andrea Nelson, Nicky Cullum, and June Jones

What are the effects of treatments?

BENEFICIAL

Compression

One systematic review has found that compression versus no compression significantly increases the proportion of venous leg ulcers healed.

Pentoxifylline

One systematic review has found that oral pentoxifylline (oxpentifylline) versus placebo significantly increases the proportion of ulcers healed at 6 months.

LIKELY TO BE BENEFICIAL

Cultured allogenic bilayer skin replacement

One RCT found that cultured allogenic bilayer skin replacement**G** versus a non-adherent dressing significantly increased the proportion of ulcers healed after 6 months.

Flavonoids

Two RCTs have found that flavonoids versus placebo or versus standard care significantly increase the proportion of ulcers healed.

Peri-ulcer injection of granulocyte–macrophage colony stimulating factor (GM-CSF)

One RCT found that peri-ulcer injection of GM-CSF versus placebo significantly increased the proportion of ulcers healed after 13 weeks' treatment.

Systemic mesoglycan

One RCT found that systemic mesoglycan plus compression versus compression alone significantly increased the proportion of ulcers healed after 24 weeks' treatment.

UNKNOWN EFFECTIVENESS

Antimicrobial agents; aspirin; debriding agents; foam, film, or alginate (semi-occlusive) dressings versus simple dressings in the presence of compression; intermittent pneumatic compression; low level laser treatment; oral zinc; skin grafting; thromboxane α_2 antagonists; topical calcitonin gene related peptide plus vasoactive intestinal polypeptide; topical mesoglycan; topical negative pressure; therapeutic ultrasound; vein surgery

We found insufficient evidence on the effects of these interventions on ulcer healing.

Sulodexide

One RCT found limited evidence that sulodexide plus compression versus compression alone significantly increased the proportion of ulcers healed after 60 days' treatment.

UNLIKELY TO BE BENEFICIAL

Hydrocolloid (occlusive) dressings versus simple low adherent dressings in the presence of compression

One systematic review found that, in the presence of compression, hydrocolloid dressings did not heal more venous leg ulcers than simple, low adherent dressings.

Clin Evid Concise 2003;9:410–411.

Topically applied autologous platelet lysate

One RCT found no significant difference after 9 months in time to healing of ulcers with topically applied autologous platelet lysate versus placebo.

What are the effects of interventions to prevent recurrence?

LIKELY TO BE BENEFICIAL

Compression

One RCT found that compression stockings versus no stockings significantly reduced the risk of ulcer recurrence after 6 months.

UNKNOWN EFFECTIVENESS

Rutoside; stanozolol; vein surgery

We found insufficient evidence on the effects of these interventions on ulcer recurrence.

DEFINITION Definitions of leg ulcers vary, but the following is widely used: loss of skin on the leg or foot that takes more than 6 weeks to heal. Some definitions exclude ulcers confined to the foot, whereas others include ulcers on the whole of the lower limb. This review deals with ulcers of venous origin in people without concurrent diabetes mellitus, arterial insufficiency, or rheumatoid arthritis.

INCIDENCE/ PREVALENCE Between 1.5 and 3/1000 people have active leg ulcers. Prevalence increases with age to about 20/1000 in people aged over 80 years.[1]

AETIOLOGY/ RISK FACTORS Leg ulceration is strongly associated with venous disease. However, about a fifth of people with leg ulceration have arterial disease, either alone or in combination with venous problems, which may require specialist referral.[1] Venous ulcers (also known as varicose or stasis ulcers) are caused by venous reflux or obstruction, both of which lead to poor venous return and venous hypertension.

PROGNOSIS People with leg ulcers have a poorer quality of life than age matched controls because of pain, odour, and reduced mobility.[2] In the UK, audits have found wide variation in the types of care (hospital inpatient care, hospital clinics, outpatient clinics, home visits), in the treatments used (topical agents, dressings, bandages, stockings), in healing rates, and in recurrence rates (26–69% in 1 year).[3,4]

Please refer to CD-ROM for full text and references.

Note

When looking up a class of drug, the reader is advised to also look up specific examples of that class of drug where additional entries may be found. The reverse situation also applies. Abbreviations used: CVD, cardiovascular disease; HRT, hormone replacement therapy; IVF, in vitro fertilisation; MI, myocardial infarction; NSAIDs, non-steroidal anti-inflammatory drugs; STD, sexually transmitted disease.

INDEX

Subject index

Subject index

Subject index

Subject index

Subject index

Estimating cardiovascular risk and treatment benefit

Adapted from the New Zealand guidelines on management of dyslipidaemia[1] and raised blood pressure[2] by Rod Jackson

How to use these colour charts

The charts help the estimation of a person's absolute risk of a cardiovascular event and the likely benefit of drug treatment to lower cholesterol or blood pressure. For these charts, cardiovascular events include: new angina, myocardial infarction, coronary death, stroke or transient ischaemic attack (TIA), onset of congestive cardiac failure, or peripheral vascular syndrome.

There is a group of patients in whom risk can be assumed to be high (>20% in 5 years) without using the charts. They include those with symptomatic cardiovascular disease (angina, myocardial infarction, congestive heart failure, stroke, TIA, and peripheral vascular disease), or left ventricular hypertrophy on ECG.

To estimate a person's absolute 5 year risk:

- Find the table relating to their sex, diabetic status (on insulin, oral hypoglycaemics, or fasting blood glucose over 8 mmol/L), smoking status, and age. The age shown in the charts is the mean for that category, i.e. age 60 = 55 to 65 years.
- Within the table find the cell nearest to the person's blood pressure and total cholesterol : HDL ratio. For risk assessment it is enough to use a mean blood pressure based on two readings on each of two occasions, and cholesterol measurements based on one laboratory or two non-fasting Reflotron measurements. More readings are needed to establish the pre-treatment baseline.
- The colour of the box indicates the person's 5 year cardiovascular disease risk (see below).

Notes: (1) People with a strong history of CVD (first degree male relatives with CVD before 55 years, female relatives before 65 years) or obesity (body mass index above 30 kg/m^2) are likely to be at greater risk than the tables indicate. The magnitude of the independent predictive value of these risk factors remains unclear — their presence should influence treatment decisions for patients at borderline treatment levels. (2) If total cholesterol or total cholesterol : HDL ratio is greater than 8 then the risk is at least 15%. (3) Nearly all people aged 75 years or over also have an absolute cardiovascular risk over 15%.

Charts reproduced with permission from The National Heart Foundation of New Zealand. Also available on http://www.nzgg.org.nz/library/gl_complete/bloodpressure/table1.cfm.

REFERENCES

1. Dyslipidaemia Advisory Group. 1996 National Heart Foundation clinical guidelines for the assessment and management of dyslipidaemia. *NZ Med J* 1996;109:224–232.
2. National Health Committee. Guidelines for the management of mildly raised blood pressure in New Zealand: Ministry of Health National Health Committee Report, Wellington, 1995.

RISK LEVEL 5 year CVD risk (non-fatal and fatal)		**BENEFIT (1)** CVD events prevented per 100 treated for 5 years*	**BENEFIT (2)** Number needed to treat for 5 years to prevent one event*
Very High	>30%	>10 per 100	<10
	25–30%	9 per 100	11
	20–25%	7.5 per 100	13
High	15–20%	6 per 100	16
Moderate	10–15%	4 per 100	25
Mild	5–10%	2.5 per 100	40
	2.5–5%	1.25 per 100	80
	<2.5%	<0.8 per 100	>120

*Based on a 20% reduction in total cholesterol or a reduction in blood pressure of 10–15 mm Hg systolic or 5–10 mm Hg diastolic, which is estimated to reduce CVD risk by about a third over 5 years.

Estimating cardiovascular risk and treatment benefit

RISK LEVEL: MEN

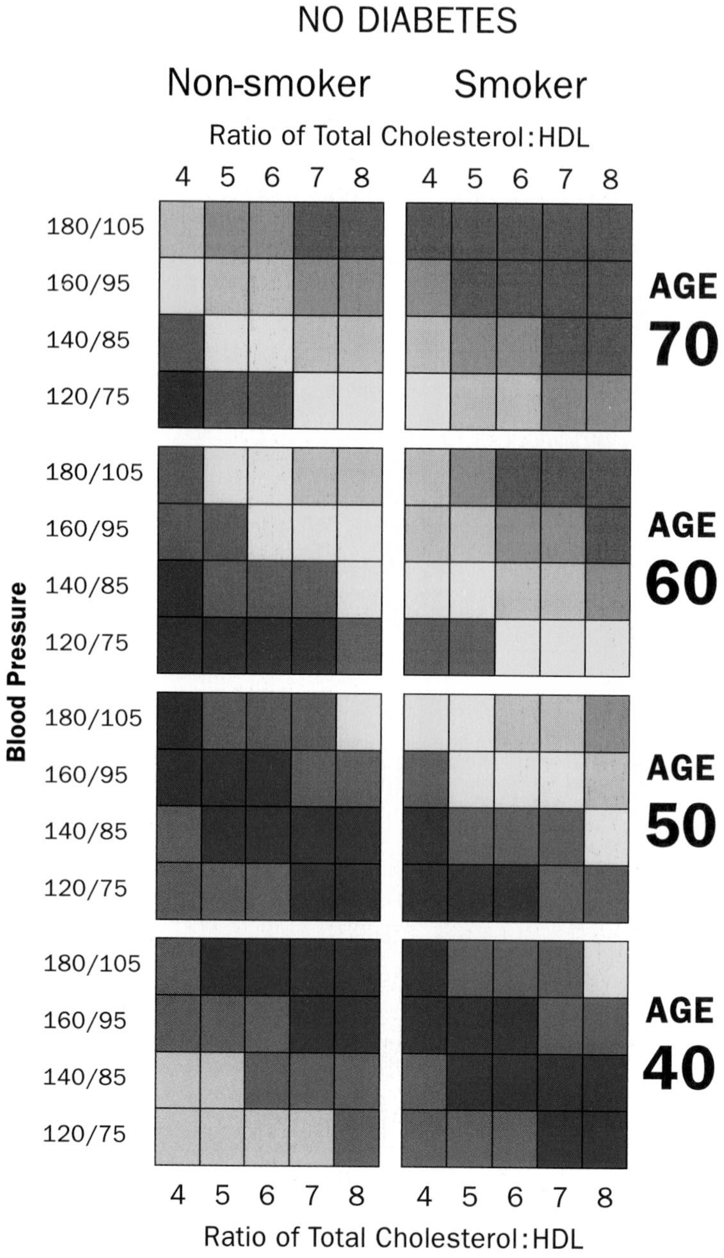

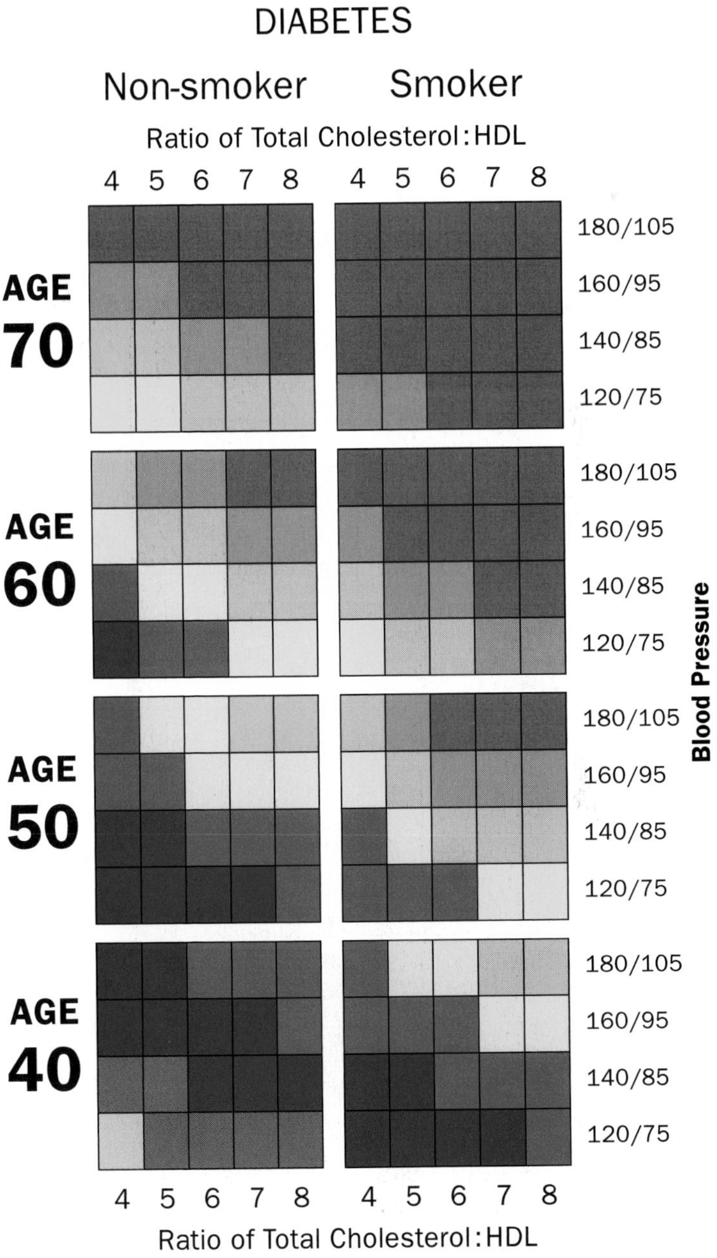
DIABETES
Non-smoker
Smoker
Ratio of Total Cholesterol : HDL
4 5 6 7 8 4 5 6 7 8
AGE 70
AGE 60
AGE 50
AGE 40
180/105
160/95
140/85
120/75
Blood Pressure
4 5 6 7 8 4 5 6 7 8
Ratio of Total Cholesterol : HDL

Estimating cardiovascular risk and treatment benefit

RISK LEVEL: WOMEN

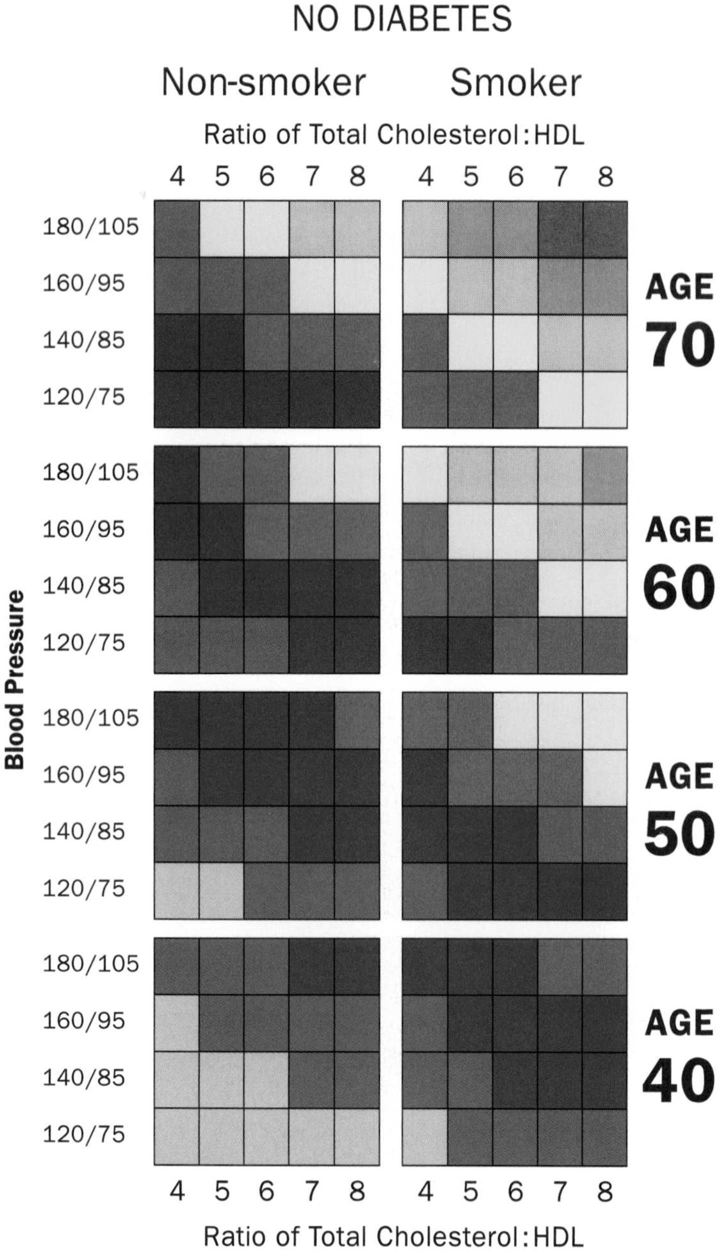

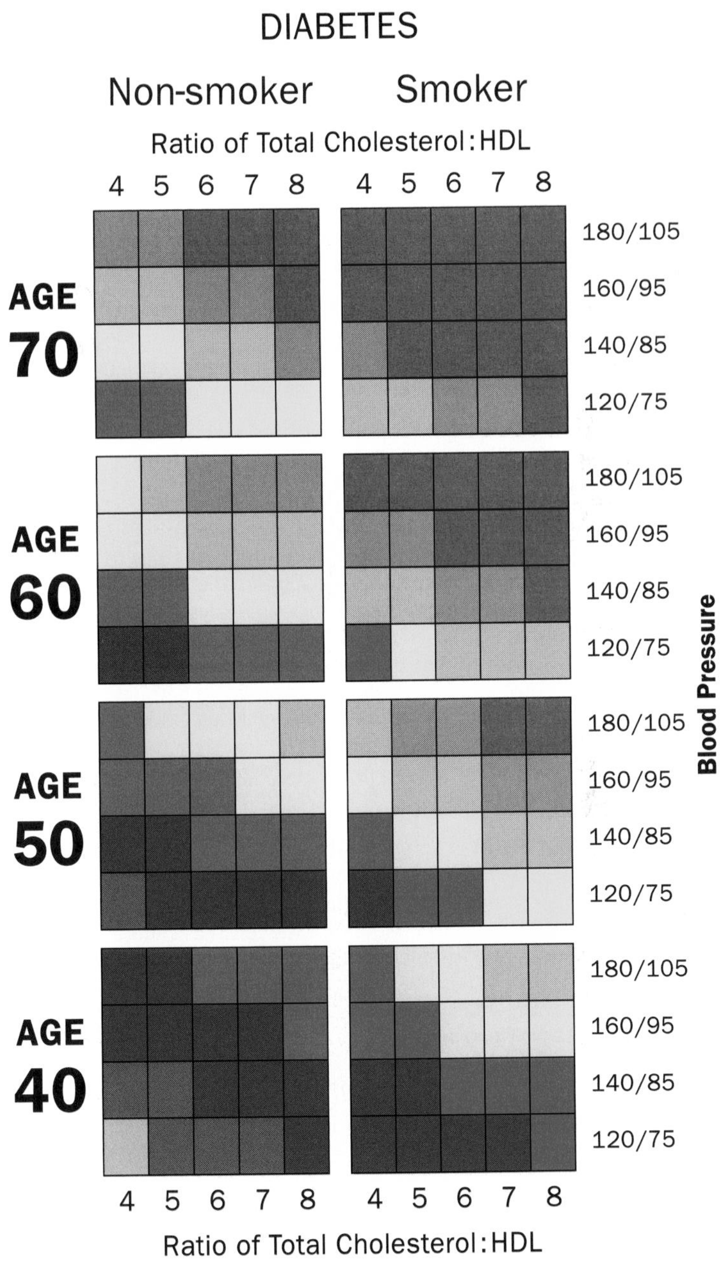
DIABETES
Non-smoker
Smoker
Ratio of Total Cholesterol:HDL
4 5 6 7 8
AGE 70
AGE 60
AGE 50
AGE 40
180/105
160/95
140/85
120/75
Blood Pressure

Appendix 2

The number needed to treat: adjusting for baseline risk

Adapted with permission from Chatellier et al, 1996[1]

BACKGROUND

The number needed to treat (NNT) to avoid a single additional adverse outcome is a meaningful way of expressing the benefit of an active treatment over a control. It can be used both to summarise the results of a therapeutic trial or series of trials and to help medical decision making about an individual patient.

If the absolute risk of adverse outcomes in a therapeutic trial is ARC in the control group and ART in the treatment group, then the absolute risk reduction (ARR) is defined as (ARC – ART). The NNT is defined as the inverse of the ARR:

$$\text{NNT} = 1/(\text{ARC} - \text{ART})$$

Since the Relative Risk Reduction (RRR) is defined as (ARC – ART)/ARC, it follows that NNT, RRR, and ARC are related by their definitions in the following way:

$$\text{NNT} \times \text{RRR} \times \text{ARC} = 1$$

This relationship can be used to estimate the likely benefits of a treatment in populations with different levels of baseline risk (that is different levels of ARC). This allows extrapolation of the results of a trial or meta-analysis to people with different baseline risks. Ideally, there should be experimental evidence of the RRR in each population. However, in many trials, subgroup analyses show that the RRR is approximately constant in groups of patients with different characteristics. Cook and Sackett therefore proposed that decisions about individual patients could be made by using the NNT calculated from the RRR measured in trials and the baseline risk in the absence of treatment estimated for the individual patient.[2]

The method may not apply to periods of time different to that studied in the original trials.

USING THE NOMOGRAM

The nomogram shown on the next page allows the NNT to be found directly without any calculation: a straight line should be drawn from the point corresponding to the estimated absolute risk for the patient on the left hand scale to the point corresponding to the relative risk reduction stated in a trial or meta-analysis on the central scale. The intercept of this line with the right hand scale gives the NNT. By taking the upper and lower limits of the confidence interval of the RRR, the upper and lower limits of the NNT can be estimated.

REFERENCES

1. Chatellier G, Zapletal E, Lemaitre D, *et al*. The number needed to treat: a clinically useful nomogram in its proper context. *BMJ* 1996;321:426–429.
2. Cook RJ, Sackett DL. The number needed to treat: a clinically useful measure of treatment effect. *BMJ* 1995;310:452–454.

The number needed to treat

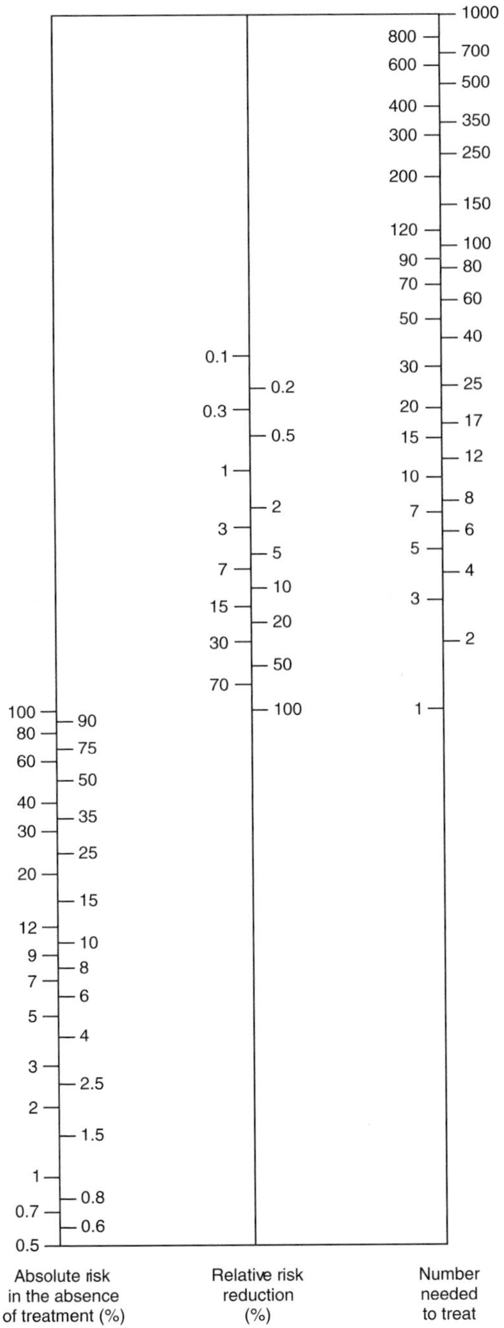

FIGURE **Nomogram for calculating the number needed to treat. Published with permission.[1]**

Clinical Evidence mini CD-ROM

The *Clinical Evidence* mini CD-ROM allows you to:

- Refer to the full *Clinical Evidence* content, including clinical questions, summary, and background information, evidence detail, figures, tables and appendices
- Choose the method of navigation you prefer, through the table of contents, topic sections, or the search engine
- Hyperlink references to abstracts where they appear on PubMed and Cochrane (Internet access required)
- Hyperlink to the glossary, figures, tables, and references
- Print the full text of any of the 170 topics

To access *Clinical Evidence* help:

- From within the *Clinical Evidence* CD-ROM, simply click on the link at the top of the screen or from within Windows, select Programs > Clinical Evidence > Help (if you have already installed *Clinical Evidence*)
- For technical help, please go to the FAQs at www.clinicalevidence.com
- For damaged CD-ROMs please contact:
  BMJ Publishing Group • Tel: +44(0) 207 383 6270 • subscriptions@bmjgroup.com (UK/ROW)
  For individual subscriptions • Tel: +1 800 373 2897/+1 240 646 7000 • clinevid@pmds.com (USA)
  For individuals receiving *Clinical Evidence* courtesy of United Health Foundation: ce@unitedhealthfoundation.org

To install *Clinical Evidence*

(i) Exit from any programs you have running.
(ii) Insert the *Clinical Evidence* Installation CD-ROM into the CD-ROM drive. The installation starts automatically (if it does not, select Run from the Start menu and enter d:\setup (where d: is your CD-ROM drive letter).
(iii) Follow the on-screen instructions. As part of this process, you can install Adobe Acrobat Reader so you can efficiently print *Clinical Evidence* topics — this can also be installed later by following the instructions below. An additional 20 Mbytes of hard disk space is required for this.

Minimum system requirements

An IBM compatible PC with at least this specification:

- 60 MBytes hard disk space
- 90 MHz processor
- 32 MBytes of RAM
- CD-ROM drive
- Modem, if you want to access the Internet for updates, etc.
- SVGA monitor recommended

Operating systems

This software has been tested with the following operating systems:

- Microsoft Windows 95
- Microsoft Windows 98
- Microsoft Windows 2000 Professional
- Microsoft Windows XP Professional
- Microsoft Windows NT SP6
- Microsoft Windows 2000 Server

Please note

Windows XP Home Edition may require special handling. Please refer to the appropriate section in the Readme file, or access the full text at www.clinicalevidence.com. The Readme file is located at:
Start > Programs > Clinical Evidence > Readme (if you have already installed *Clinical Evidence*) or contact technical help.

Browsers

Microsoft Internet Explorer 5.5 is the recommended browser, and should be your default browser when installing *Clinical Evidence*.
This software has been tested with the following browsers:

- Microsoft Internet Explorer 5.0 (English)
- Microsoft Internet Explorer 5.5 (English)
- Microsoft Internet Explorer 6.0 (English)
- Netscape 4.7 (English)
- Netscape 6.0 (English)

Please note

Microsoft Internet Explorer 4 is not a supported browser.
Microsoft Internet Explorer 6 is not compatible with Windows 95.
Internet Explorer 5.5 and 6.0 are available on the installation CD-ROM — see below for details.

To install Microsoft Internet Explorer v5.5

(i) With the *Clinical Evidence* Installation CD-ROM in the CD-ROM drive, select Run from the Start menu.
(ii) Type d:\other\ie5.5\ie5setup and click OK (where d: is your CD-ROM drive letter).
(iii) Follow the on-screen instructions. The typical installation requires approximately 17 Mbytes of hard disk space.

To install Microsoft Internet Explorer v6.0

(i) With the *Clinical Evidence* Installation CD-ROM in the CD-ROM drive, select Run from the Start menu.
(ii) Type d:\other\ie6.0\ie6setup and click OK (where d: is your CD-ROM drive letter).
(iii) Follow the on-screen instructions. The typical installation requires approximately 25 Mbytes of hard disk space.

To install Adobe Acrobat Reader v5.0.5

(i) With the *Clinical Evidence* Installation CD-ROM in the CD-ROM drive, select Run from the Start menu.
(ii) Type d:\Adobe\ar505enu and click OK (where d: is your CD-ROM drive letter).
(iii) Follow the on-screen instructions.